T0205796

Surgical Neuro-Oncology

Samer S. Hoz • Oday Atallah • Li Ma • Zaid Aljuboori
Mayur Sharma • Mustafa Ismail • Maliya Delawan
Editors

Surgical Neuro-Oncology

In Multiple Choice Questions

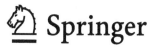 Springer

Editors
Samer S. Hoz
Department of Neurosurgery
University of Pittsburgh Medical Center
Pittsburgh, PA, USA

Li Ma
Department of Neurosurgery
University of Pittsburgh Medical Center
Pittsburgh, PA, USA

Mayur Sharma
Department of Neurosurgery
University of Minnesota
Minneapolis, MN, USA

Maliya Delawan
College of Medicine,
Gulf Medical University
Al Jurf, Ajman, United Arab Emirates

Oday Atallah
Department of Neurosurgery
Hannover Medical School
Hannover, Germany

Zaid Aljuboori
Department of Neurosurgery
Geisinger Commonwealth School
of Medicin
Scranton, PA, USA

Mustafa Ismail
Department of Neurosurgery
Neurosurgery Teaching Hospital
Baghdad, Iraq

ISBN 978-3-031-53641-0   ISBN 978-3-031-53642-7   (eBook)
https://doi.org/10.1007/978-3-031-53642-7

This Springer imprint is published by the registered company Springer Nature Switzerland AG
The registered company address is: Gewerbestrasse 11, 6330 Cham, Switzerland

Paper in this product is recyclable.

"To my lovely family: Sawsan, Saad, Arwa, Farah, Ward, Samhar, Anoona, Sanaa, Faris, and Luay. To the GYL team, Prof. Andaluz, Kathleen Smith, and Paolo Palmisciano."

Samer S. Hoz

"To my parents: Emad and Khuloud. To my adorable wife Aseel and my darling daughter Lara. To my country Palestine as well."

Oday Atallah

"To my beloved family, for their unwavering support, understanding, and love that have fueled my journey. To my exceptional colleagues, your collaboration, dedication, and camaraderie have enriched my professional life and been the pillars of my inspiration."

Li Ma

"I would like to dedicate this book to my mentors for their support and guidance."

Zaid Aljuboori

"To my mentors, parents (mother and late father), wife (Smita), daughters (Riya and Shreya), friends, and my patients who have given me the opportunity to learn."

Mayur Sharma

"To my mentors and teachers, for their constant support and ongoing encouragement."

Mustafa Ismail

"To my mom Zhijun, my dad Ghassan, my sister Judi, and my mentors who guided me through my medical journey."

Maliya Delawan

Foreword 1

Thorough knowledge and understanding of surgical neuro-oncology are sine qua non for gaining the incomparable privilege of caring for those who suffer from the daunting diseases that affect the organs that define our very human condition. For those of us who embarked on the humbling mission of performing neurosurgical procedures several years ago, the learning process in surgical neuro-oncology remains with no end in sight. For those beginning this fascinating journey, who are the intended readership of this work, you will find this book a valuable tool for immersion and recurrent assessment of acquired milestones in surgical neuro-oncology knowledge.

Mustafa K. Baskaya
University of Wisconsin Medical School and Public Health
Madison, WI, USA

Foreword 2: A Pathway to Mastery

In the ever-evolving field of neurosurgery, the pursuit of knowledge and excellence is a lifelong journey. As the understanding of neurosurgical oncology continues to expand, so too does the need for innovative and effective tools to aid in the acquisition and retention of essential knowledge.

It is with great pleasure and anticipation that I introduce you to *Surgical Neuro-Oncology: In Multiple Choice Questions*, the latest addition to the esteemed neurosurgery subspecialty series by Springer International.

This ground-breaking book is the first of its kind, introducing the multiple-choice question (MCQ) format to the realm of neurosurgical oncology. The mission of this book transcends the mere provision of answers; it is a dedicated effort to enhance comprehension and maintain knowledge, ultimately fostering the growth and development of neurosurgical practitioners.

The chapters within this book are meticulously crafted to offer comprehensive coverage of the core concepts in neurosurgical oncology. They mirror the MCQ format embraced by the majority of shelf and board examinations, ensuring that readers are well prepared to face these critical assessments.

With more than 800 thoughtfully designed MCQs, this study companion is ideal for self-study, enabling learners to embark on a journey of exploration and mastery at their own pace. The questions are structured to provide a step-by-step elucidation of each disease, guiding readers from its definition and associated anatomy, through pathology, clinical features, radiology, and surgical decision-making, all the way to surgical techniques and tricks. The immediate availability of answers and definitions beneath each question fosters effective information retention, making this book an indispensable resource for those seeking to solidify their knowledge.

It is important to emphasize that *Surgical Neuro-Oncology: In Multiple Choice Questions* is intended to be an adjunct to existing texts, complementing the rich body of neurosurgical literature. It serves as a means for readers to identify their strengths and weaknesses in the field, facilitating targeted learning and continuous improvement.

This book is designed to be flexible, catering to both long and shorter study sessions. Whether you are a neurosurgical resident preparing for certification tests or a seasoned practitioner looking to refresh and reinforce your knowledge, this book is a valuable asset that can adapt to your learning needs.

As the final volume in the esteemed neurosurgery subspecialty series by Springer International, *Surgical Neuro-Oncology: In Multiple Choice Questions* brings the series to a culmination. It follows in the footsteps of *Vascular Neurosurgery in Multiple Choice Questions, Neurotrauma in Multiple Choice Questions, Cerebral Ventricles in Multiple Choice Questions,* and *Pediatric Neurosurgery in Multiple Choice Questions.* Together, these volumes represent a comprehensive resource for neurosurgical education and certification.

In closing, it is my hope that this book becomes a trusted companion on your journey through the intricacies of surgical neuro-oncology. May it empower you to navigate the complexities of this field with confidence and expertise. Whether you are embarking on the path of knowledge acquisition or seeking to enhance your existing skills, *Surgical Neuro-Oncology: In Multiple Choice Questions* stands ready to guide you toward mastery.

As I know, there is a good tradition that young fellows and residents in neurosurgery edited a series of reference books in different subspecialties with up-to-date knowledge and first-hand clinical cases. Here is another excellent example. I am quite sure the authors, i.e., the next-generation young neurosurgeons will become the pioneers in twenty-first century, just as Harvey Cushing and Walter Dandy in twentieth century.

Yuanli Zhao
Department of Neurological Surgery
Peking Union Medical College Hospital
Beijing, China

Department of Neurological Surgery
Peking Union Medical College and Chinese Academy of Medical Sciences
Beijing, China

Beijing Tiantan Hospital, Capital Medical University
Beijing, China

Preface

Dear reader,

The journey toward mastering a neurosurgical specialty can be a formidable task. Surgical neuro-oncology is a multifaceted field that requires precision, an extensive knowledge base, and a profound grasp of the diverse features and behaviors exhibited by central nervous system tumors. To aid you in this remarkable journey, we introduce to you *Surgical Neuro-Oncology: In Multiple Choice Questions* as your study companion.

Our MCQ book covers the breadth of the field and delves into the nuances of specific tumors. It serves as a guide to understanding the molecular basis of these conditions, the role of radiology in diagnosis and differentiation, the clinical behavior of these tumors, and the practical aspects of their management. Furthermore, it provides insights into the nuances of surgical procedures and the pre-, peri-, and postoperative considerations.

This is the first review book to use the multiple-choice question format in surgical neuro-oncology, and it contains over 700 board-favorite questions for students, residents, fellows, and junior neurosurgeons. The choice to present in an MCQ format promotes active engagement and ensures that essential knowledge becomes an integral part of your practice in the field of surgical neuro-oncology.

As you delve into these pages, we hope for this book to serve as both a valuable resource on your journey to expertise in the field and an inspiration for excellence in patient care.

Samer S. Hoz
Pittsburgh, PA, USA

Oday Atallah
Hannover, Germany

Li Ma
Pittsburgh, PA, USA

Zaid Aljuboori
Scranton, PA, USA

Mayur Sharma
Minneapolis, MN, USA

Mustafa Ismail
Baghdad, Iraq

Maliya Delawan
Ajman, United Arab Emirates

Key Features

- *Surgical Neuro-Oncology in Multiple Choice Questions* is the first review book to use the multiple-choice question format in neurosurgical oncology.
- The mission of the book is to help readers understand the content and maintain the knowledge, rather than merely finding answers to complicated questions.
- The chapters of this book provide comprehensive coverage of the core concepts in neurosurgical oncology.
- This essential review mirrors the multiple-choice format adopted by the majority of shelf and board examinations.
- This study companion provides more than 800 MCQs in a convenient format that is suitable for self-study.
- The strategy and the format of the questions provide a step-by-step, thorough explanation of each disease from the definition, associated anatomy, pathology, clinical features, radiology to surgical decision-making, and surgical tricks, providing a comprehensive and concise overview.
- Answers and definitions appear immediately below the questions to facilitate information retention.
- This book is an adjunct to the existing texts and does not intend to be the primary source of information; it rather aims to help readers identify their relevant strengths and weaknesses in the area.
- These questions are structured as a refresher course for both long and shorter study sessions.
- The book is an important asset for residents across neurosurgical disciplines as it includes much of the neuro-oncology knowledge that neurosurgical residents need to prepare for their certification tests. It is also useful for those seeking ways to solidify their knowledge or maintain their current certification.

Contents

III   High Yield Facts on CNS Tumors

Contributors

Husain A. Abdali Department of Neurosurgery, Salmaniya Medical Complex, Manama, Bahrain

Ebtesam Abdulla Neurosurgery, Salmaniya Medical Complex, Manama, Bahrain

Muthanna N. Abdulqader Neurosurgery Teaching Hospital, Baghdad, Iraq

Alkawthar M. Abdulsada Azerbaijan Medical University, Baku, Azerbaijan

Fatimah O. Ahmed College of Medicine, University of Mustansiriyah, Baghdad, Iraq

Mays S. Ahmed College of Medicine, University of Baghdad, Baghdad, Iraq

Awfa Aktham Department of Neurosurgery, Tokyo General Hospital, Nakano, Japan

Arwa S. Alabedi Faculty of Medicine, Al Kufa University, Najaf, Iraq

Ammar S. Al-Adhami Saad Al-Witry Teaching Hospital, Baghdad, Iraq

Teeba A. Al-Ageely College of Medicine, University of Baghdad, Baghdad, Iraq

Abdulaziz Y. Alahmed Department of Neurosurgery, Aceer Central Hospital, Aceer, Saudi Arabia

Zinah A. Alaraji College of Medicine, Al-Nahrain University, Baghdad, Iraq

Osama M. Al-Awadi Neurosurgery Teaching Hospital, Baghdad, Iraq

Sajjad G. Al-Badri College of Medicine, University of Baghdad, Baghdad, Iraq

Sama Albairmani College of Medicine, University of Al-Iraqia, Baghdad, Iraq

Sadeem A. Albulaihed College of Medicine, Alfaisal University, Riyadh, Saudi Arabia

Usama AlDallal   School of Medicine, Royal College of Surgeons In Ireland—Medical University of Bahrain, Manama, Bahrain

Mohammed A. Al-Dhahir   Yemeni German Hospital, Sana'a, Yemen

Mostafa H. Algabri   College of Medicine, University of Baghdad, Baghdad, Iraq

Sami Al-Horani   Faculty of Medicine, Jordan University of Science and Technology, Irbid, Jordan

Zaid Aljuboori   Department of Neurosurgery, Geisinger Commonwealth School of Medicine, Scranton, PA, USA

Younus M. Al-Khazaali   College of Medicine, Al-Nahrain University, Baghdad, Iraq

Khalil Al-Qadasi   Department of Neurosurgery, University of Montreal, Montreal, QC, Canada

Abdullah K. Al-Qaraghuli   MedStar Health Research, MedStar Washington Hospital Center, Washington, DC, USA

Mohammed A. Alrawi   Neurosurgery Teaching Hospital, Baghdad, Iraq

Khalid M. Alshuqayfi   Faculty of Medicine, King Abdulaziz University, Jeddah, Saudi Arabia

Zahraa A. Alsubaihawi   College of Medicine, University of Baghdad, Baghdad, Iraq

Rania H. Al-Taie   College of Medicine, University of Mustansiriyah, Baghdad, Iraq

Noor K. Al-Waely   College of Medicine, Al-Nahrain University, Baghdad, Iraq

Rasha A. Al-Youzbaki   Ibn Sina Teaching Hospital, Mosul, Iraq

Mahmood F. Alzaidy   College of Medicine, University of Baghdad, Baghdad, Iraq

Giulio Anichini   Imperial College Healthcare NHS Trust, London, UK

Mohamed M. Arnaout Faculty of Medicine, Neurosurgery Department, Zagazig University, Zagazig, Egypt

Neurosurgery Division, Surgery Institute, Sheikh Khalifa Medical City, Abu Dhabi, United Arab Emirates

Oday Atallah Hannover Medical School, Hannover, Germany

Leen Azzam School of Medicine, Royal College of Surgeons In Ireland—Medical University of Bahrain, Manama, Bahrain

Sara Benchekroun Université de Laval, Quebec, QC, Canada

Maliya Delawan College of Medicine, Gulf Medical University, Ajman, United Arab Emirates

Ali A. Dolachee Department of Surgery, Al-Kindy College of Medicine, University of Baghdad, Baghdad, Iraq

Osman Elamin Neurosurgery Department, Jordan Hospital and Medical Center, Amman, Jordan

Ahmed M. N. ElGhamry St George's University Hospital, London, UK

Ignatius N. Esene Neurosurgery Division, Faculty of Health Sciences, University of Bamenda, Bambili, Cameroon

Almutasimbellah K. Etaiwi Saudi German Hospital Ajman, Ajman, United Arab Emirates

Ahmed A. Farag King Abdullah Medical City, Makkah, Saudi Arabia

Minaam Farooq New York Presbyterian Hospital/Och Spine, Weill Cornell Medicine, New York, NY, USA

Noor A. Fayadh College of Medicine, Al-Nahrain University, Baghdad, Iraq

Farah M. Hameed Ibn Sina Teaching Hospital, Mosul, Iraq

Waeel O. Hamouda   Neurological and Spinal Surgery Department, Cairo University Faculty of Medicine, Teaching and Research Hospitals, Cairo, Egypt

Viraat Harsh   Department of Neurosurgery, Rajendra Institute of Medical Sciences, Ranchi, Jharkhand, India

Hussein M. Hasan   College of Medicine, University of Baghdad, Baghdad, Iraq

Samer S. Hoz   Department of Neurosurgery, University of Pittsburgh Medical Center (UPMC), Pittsburgh, PA, USA

Mustafa Ismail   Neurosurgery Teaching Hospital, Baghdad, Iraq

Sanad M. A. Kamal   School of Medicine, Royal College of Surgeons in Ireland—Medical University of Bahrain, Manama, Bahrain

Ameya S. Kamat   Macquarie University Hospital, Sydney, Australia

Ruqaya A. Kassim   College of Medicine, University of Baghdad, Baghdad, Iraq

Anil Kumar   Department of Neurosurgery, Rajendra Institute of Medical Sciences, Ranchi, Jharkhand, India

Manoj Kumar   Department of Neurosurgery, Rajendra Institute of Medical Sciences, Ranchi, Jharkhand, India

Issa A. M. Lahirish   Neurosurgical Oncology Fellow, Cleveland Clinic, Cleveland, OH, USA

Hazem Madi   Jordan Hospital and Medical Center, Amman, Jordan

Dominic E. Mahoney   United Lincolnshire Hospitals NHS Trust, Lincolnshire, UK

Li Ma   Department of Neurosurgery, University of Pittsburgh Medical Center (UPMC), Pittsburgh, PA, USA

Saad Mallah   School of Medicine, Royal College of Surgeons In Ireland—Medical University of Bahrain, Manama, Bahrain

Wamedh E. Matti   Saad Al-Witry Teaching Hospital, Baghdad, Iraq

Iman Mohamoud College of Medicine, Gulf Medical University, Ajman, United Arab Emirates

Mohamed J. Mubarak Salmaniya Medical Complex, Manama, Bahrain

Baha'eddin A. Muhsen Rose Ella Burkhardt Brain Tumor and Neuro-Oncology Center, Neurological Institute, Cleveland Clinic, Cleveland, OH, USA

Ahmed Muthana College of Medicine, University of Baghdad, Baghdad, Iraq

Kevin O'Neill Imperial College Healthcare NHS Trust, London, UK

Abdullah H. Al Ramadan Department of Neurosurgery and Spine Surgery, Qatif Central Hospital, First Eastern Health Cluster, Al-Qatif, Saudi Arabia

Hatem Sadik Department of Intensive Care, Hammersmith Hospital, Imperial College Healthcare NHS Trust, London, UK

Saleh A. Saleh College of Medicine, University of Baghdad, Baghdad, Iraq

Hayder R. Salih Neurosurgery Teaching Hospital, Baghdad, Iraq

Mayur Sharma Department of Neurosurgery, University of Minnesota, Minneapolis, MN, USA

Wardan A. Tamer Faculty of Medicine, Neurosurgery Department, National Hospital, University of Hama, Hama, Syria

Muhammad S. Umerani Department of Neurosurgery, Royal Commission Hospital, Jubail, Saudi Arabia

Abbreviations

5-ALA	5-Aminolevulinic acid	CPC	Choroid plexus carcinoma
ABC	Aneurysmal bone cyst	CPP	Choroid plexus papilloma
ACP	Adamantinomatous Craniopharyngioma	CS	Cavernous sinus
		CSF	Cerebrospinal fluid
ACTH	Adrenocorticotropic hormone	CT	Computed tomography
		CUSA	Cavitational ultrasonic surgical aspiration
ADC	Apparent diffusion coefficient		
AFP	Alpha-fetoprotein	DC	Dermoid cyst
AG	Angiocentric glioma	DI	Diabetes insipidus
AIDS	Acquired immunodeficiency syndrome	DIA	Desmoplastic infantile astrocytoma
ASL	Arterial spin labeling	DIC	Disseminated intravascular coagulation
AT/RT	Atypical teratoid/rhabdoid		
		DIG	Desmoplastic infantile ganglioglioma
BAER	Brainstem auditory evoked response	DLBCL	Diffuse large B-cell lymphoma
BST	Brainstem tumor		
		DLGG	Diffuse low-grade glioma
CC	Colloid cysts	DNA	Deoxyribonucleic acid
CCA	Common carotid artery	DNET	Dysembryoplastic neuroepithelial tumor
CD	Cushing disease		
CDS	Cranial dermal sinus	DTI	Diffusion tensor imaging
CEA	Carcinoembryonic antigen	DVT	Deep vein thrombosis
cEBRT	Conventional external beam radiotherapy	DWI	Diffusion-weighted imaging
CM	Carcinomatous meningitis	EBV	Epstein–barr virus
CMF	Chondromyxoid fibroma	EC	Epidermoid cyst
CN	Cranial nerve	ECOG	Eastern Cooperative Oncology Group
CNS	Central nervous system		
CPA	Cerebellopontine angle	EEG	Electroencephalogram

EG	Eosinophilic granuloma		HGG	High-grade glioma
EGFR	Epidermal Growth Factor Receptor		HIF	Hypoxia-inducible factor
EMA	Epithelial membrane antigen		HIV	Human immunodeficiency virus
EMG	Electromyography		HNST	Hybrid nerve sheath tumor
ESCC	Epidural spinal cord compression		HP	Hearing preservation
ETANTR	Embryonal tumor with abundant neuropil and true rosettes		IAC	Internal acoustic canal
			ICA	Internal carotid artery
			ICP	Intracranial pressure
ETMR	Embryonal tumors with multi-layered rosettes		IDEM	Intradural extramedullary
			IDH	Isocitrate dehydrogenase
ETV	Endoscopic third ventriculostomy		IDIM	Intradural intramedullary
			IELSG	International Extranodal Lymphoma Study Group
FLAIR	Fluid-attenuated inversion recovery		IGF-I	Insulin-like Growth Factor 1
			INR	International normalized ratio
GABA	Gamma-aminobutyric acid		IPCG	International PCNSL Collaboration Group
GBM	Glioblastoma multiforme			
GCT	Germ cell tumor			
GFAP	Glial fibrillary acidic protein		JPA	Juvenile pilocytic astrocytoma
GH	Growth hormone			
GKS	Gamma knife surgery		KPS	Karnofsky performance scale
GTR	Gross total resection			
Gy	Gray			
			L1CAM	L1 cell adhesion molecule
HAART	Highly active antiretroviral therapy		LDH	Lactate dehydrogenase
			LINAC	Linear accelerator
HCG	Human chorionic gonadotropin		LP	Lumbar puncture
HDC/ ASCT	High-dose chemotherapy supported by autologous stem-cell transplantation		MAP	Mitogen-activated protein
			MCS	Multiple chondromatosis syndrome

MGMT	O6-methylguanine-DNA methyltransferase	PNET	Primitive neuroectodermal tumors
MPNST	Malignant peripheral nerve sheath tumors	PNST	Peripheral nerve sheath tumor
MRI	Magnetic resonance imaging	PPTID	Pineal parenchymal tumor of intermediate differentiation
MRN	MR neurography		
MVNT	Multinodular and vacuolating neuronal tumor	PSR	Percentage signal recovery
		PXA	Pleomorphic xanthoastrocytoma
NC	Nucleus:cytoplasm		
NAA	N-acetylaspartate	rCBF	Relative cerebral blood flow
NCS	Nerve Conduction Study		
NF1	Neurofibromatosis 1	RGNT	Rosette-forming glioneuronal tumor
NF2	Neurofibromatosis 2	RPA	Recursive partitioning analysis
NHL	Non-hodgkin lymphoma		
NSAIDs	Non-steroidal anti-inflammatory drugs	rTBV	Relative tumor blood volume
		RTOG	Radiation Therapy Oncology Group
OPG	Optic pathway glioma		
ORI	Oswestry risk index		
OS	Overall survival	SARC	Sarcoma Alliance for Research Through Collaboration
PC	Pineal cysts		
PCA	Pilocytic astrocytoma	SCNSL	Secondary CNS lymphoma
PCC	Prothrombin complex concentrate	SCO	Spindle cell oncocytoma
		SCT	Spinal cord tumors
PCNL	Primary Central Nervous System Lymphoma	SDS	Spinal dermal sinus
		SEGA	Subependymal giant cell astrocytoma
PCP	Papillary craniopharyngioma		
		SEN	Subependymal nodules
PCR	Polymerase chain reaction	SINS	Spinal instability neoplastic score
PET	Positron emission tomography		
		SORG	Skeletal Oncology Research Group
PI	Proliferation index		
PMA	Pilomyxoid astrocytoma	SRS	Stereotactic radiosurgery

Abbreviations

SRT	Stereotactic radiotherapy	VHL	Von Hippel-Lindau
STIR	Short tau inversion recovery	VoG	Vein of Galen
		VR	Virchow-Robin
TB	Tuberculosis	VS	Vestibular schwannoma
TCR	Trigeminocardiac reflex		
TLL	Tumor-like lesion	WBRT	Whole brain radiation therapy
TSC	Tuberous sclerosis complex		
		WHO	World Health Organization
VCF	Vertebral compression fractures	WI	Weighted image
VEGF	Vascular endothelial growth factor	XRT	Radiotherapy

CNS Tumors' Essential Principles

Contents

Epidemiology and Presentation of CNS Tumors

Hatem Sadik, Alkawthar M. Abdulsada,
Osman Elamin, Hussein M. Hasan, Maliya Delawan,
and Samer S. Hoz

© The Author(s), under exclusive license to Springer Nature Switzerland AG 2024
S. S. Hoz et al. (eds.), *Surgical Neuro-Oncology*,
https://doi.org/10.1007/978-3-031-53642-7_1

1

? 1. Diffuse low-grade gliomas (DLGGs). The FALSE answer is:
   A. Account for 10–15% of all primary brain tumors.
   B. Are diagnosed in patients typically between the ages of 50 and 65 years.
   C. Are gliomas of a grade lower than anaplastic according to the WHO classification of tumors of the CNS.
   D. Are frequently located in eloquent areas of the brain.
   E. Undergo evolution into biologically more aggressive entities.

✔ Answer B
– Diffuse low-grade gliomas are diagnosed in patients typically between the ages of 30 and 45 years.

? 2. Diffuse low-grade gliomas. The FALSE answer is:
   A. More than 80% of patients with DLGGs present with seizures.
   B. 50% of patients who present with seizures have intractable seizures.
   C. Gross neurological deficits are common at presentation.
   D. Patients may experience associated neuropsychological disorders.
   E. The incidence, based on data from Europe and the US is 1–1.5/100,000 patients/year.

✔ Answer C
– Gross neurological deficits are rare at presentation mostly because of the slow-growing nature which allows for brain plasticity.

? 3. High-grade gliomas (HGGs). The FALSE answer is:
   A. Are the most common primary intrinsic brain tumor.
   B. Account for 85% of all newly diagnosed primary malignant brain tumors.
   C. The incidence is approximately 5/100,000 patients/year in Europe and North America.
   D. Glioblastomas account for 30–40% of HGGs.
   E. The peak incidence of glioblastomas is between 65 and 75 years of age.

✔ Answer D
– Glioblastomas account for 60–70% of HGGs.

? 4. **High-grade gliomas. The FALSE answer is:**
  A. Mostly present with signs and symptoms of raised intracranial pressure.
  B. Approximately 25–50% of grade III and grade IV tumors present with seizures.
  C. Tumors located in the posterior fossa may present with ataxia, dizziness, and incoordination.
  D. Clinical findings often vary depending on the specific tumor type.
  E. Associated headache is usually worse in the morning and decreases throughout the day.

✓ Answer D
▬ There are no clinical findings unique to the various tumor types. However, more aggressive, rapidly progressing lesions tend to have a more rapid onset with more severe symptoms, whereas lower-grade tumors have a more insidious course.

? 5. **Intracranial metastases. The FALSE answer is:**
  A. The annual age-adjusted incidence is reported to be around 7–14 per 100,000.
  B. Most patients present with polymetastatic disease (>4 intracranial lesions).
  C. Up to 20% of patients with lung cancer develop brain disease.
  D. Less than 1% of patients with thyroid, prostate, stomach, or ovarian cancer develop brain disease.
  E. Nonsmall cell lung cancer is the most prevalent cancer type in patients with intracranial metastases.

✓ Answer B
▬ Approximately one-third of patients present with a solitary lesion, one-third with oligometastatic disease (2–3 lesions), and a third with polymetastatic disease (>4 lesions).

? 6. **Intracranial metastases. The FALSE answer is:**
  A. 40–60% of patients with malignant melanoma develop brain metastases.
  B. On gross examination, they have an infiltrative appearance.
  C. Are most often located at the junction of the gray and white matter.

    D. 80–85% of lesions are in the cerebrum, while 10–15% are in the cerebellum.

    E. In breast cancer, both triple-negative and HER receptor-positive subtypes are associated with a higher risk of brain metastasis.

✅ **Answer B**

- On gross examination, most metastases are spheroid and well-demarcated from the surrounding brain tissue. However, on microscopic examination, these tumors may have an infiltrative appearance.

❓ 7. **Primary central nervous system lymphoma (PCNSL). The FALSE answer is:**
    A. Is a rare form of non-Hodgkin's lymphoma confined to the CNS.
    B. Comprises approximately 2–3% of primary CNS tumors.
    C. The vast majority are of the diffuse large B-cell type (DLBCL).
    D. The peak incidence in the immunocompetent population is 60 years and above.
    E. HIV-associated PCNSL is almost always associated with cytomegalovirus.

✅ **Answer E**

- HIV-associated PCNSL is almost always associated with Epstein-Barr virus (EBV).

❓ 8. **Meningiomas. The FALSE answer is:**
    A. Meningiomas account for about 36% of all primary intracranial neoplasms.
    B. The most affected age range is 20–40 years.
    C. There is a predilection for women with a female-to-male ratio of 1.8:1.
    D. Meningiomas are uncommon in children, accounting for only 1.5% of total cases.
    E. Up to 15–25% of childhood cases are associated with neurofibromatosis type 1 or 2.

✅ **Answer B**

- The risk of developing meningiomas increases with age, with the most affected age range being 40–70 years.

9. **Sporadic vestibular schwannoma. The FALSE answer is:**
   A. Is the most common cerebellopontine angle tumor.
   B. Comprises 6–8% of all intracranial tumors.
   C. Arises from the inferior branch of the vestibular branch of cranial nerve VIII in 65–75% of cases.
   D. The most common age at diagnosis is between 50 and 64 years.
   E. At diagnosis, most have one or more of the following: hearing deficit, vertigo, and facial nerve palsy.

✓ **Answer E**
- At diagnosis, most have one or more of the following: hearing deficit, vertigo, and tinnitus. The facial and trigeminal nerves are more affected by treatment.

10. **Pituitary adenomas. The FALSE answer is:**
    A. Account for 15% of all intracranial tumors.
    B. Microadenomas are less than 10 mm in diameter, generally enclosed, and less frequently invasive.
    C. Up to 5% are discovered incidentally and many remain asymptomatic.
    D. Pituitary hemorrhage occurs in up to 27% of cases.
    E. May present with headaches due to compression or stretching of the dura lining of the sella or of the diaphragm.

✓ **Answer C**
- Up to 20% of pituitary adenomas are discovered incidentally and many remain asymptomatic.

11. **Prolactinomas. The FALSE answer is:**
    A. Account for 30–60% of pituitary tumors.
    B. Can be associated with anxiety, depression, fatigue, and emotional instability.
    C. In women of reproductive age symptoms include amenorrhea, galactorrhea, infertility, seborrhea, and hirsutism.
    D. In men, the most common presentation is a loss of libido and impotency, and less commonly oligospermia and hypogonadism.
    E. Galactorrhea or gynecomastia is present in 15–30% of male patients.

✓ **Answer E**
- Galactorrhea or gynecomastia is present in 50% of male patients.

1

❓ 12. Acromegaly. The FALSE answer is:
  A. A disease of chronic overproduction of growth hormone (GH).
  B. Upper airway obstruction affects up to 40% of patients.
  C. Some features of acromegaly include facial changes, laryngeal hypertrophy, bony hypertrophy, hypertension, cardiomyopathy, and high adrenocorticoid output.
  D. Can be diagnosed by clinical features and an elevated serum IGF-I level.
  E. GH following oral glucose tolerance test (OGTT) has increased false-positive results in patients with diabetes.

✅ Answer B
— Upper airway obstruction affects up to 70% of patients.

❓ 13. Cushing's disease. The FALSE answer is:
  A. Results from the unregulated hypersecretion of ACTH by a pituitary adenoma and consequent hypercortisolism.
  B. Up to 80% of patients have systemic hypertension.
  C. Features include weight gain, centripetal obesity, and fat deposits over the cheeks and temporal regions.
  D. Glucose intolerance occurs in at least 60% of patients.
  E. 5% of patients with a pituitary adenoma causing Cushing's disease have no visible lesion on MRI.

✅ Answer E
— 50% of patients with a pituitary adenoma causing Cushing's disease have no visible lesion on MRI.

❓ 14. Craniopharyngiomas. The FALSE answer is:
  A. Are benign epithelial neoplasms of the sellar region that arise from embryonic squamous cells of the hypophysio-pharyngeal duct.
  B. Have a bimodal age distribution, at 5–14 years and in the fifth decade of life.
  C. Are regarded as histopathologically benign intracranial tumors.
  D. Classically, a bitemporal hemianopia occurs due to compression of the optic chiasm from below.
  E. Subjective visual symptoms at presentation occur in around 90% of cases.

✅ **Answer E**

- Subjective visual symptoms at the time of presentation are encountered in approximately 47% of patients but ophthalmological findings at the time of presentation occur in 75%.

❓ 15. **Brainstem tumors (BST). The FALSE answer is:**
   A. Patients have a mean age at presentation ranging between 7 and 9 years.
   B. Account for 10–15% of pediatric brain tumors.
   C. It is estimated that 58–75% are focal and 25% are diffuse.
   D. Diffuse tumors originate from the pons and are now often referred to as diffuse intrinsic pontine gliomas.
   E. Children with diffuse BSTs typically present with a triad of cerebellar dysfunction, cranial neuropathies, and long-tract signs.

✅ **Answer C**

- It is estimated that 58–75% of brainstem tumors are diffuse and 25% are focal.

❓ 16. **Medulloblastomas. The FALSE answer is:**
   A. Are the most common malignant brain tumor of childhood.
   B. More than half occur in the first 10 years of life but are uncommon under the age of 1 year.
   C. Most patients present with a short history.
   D. Typically, a posterior fossa midline tumor causes obstructive hydrocephalus and increased intracranial pressure.
   E. Older children typically suffer from evening headaches and vomiting episodes that relieve the headache.

✅ **Answer E**

- Older children typically suffer from morning headaches and vomiting episodes that relieve the headache. Possibly, the accumulation of CO_2 during sleep causes vasodilation and further increase of the intracranial pressure.

❓ 17. **Ependymomas. The FALSE answer is:**
   A. Are slow-growing tumors believed to arise from radial glial stem cells within the ependymal surface.
   B. The peak incidence of presentation is 6 years of age.

1

C. They account for 10% of all pediatric tumors and approximately 30% of tumors in children younger than 3 years of age.
D. In children, 70% are supratentorial lesions.
E. Adults present with an almost equal incidence of intracranial and spinal cord tumors.

✔ **Answer D**
— In children, 70% of ependymomas are infratentorial lesions.

❓ 18. **Ganglioglioma. The FALSE answer is:**
   A. The incidence is around 0.3–5.2% in adults and up to 14% in the pediatric group with brain tumors.
   B. The most common tumor location is the frontal lobe followed by the brainstem.
   C. Typically presents with epilepsy that is often resistant to pharmacotherapy.
   D. Deep-seated, cerebellar, brainstem, and spinal gangliogliomas present with location-dependent signs and symptoms.
   E. A nonepileptic presentation in a case with a presumed ganglioglioma should alert the treating clinician to the possibility of a nonbenign clinical course.

✔ **Answer B**
— The most common tumor location is the temporal followed by the frontal lobe.

❓ 19. **Chordomas and chondrosarcomas. The FALSE answer is:**
   A. Make up 0.1% of all brain tumors and have a combined incidence of 0.02 per 100,000.
   B. Chordomas may occur in the skull base, mobile spine, or sacrum.
   C. Chordomas exhibit a male predominance, possibly as high as 2:1.
   D. Cranial chordomas present at a later age than chordomas at other sites.
   E. In adults, skull base chordomas most commonly occur in the third and fourth decades.

✔ **Answer D**
— Cranial chordomas often present at an earlier age than chordomas at other sites.

❓ 20. Glomus tumors (paragangliomas). The FALSE answer is:

    A. Are slow-growing vascular tumors that occur in the anatomically complex jugulotympanic region of the lateral skull base.

    B. Are generally indolent and can progress to a significant size before diagnosis due to a lack of symptoms or subtle symptoms.

    C. They produce pulsatile tinnitus in 90% of patients and lead to local invasion, resulting in conductive hearing loss in 80% of patients.

    D. Otalgia and aural fullness occur in around 10% of symptomatic patients.

    E. Otoscopy classically reveals a red mass in the middle ear in up to 50% of cases.

✔ Answer E

▬ Otoscopy classically reveals a red mass in the middle ear in more than 90% of cases.

Bibliography

1. Smits A, Jakola AS. Clinical presentation, natural history, and prognosis of diffuse low-grade gliomas. Neurosurg Clin. 2019;30(1):35–42.
2. Pallud J, McKhann GM. Diffuse low-grade glioma-related epilepsy. Neurosurg Clin. 2019;30(1):43–54.
3. Di Carlo DT, Cagnazzo F, Benedetto N, Morganti R, Perrini P. Multiple high-grade gliomas: epidemiology, management, and outcome. A systematic review and meta-analysis. Neurosurg Rev. 2019;42:263–75.
4. Rasmussen BK, Hansen S, Laursen RJ, Kosteljanetz M, Schultz H, Nørgård BM, Guldberg R, Gradel KO. Epidemiology of glioma: clinical characteristics, symptoms, and predictors of glioma patients grade I–IV in the the Danish Neuro-Oncology Registry. J Neurooncol. 2017;135:571–9.
5. Sacks P, Rahman M. Epidemiology of brain metastases. Neurosurg Clin. 2020;31(4):481–8.
6. Gavrilovic IT, Posner JB. Brain metastases: epidemiology and pathophysiology. J Neurooncol. 2005;75:5–14.
7. Gerstner ER, Batchelor TT. Primary central nervous system lymphoma. In: Primary central nervous system tumors: pathogenesis and therapy. Humana Press; 2011. p. 333–53.
8. Baldi I, Engelhardt J, Bonnet C, Bauchet L, Berteaud E, Grüber A, Loiseau H. Epidemiology of meningiomas. Neurochirurgie. 2018;64(1):5–14.
9. Berkowitz O, Iyer AK, Kano H, Talbott EO, Lunsford LD. Epidemiology and environmental risk factors associated with vestibular schwannoma. World Neurosurg. 2015;84(6):1674–80.

10. Gittleman H, Ostrom QT, Farah PD, Ondracek A, Chen Y, Wolinsky Y, Kruchko C, Singer J, Kshettry VR, Laws ER, Sloan AE. Descriptive epidemiology of pituitary tumors in the United States, 2004–2009. J Neurosurg. 2014;121(3):527–35.
11. Vroonen L, Daly AF, Beckers A. Epidemiology and management challenges in prolactinomas. Neuroendocrinology. 2019;109(1):20–7.
12. Lavrentaki A, Paluzzi A, Wass JA, Karavitaki N. Epidemiology of acromegaly: review of population studies. Pituitary. 2017;20:4–9.
13. Ahn CH, Kim JH, Park MY, Kim SW. Epidemiology and comorbidity of adrenal Cushing syndrome: a nationwide cohort study. J Clin Endocrinol Metabol. 2021;106(3):e1362–72.
14. Zacharia BE, Bruce SS, Goldstein H, Malone HR, Neugut AI, Bruce JN. Incidence, treatment and survival of patients with craniopharyngioma in the surveillance, epidemiology and end results program. Neuro Oncol. 2012;14(8):1070–8.
15. Darlix A, Zouaoui S, Rigau V, Bessaoud F, Figarella-Branger D, Mathieu-Daudé H, Trétarre B, Bauchet F, Duffau H, Taillandier L, Bauchet L. Epidemiology for primary brain tumors: a nationwide population-based study. J Neurooncol. 2017;131:525–46.
16. Khanna V, Achey RL, Ostrom QT, Block-Beach H, Kruchko C, Barnholtz-Sloan JS, de Blank PM. Incidence and survival trends for medulloblastomas in the United States from 2001 to 2013. J Neurooncol. 2017;135:433–41.
17. McGuire CS, Sainani KL, Fisher PG. Incidence patterns for ependymoma: a surveillance, epidemiology, and end results study. J Neurosurg. 2009;110(4):725–9.
18. Diwanji TP, Engelman A, Snider JW, Mohindra P. Epidemiology, diagnosis, and optimal management of glioma in adolescents and young adults. Adolesc Health Med Ther. 2017;8:99–113.
19. Bakker SH, Jacobs WC, Pondaag W, Gelderblom H, Nout RA, Dijkstra PD, Peul WC, Vleggeert-Lankamp CL. Chordoma: a systematic review of the epidemiology and clinical prognostic factors predicting progression-free and overall survival. Eur Spine J. 2018;27:3043–58.
20. Young WF, Wen PY. Paragangliomas: epidemiology, clinical presentation, diagnosis, and histology. 2021. Available at: https://www.uptodate.com/contents/paragangliomas-epidemiology-clinical-presentation-diagnosis-andhistology.

Tumors Molecular and Genomic Mechanism and Diagnostics of CNS Tumors

*Oday Atallah, Teeba A. Al-Ageely,
Younus M. Al-Khazaali, Fatimah O. Ahmed,
Alkawthar M. Abdulsada, Maliya Delawan,
and Samer S. Hoz*

© The Author(s), under exclusive license to Springer Nature Switzerland AG 2024
S. S. Hoz et al. (eds.), *Surgical Neuro-Oncology*,
https://doi.org/10.1007/978-3-031-53642-7_2

2

❓ 1. **Glioma: IDH1/IDH2 mutations. The FALSE answer is:**
A. They are associated with the development of secondary glioblastomas.
B. The R132H substitution in the IDH1 gene is the most frequent mutation in gliomas.
C. All gliomas have IDH1/IDH2 mutations.
D. They can be exploited therapeutically.
E. They result in a neomorphic enzyme activity producing D-2-hydroxyglutarate.

✅ **Answer C**
— Not all gliomas have IDH1/IDH2 mutations.

❓ 2. **Glioma: MGMT methylation. The FALSE answer is:**
A. It is present in approximately 50% of grade IV gliomas.
B. It predicts a greater survival advantage.
C. It is typically associated with a positive response to alkylating agents.
D. It decreases the effectiveness of radiation monotherapy.
E. Standard PCR techniques allow for determining the status of MGMT.

✅ **Answer D**
— It increases the effectiveness of radiation monotherapy.

❓ 3. **Diffuse midline glioma with H3 K27M mutation. The FALSE answer is:**
A. Classified as a WHO Grade IV tumor.
B. The mutation predominantly affects the HIST1H3B/C or H3F3A genes.
C. Correlates to a lower overall survival rate.
D. Most commonly occurs in the pons and the thalamus.
E. Is more common in adults than in children.

✅ **Answer E**
— Diffuse midline glioma with H3 K27M mutation is more common in children than in adults.

❓ 4. **Ependymoma: molecular subgroups. The FALSE answer is:**
A. Myxopapillary ependymoma predominantly arises in the most caudal part of the spinal cord.

B. PF-A and PF-B ependymomas are supratentorial in location.

C. *ZFTA*-fusion and *YAP1*-fusion positive ependymomas are normally located supratentorially.

D. Subependymomas may arise in all CNS compartments.

E. Subependymomas most frequently originate from the fourth and lateral ventricles.

✅ **Answer C**

– PF-A and PF-B ependymomas are infratentorial in location.

❓ 5. **Medulloblastoma: molecular subgroups include the following. The FALSE answer is:**

A. WNT subgroup.

B. SHH subgroup with TP3-mutant.

C. SHH-subgroup with TP53 wild-type.

D. Group 3 non-WNT and non-SHH group.

E. Loss of FUBP1 subgroup.

✅ **Answer E**

– Loss of FUBP1 expression is seen in low-grade glioma, not medulloblastoma.

❓ 6. **Medulloblastoma: WNT and SHH subgroup. The FALSE answer is:**

A. The prognosis for the WNT subgroup is more favorable than for the other subgroups.

B. Most cases from the WNT subgroup affect children.

C. Immunohistochemistry makes it simple to identify WNT and SHH subgroups.

D. SHH medulloblastomas with TP53 mutations are associated with a poor prognosis.

E. All SHH medulloblastomas have TP53 mutations.

✅ **Answer E**

– SHH medulloblastomas can be TP53 wild-type or TP53-mutant.

❓ 7. **Medulloblastoma: group 3 and 4. The FALSE answer is:**

A. Group 3 and 4 medulloblastomas constitute the greatest cohort.

B. Group 3 medulloblastomas generally have a good prognosis.

2

C. Group 3 medulloblastomas are most prevalent in infants.
D. Group 4 medulloblastomas are the most prevalent, particularly in adolescents and adults.
E. MYC or MYCN/CDK6 amplification is characteristic of group 3 and 4.

✅ **Answer B**
- Group 3 medulloblastomas are associated with a poor prognosis.

❓ 8. **Atypical teratoid/rhabdoid tumor (AT/RT): molecular mechanism. The FALSE answer is:**
A. Loss of function of the SMARCB1 (INI1) gene is a crucial molecular event.
B. The majority of cases have inactivation of SMARCA4.
C. There are three subgroups of AT/RTs: TYR, MYC, and SHH.
D. Biallelic mutations in the SMARCA4 genes are characteristic of AT/RTs.
E. AT/RTs can be histologically mistaken for medulloblastomas.

✅ **Answer B**
- Only a minority of cases (<5%) have inactivation of SMARCA4; the majority of AT/RTs exhibit inactivation of both copies of SMARCB1.

❓ 9. **Tumors of the pineal region: molecular mechanism. The FALSE answer is:**
A. Pineoblastomas have fewer cytogenetic alterations.
B. There are no distinctive diagnostic molecular characteristics for these tumors.
C. DICER1 mutations are associated with germinomas.
D. They are associated with heterologous differentiation.
E. RP1 mutations are associated with pineoblastomas.

✅ **Answer C**
- DICER1 mutations are associated with pineoblastomas.

❓ 10. **Meningioma: molecular and genomic mechanism. The FALSE answer is:**
A. NF2 gene mutations are the most common genetic alterations in meningiomas.
B. The TERT promoter mutation indicates a more aggressive clinical phenotype.
C. KLF4 mutations frequently accompany TRAF5 mutations.

    D. AKT1 mutations are often found in meningothelial and transitional meningiomas.

    E. Loss of chromosome 22q commonly occurs in meningiomas.

✅ **Answer C**

➖ TRAF7 mutations frequently occur alongside KLF4 mutations in meningiomas.

❓ 11. **Central nervous system solitary fibrous tumors/hemangiopericytomas: molecular and genomic mechanism. The FALSE answer is:**

    A. NAB2-STAT6 gene fusion is a characteristic molecular feature.

    B. The high MIB-1 labeling index correlates with a more aggressive clinical course.

    C. The NAB2-STAT6 fusion gene is a result of a chromosome 12q inversion.

    D. BRAF gene mutation is typical for these tumors.

    E. Immunohistochemistry frequently reveals robust nuclear positivity for STAT6.

✅ **Answer D**

➖ BRAF mutations are most commonly found in melanomas.

❓ 12. **Hemangioblastoma: molecular and genomic mechanism. The FALSE answer is:**

    A. Mutations in IDH1/2 genes are a common feature in hemangioblastomas.

    B. It is frequently associated with Von Hippel-Lindau (VHL) disease.

    C. It is characterized by the overexpression of vascular endothelial growth factor (VEGF).

    D. Hemangioblastomas can occur sporadically.

    E. It shows the overexpression of hypoxia-inducible factor (HIF).

✅ **Answer A**

➖ Mutations in IDH1/2 genes are common in gliomas.

2

? 13. **Craniopharyngioma: molecular and genomic mechanism. The FALSE answer is:**
   A. Mutations in the CTNNB1 gene are linked with the adamantino-matous type.
   B. BRAF V600E mutations are prevalent in the papillary type.
   C. It often shows disrupted WNT signaling pathway due to CTNNB1 mutations.
   D. The BRAF V600E mutation activates the MAP kinase pathway in the papillary type.
   E. EGFR mutations are a characteristic feature.

✅ **Answer E**
– EGFR mutations are a defining characteristic of adenocarcinoma, not craniopharyngioma.

? 14. **Vestibular schwannoma: molecular and genomic mechanism. The FALSE answer is:**
   A. Mutations in the NF1 gene are a frequent occurrence.
   B. Mutations in the NF2 gene are commonly observed.
   C. The NF2 gene encodes a protein called Merlin that acts as a tumor suppressor.
   D. Vestibular schwannomas can occur sporadically.
   E. The loss of function of the NF2 gene results in uncontrolled cell growth.

✅ **Answer A**
– Mutations in the NF2 gene, not the NF1 gene, are frequently encountered in vestibular schwannoma.

Bibliography

1. Routman DM, Raghunathan A, Giannini C, Mahajan A, Beltran C, Nagib MG, Nageswara Rao AA, Skrypek MM, Laack NNI. Anaplastic ependymoma and posterior fossa grouping in a patient with H3K27ME3 loss of expression but chromosomal imbalance. Adv Radiat Oncol. 2019;4(3):466–72.
2. Kristensen BW, Priesterbach-Ackley LP, Petersen JK, Wesseling P. Molecular pathology of tumors of the central nervous system. Ann Oncol. 2019;30(8):1265–78.
3. Spiegl-Kreinecker S, Lötsch D, Neumayer K, Kastler L, Gojo J, Pirker C, Pichler J, Weis S, Kumar R, Webersinke G, Gruber A, Berger W. TERT promoter mutations are associ-

ated with poor prognosis and cell immortalization in meningioma. Neuro Oncol. 2018;20(12):1584–93.

4. Koczkodaj D, Muzyka-Kasietczuk J, Chocholska S, Podhorecka M. Prognostic significance of isochromosome 17q in hematologic malignancies. Oncotarget. 2021;12(7): 708–18.

5. Park SH, Won J, Kim SI, Lee Y, Park CK, Kim SK, Choi SH. Molecular testing of brain tumor. J Pathol Transl Med. 2017;51(3):205–23.

6. Shan FY, Castro E, Sybenga A, Mukherjee S, Wu E, Fung K, Li T, Fonkem E, Huang JH, Rao A. Molecular diagnostics and pathology of major brain tumors. In: Primary intracranial tumors. IntechOpen; 2019.

7. Louis DN, Perry A, Wesseling P, Brat DJ, Cree IA, Figarella-Branger D, Hawkins C, Ng HK, Pfister SM, Reifenberger G, Soffietti R, von Deimling A, Ellison DW. The 2021 WHO classification of tumors of the central nervous system: a summary. Neuro Oncol. 2021;23(8):1231–51.

8. Rodriguez FJ, Vizcaino MA, Lin MT. Recent advances on the molecular pathology of glial neoplasms in children and adults. J Mol Diagn. 2016;18(5):620–34.

9. Wood MD, Halfpenny AM, Moore SR. Applications of molecular neuro-oncology—a review of diffuse glioma integrated diagnosis and emerging molecular entities. Diagn Pathol. 2019;14(1):29.

10. Meredith DM, Alexandrescu S. Embryonal and non-meningothelial mesenchymal tumors of the central nervous system—advances in diagnosis and prognostication. Brain Pathol. 2022;32(4):e13059.

11. Cohen AL, Colman H. Glioma biology and molecular markers. Cancer Treat Res. 2015;163:15–30.

12. Chan KM, Fang D, Gan H, Hashizume R, Yu C, Schroeder M, Gupta N, Mueller S, James CD, Jenkins R, Sarkaria J, Zhang Z. The histone H3.3K27M mutation in pediatric glioma reprograms H3K27 methylation and gene expression. Genes Dev. 2013;27(9):985–90.

13. Yang P, Cai J, Yan W, Zhang W, Wang Y, Chen B, Li G, Li S, Wu C, Yao K, Li W, Peng X, You Y, Chen L, Jiang C, Qiu X, Jiang T, CGGA Project. Classification based on mutations of TERT promoter and IDH characterizes subtypes in grade II/III gliomas. Neuro Oncol. 2016;18(8):1099–108.

14. Masliah-Planchon J, Machet MC, Fréneaux P, Jourdain A, Mortemousque I, Raïs KA, Ballet S, Jouvet A, Figarella-Branger D, Delattre O, Bourdeaut F. SMARCA4-mutated atypical teratoid/rhabdoid tumor with retained BRG1 expression. Pediatr Blood Cancer. 2016;63(3):568–9.

Imaging of CNS Tumors

*Noor A. Fayadh, Noor K. Al-Waely,
Khalid M. Alshuqayfi, and Samer S. Hoz*

3

? 1. **General imaging principles.**
   **Tumor location: imaging findings in extra-axial brain tumors. The
   FALSE answer is:**
   A. White matter buckling sign.
   B. Spoke-wheel or sunburst pattern of vascularity.
   C. Should have intact gray matter deep to the lesion.
   D. Dural tail is not completely specific for extra-axial origin.
   E. Corpus callosum is not thickened in midline tumors.

✓ Answer C
— While an intact cortex deep to the mass suggests extra-axial origin, the
   lack of an intact cortex does not exclude extra-axial origin, as the gray
   matter may be markedly thinned and not visible on imaging.

? 2. **General imaging principles.**
   **Tumor location: imaging signs of extra-axial brain tumors. The
   FALSE answer is:**
   A. Cleft sign.
   B. Claw sign.
   C. Broad dural base.
   D. Dural tail sign.
   E. Hyperostosis of the overlying bone.

✓ Answer B
— The claw sign refers to sharp angles of the normal brain parenchyma
   around the mass and is seen in intra-axial tumors.

? 3. **General imaging principles.**
   **Tumor location: intra-axial brain tumors' imaging features. The
   FALSE answer is:**
   A. Expand the cortex of the brain.
   B. No expansion of the subarachnoid space.
   C. Dura lateral to the lesion.
   D. Pial vessels lateral to the lesion.
   E. The presence of gray matter between the lesion and the white
      matter.

✓ Answer E
— The presence of gray matter between the lesion and the white matter is
   suggestive of extra-axial origin.

? 4. **General imaging principles.**
   Tumor location: cortical tumors. The FALSE answer is:
   A. PXA.
   B. DNET.
   C. Primary CNS lymphoma.
   D. Oligodendroglioma.
   E. Ganglioglioma.

✓ **Answer C**
— Primary CNS lymphoma is typically a deep white or gray matter lesion.

? 5. **General imaging principles.**
   Tumor composition: the typical appearance of fat on imaging. The FALSE answer is:
   A. Bright on T1 WI.
   B. Exhibits chemical shift artifact.
   C. Low density on CT.
   D. Low signal on STIR.
   E. Low signal on T2 WI.

✓ **Answer E**
— Fat typically has bright T1 and T2 signal.

? 6. **General imaging principles.**
   Tumor composition: brain tumors that have intralesional fat. The FALSE answer is:
   A. Callosal lipoma.
   B. Dermoid.
   C. Glioblastoma.
   D. Meningioma.
   E. Teratoma.

✓ **Answer C**
— Glioblastomas do not have intralesional fat. In contrast, lipoma is typically composed of fat. Teratomas and dermoids can have intralesional macroscopic fat components. Lipomatous meningioma, a rare type of meningioma, typically has fat.

3

? 7. **General imaging principles.**
Tumor composition: imaging appearance of calcification. The FALSE answer is:
A. High density on CT.
B. High signal on T1 WI.
C. High signal on gradient sequences.
D. Low signal on T1 WI.
E. Low signal on T2 WI.

✔ **Answer C**
— Calcification typically appears as low intensity (blooming) on gradient sequences. Although calcification typically exhibits low T1 and T2 signals, in special conditions it can exhibit bright T1 and even bright T2 signals.

? 8. **General imaging principles.**
Tumor composition: intra-axial tumors that exhibit calcification. The FALSE answer is:
A. Astrocytoma.
B. Choroid plexus papilloma.
C. Ganglioglioma.
D. Glioblastoma.
E. Oligodendroglioma.

✔ **Answer D**
— Glioblastoma does not typically show calcification.

? 9. **General imaging principles.**
Tumor composition: intra-axial tumors that are likely to exhibit calcification radiologically. The FALSE answer is:
A. Callosal lipoma.
B. Dysembryoplastic neuroepithelial tumors (DNET).
C. Ependymoma.
D. Medulloblastoma.
E. Teratoma.

✔ **Answer B**
— Although calcification is described in DNET, it is more likely to appear histologically than radiologically.

? 10. **General imaging principles.**
Tumor composition: extra-axial tumors that commonly show calcification. The FALSE answer is:
A. Chondrosarcoma.
B. Chordoma.
C. Craniopharyngioma.
D. Meningioma.
E. Virchow Robin spaces.

✔ **Answer E**
— Virchow Robin spaces are extensions of CSF and exhibit identical signals and densities to CSF. They do not show calcification.

? 11. **General imaging principles.**
Tumor composition-MRI: brain tumors that may exhibit a bright T1 signal. The FALSE answer is:
A. Arachnoid cyst.
B. Glioblastoma.
C. Melanoma metastasis.
D. Pituitary adenoma.
E. Teratoma.

✔ **Answer A**
— Arachnoid cyst typically has signal criteria identical to CSF appearing low on T1 and bright on T2 WI. Pituitary adenoma and glioblastoma may have hemorrhagic components which typically appear bright on T1. Melanoma metastasis typically has a bright T1 signal due to the paramagnetic effect of melanin. Teratoma may show fat, which is typically bright on T1.

? 12. **General imaging principles.**
Tumor composition-MRI: cellular tumors that show low T2 signals. The FALSE answer is:
A. DNET.
B. Lymphoma.
C. Meningioma.
D. Oligodendroglioma.
E. PNET.

✔ **Answer A**
— DNET usually exhibits a bubbly bright T2 signal.

? 13. **General imaging principles.**
Multifocal brain tumors and tumor-like lesions. The FALSE answer is:
   A. GBM.
   B. Metastasis.
   C. Hemangioblastoma.
   D. Meningioma.
   E. Ganglioglioma.

✓ Answer E
− Ganglioglioma, like all neuronal tumors, is usually a solitary tumor.

? 14. **General imaging principles.**
Enhancement patterns: extra-axial enhancement pattern. The FALSE answer is:
   A. Either pachymeningeal or leptomeningeal.
   B. Pachymeningeal enhancement follows the bone or dural reflection.
   C. Leptomeningeal enhancement follows the pial surface of the brain.
   D. Pachymeningeal enhancement fills the subarachnoid space, sulci, and cisterns.
   E. Leptomeningeal enhancement has a serpentine appearance.

✓ Answer D
− Leptomeningeal enhancement fills the subarachnoid space, sulci, and cisterns.

? 15. **General imaging principles.**
Enhancement pattern: neoplasms and conditions causing a pachymeningeal pattern of enhancement. The FALSE answer is:
   A. TB meningitis.
   B. Metastasis.
   C. Viral meningitis.
   D. Lymphoma.
   E. Granulomatous meningitis.

✓ Answer C
− Viral meningitis causes a leptomeningeal pattern of enhancement.

16. General imaging principles.
Enhancement pattern: neoplasms and conditions associated with leptomeningeal enhancement. The FALSE answer is:
A. Glioblastoma.
B. Meningioma.
C. TB meningitis.
D. Oligodendroglioma.
E. Lymphoma.

Answer B
— Meningioma causes a pachymeningeal pattern of enhancement.

17. General imaging principles.
Enhancement pattern: carcinomatous leptomeningeal enhancement. The FALSE answer is:
A. Can be seen along the ependymal line of ventricles.
B. May coexist with pachymeningeal enhancement in metastasis.
C. May appear exquisitely thin and regular.
D. May appear thick and lumpy.
E. Normal cranial nerves may enhance in the subarachnoid space.

Answer E
— Cisternal portions of cranial nerves do not show contrast enhancement.

18. General imaging principles.
Enhancement pattern: intra-axial enhancement. The FALSE answer is:
A. Gyral enhancement is generally nonneoplastic.
B. Gyral enhancement is inflammatory or vascular.
C. Nodular cortical and subcortical enhancement is seen with metastatic deposits.
D. Nodular cortical and subcortical enhancement is seen in septic emboli.
E. Periventricular enhancement is pathognomonic for primary CNS lymphoma.

Answer E
— While periventricular/ependymal enhancement is commonly seen in CNS lymphoma, it can be seen with glial tumors as well.

? 19. **General imaging principles.**

Enhancement pattern: ring-enhancing lesions. The FALSE answer is:

A. Glioma.

B. Metastasis.

C. Cerebritis.

D. Abscesses.

E. Inactive demyelination.

✓ Answer E

— Active demyelination plaques cause this pattern of enhancement.

? 20. **General imaging principles.**

Enhancement pattern: ring-enhancing lesions. The FALSE answer is:

A. Necrotic metastases are usually cortical/subcortical.

B. Abscesses and cerebritis can be superficial or deep.

C. Deep white matter location is seen in primary tumors.

D. Location in corpus callosum favors abscess.

E. Location in the thalamus favors primary tumors.

✓ Answer D

— Location in the corpus callosum favors glial tumors or lymphomas.

? 21. **General imaging principles.**

Enhancement pattern: ring-enhancing lesions. The FALSE answer is:

A. Extensive vasogenic edema for lesion size favors a primary tumor.

B. Metastases may present as similarly sized multiple lesions.

C. Abscesses may present as similarly sized multiple lesions.

D. An open ring of enhancement is seen in tumefactive demyelination.

E. A multilocular complex ring pattern is seen in primary tumors.

✓ Answer A

— Extensive vasogenic edema for lesion size favors an abscess.

? 22. **General imaging principles.**
   **Enhancement pattern: ring-enhancing lesions. The FALSE
   answer is:**
   A. Shaggy inner margins are seen in primary tumors.
   B. Abscesses have smooth inner and outer walls.
   C. Walls thicker than 10 mm are seen in primary tumors.
   D. Multiple lesions in the same area of edema favor a primary
      tumor.
   E. The tumor rim is typically hypointense on T2.

✅ **Answer E**
— Abscess rims usually exhibit T2 hypointensity due to their collagenous
   capsules.

? 23. **General imaging principles.**
   **Enhancement pattern: ring-enhancing lesions. The FALSE
   answer is:**
   A. Marked diffusion restriction in the lesion center favors abscess.
   B. Diffusion restriction in the lesion wall favors glioblastoma.
   C. Lack of central diffusion restriction favors a necrotic tumor.
   D. Increased perfusion favors primary or secondary neoplasm.
   E. Perfusion is high in tumefactive demyelination.

✅ **Answer E**
— Perfusion is low in tumefactive demyelination.

? 24. **General imaging principles.**
   **Enhancement pattern: solid-enhancing lesions. The FALSE
   answer is:**
   A. Primary CNS lymphoma in immunocompetent subject.
   B. Primary CNS lymphoma in immunocompromised subject.
   C. Metastasis.
   D. High-grade gliomas.
   E. Demyelination.

✅ **Answer B**
— Primary CNS lymphoma in immunocompromised subjects presents as a
   ring-enhancing lesion.

3

? 25. **General imaging principles.**
   Enhancement pattern: tumors presenting as a cyst with a mural nodule. The FALSE answer is:
   A. Pilocytic astrocytoma.
   B. PXA.
   C. Ganglioglioma.
   D. Supratentorial intraparenchymal ependymoma.
   E. Oligodendroglioma.

✓ **Answer E**
— Oligodendroglioma does not present as a cyst with a mural nodule.

? 26. **General imaging principles.**
   Enhancement pattern: tumors presenting as a cyst with a mural nodule. The FALSE answer is:
   A. Pilocytic astrocytoma is usually infratentorial.
   B. Cortical dysplasia is frequently seen with pilocytic astrocytoma.
   C. Hemangioblastoma is usually infratentorial.
   D. PXA usually occurs in the temporal lobe.
   E. Ganglioglioma usually occurs in the temporal lobe.

✓ **Answer B**
— Nearby cortical dysplasia is seen with PXA and ganglioglioma.

? 27. **General imaging principles.**
   Enhancement pattern: tumors presenting as a cyst with a mural nodule. The FALSE answer is:
   A. All lesions may show hyperintense cyst content on T1.
   B. Suppression of cyst on FLAIR suggests PXA.
   C. Edema is seen around PXA.
   D. Edema is not seen with pilocytic astrocytoma.
   E. Edema is seen with hemangioblastoma.

✓ **Answer E**
— Edema is not seen around hemangioblastomas.

? 28. **General imaging principles.**
   Enhancement pattern: tumors presenting as a cyst with a mural nodule. The FALSE answer is:
   A. Enhancement of the cyst wall is common in hemangioblastoma.
   B. Enhancement of the cyst wall is common in pilocytic astrocytoma.

C. Vivid enhancement is seen in PXA nodules.

D. Moderate enhancement is seen in ganglioglioma nodules.

E. Vivid enhancement is seen in pilocytic astrocytoma nodules.

✅ **Answer A**

— The wall of hemangioblastomas does not typically show enhancement.

❓ 29. **General imaging principles.**

Enhancement pattern: tumors presenting as a cyst with a mural nodule. The FALSE answer is:

A. Solid nodule of hemangioblastoma may show flow void.

B. Calcification is common in PXA.

C. Calcification is seen in pilocytic astrocytoma.

D. Calcification is rare in hemangioblastoma.

E. Calcification is seen in ganglioglioma.

✅ **Answer B**

— Calcification is rare in PXA.

❓ 30. **Glial tumors.**

Radiological features suggestive of grade II low-grade glial tumor. The FALSE answer is:

A. Lack of enhancement.

B. Cystic change.

C. Circumscribed border.

D. T2 FLAIR mismatch sign.

E. Expansion of the surrounding cortex.

✅ **Answer C**

— Grade II gliomas typically show ill-defined margins.

❓ 31. **Glial tumors.**

Anaplastic astrocytoma. The FALSE answer is:

A. Heterogeneous and rim enhancement.

B. Heterogeneous texture.

C. Hemorrhage.

D. T2 FLAIR mismatch.

E. Mass effect.

Answer A

- Enhancement is heterogeneous in anaplastic astrocytoma but does not typically exhibit a rim pattern. Rim enhancement suggests grade IV GBM.

3

? 32. **Glial tumors.**

Radiological features suggestive of grade IV glial tumor. The FALSE answer is:
A. Ring enhancement.
B. Perilesional edema.
C. Marked mass effect.
D. Necrosis.
E. Calcification is common.

Answer E

- While hemorrhage is seen frequently in GBM, calcification is considered uncommon.

? 33. **Glial tumors.**

CT features of oligodendroglioma. The FALSE answer is:
A. Typically located in the cerebellar hemispheres.
B. Avid enhancement.
C. Central calcification.
D. Peripheral calcification.
E. Ribbon-like calcification.

Answer A

- Typically located in the cerebral hemispheres.

? 34. **Glial tumors.**

MRI features of oligodendroglioma. The FALSE answer is:
A. Peripheral cortical location.
B. Blooming seen on T2*.
C. Lack T2 FLAIR mismatch.
D. No diffusion restriction.
E. Enhancement predicts grade.

Answer E

- Enhancement does not predict grade, as it is also normally seen in low-grade oligodendroglioma.

? 35. **Glial tumors.**
Imaging mimics for low-grade intra-axial tumors. The FALSE answer is:
A. Herpes encephalitis.
B. Subacute infarction.
C. Focal cortical dysplasia.
D. Seizure-related brain changes.
E. Cerebral abscess.

✅ **Answer E**
▬ Cerebral abscesses and cerebritis show ring enhancement and therefore mimic high-grade tumors.

? 36. **Glial tumors.**
Imaging mimics for high-grade intra-axial tumors. The FALSE answer is:
A. Abscess.
B. Tumefactive demyelination.
C. TB granulomas.
D. CNS vasculitis.
E. Tumefactive VR space.

✅ **Answer E**
▬ Tumefactive VR spaces mimic low-grade tumors.

? 37. **Supratentorial intra-axial brain tumors with ill-defined margins. The FALSE answer is:**
A. High-grade astrocytic tumors.
B. High-grade oligodendroglial tumors.
C. PNET.
D. High-grade ependymal tumors.
E. Metastasis.

✅ **Answer E**
▬ Metastatic tumors usually show well-defined borders.

? 38. **Supratentorial lesions with midline crossing. The FALSE answer is:**
A. Glioblastoma multiforme.
B. Lymphoma.

C. Neuronal/neuroglial tumors.
D. Cerebral metastasis.
E. Radiation necrosis.

✅ **Answer C**
— Neuronal/neuroglial tumors are not associated with midline crossing.

3

❓ 39. **Posterior fossa tumor.**
Tumors that classically present as posterior fossa masses in adults. The FALSE answer is:
A. Germinoma.
B. Hemangioblastoma.
C. Lhermitte Duclos disease.
D. Medulloblastoma.
E. Metastasis.

✅ **Answer A**
— Germinomas are supratentorial tumors located either in the suprasellar or pineal region.

❓ 40. **Posterior fossa tumors.**
Pediatric brain tumors typically located in the posterior fossa. The FALSE answer is:
A. Atypical teratoid/rhabdoid tumors.
B. Craniopharyngioma.
C. Ependymoma.
D. Medulloblastoma.
E. Pilocytic astrocytoma.

✅ **Answer B**
— Craniopharyngiomas are sellar/suprasellar masses.

❓ 41. **Posterior fossa tumors.**
Characteristic imaging features in pediatric posterior fossa tumors. The FALSE answer is:
A. Pilocytic astrocytoma: cyst with solid nodule.
B. Atypical teratoid/rhabdoid tumor: large and heterogeneous.
C. Diffuse midline glioma (pontine): minimal enhancement.
D. Ependymoma: extension into the foramen of Luschka.
E. Medulloblastoma: high ADC.

✅ **Answer E**

— Medulloblastomas characteristically have low ADC.

❓ 42. **Posterior fossa tumors.**
Differentiating imaging features between ependymoma and medulloblastoma. The FALSE answer is:
A. Calcification is seen in both types.
B. Ependymoma is less likely to show diffusion restriction.
C. Ependymoma typically arises from the floor of the fourth ventricle.
D. Location of the midline is described in medulloblastoma.
E. Plastic growth is typical for medulloblastoma.

✅ **Answer E**

— Plastic growth is typically seen with ependymomas and describes tumor conforming to the shape of its container (i.e., the fourth ventricle) and extending into the foramina of Luschka and foramen of Magendie. In contrast, medulloblastomas cause expansion of the fourth ventricle when they extend into it.

❓ 43. **Posterior fossa tumors.**
Classic imaging findings in medulloblastoma molecular subgroups. The FALSE answer is:
A. Group 3: early meningeal dissemination.
B. Group 3: midline location from the vermis.
C. Group 4: avid contrast enhancement.
D. WNT (wingless) subtype: bulging into the CP angle.
E. SHH (sonic hedgehog) subtype: cerebellar hemispheric location.

✅ **Answer C**

— Group 4 medulloblastomas typically show less contrast enhancement than other molecular subgroups. They represent the most common subgroup and are typically seen as a large midline vermian mass.

❓ 44. **Posterior fossa tumors.**
Imaging in brain stem glioma. The FALSE answer is:
A. High-grade gliomas (HGG) typically invade the basilar artery.
B. Pontine involvement is evocative of HGG.
C. Prepontine cistern extension is typically seen in HGG.

> D. Tumors involving the lateral medulla are typically low-grade gliomas (LGG).
> E. Variable contrast enhancement is described in LGG.

3

✅ **Answer A**

– Although extension into the prepontine cistern with engulfment of the basilar artery is described in high-grade glioma, the artery is typically not invaded and not thrombosed. Pontine involvement is the key point in the radiological assessment of brain stem glioma as it is highly suggestive of high-grade tumors. Tumors sparing the pons are typically low-grade gliomas with preferential involvement of the brachium pontis, lateral medulla, and tegmentum.

❓ 45. **Posterior fossa tumors.**
Tumors that classically have a cystic/necrotic component. The FALSE answer is:
A. Diffuse midline glioma (pontine).
B. Ependymoma.
C. Hemangioblastoma.
D. Medulloblastoma.
E. Pilocytic astrocytoma.

✅ **Answer A**

– The classic imaging appearance of diffuse midline glioma H3 K27-mutant prior to treatment is of a homogeneous minimally enhancing mass. Areas of necrosis are seen in a minority of patients.

❓ 46. **Posterior fossa tumor.**
Described imaging findings in ependymoma. The FALSE answer is:
A. Calcification.
B. Hemorrhage.
C. Heterogeneous enhancement.
D. Posterior fossa A is typically in the lateral recess of the fourth ventricle.
E. Posterior fossa B is typically in the upper part of the fourth ventricle.

✅ **Answer E**

– The molecular subgroup posterior fossa B is typically located in the lower part of the floor of the fourth ventricle near the obex.

47. Posterior fossa tumors.
   Enhancing CP angle lesions. The FALSE answer is:
   A. Epidermoid cyst.
   B. Facial schwannoma.
   C. Meningioma.
   D. Metastasis.
   E. Vestibular schwannoma.

Answer A
— Epidermoid cysts do not typically show contrast enhancement.

48. Posterior fossa tumors.
   CP angle tumors or lesions that can have a bright T1 signal. The FALSE answer is:
   A. Aneurysm.
   B. Arachnoid cyst.
   C. CP angle lipoma.
   D. Epidermoid cyst.
   E. Schwannoma.

Answer B
— Arachnoid cysts follow CSF on all pulse sequences and hence exhibit low T1 and high T2 signals. Thrombosed aneurysms exhibit a bright T1 signal. Lipomas typically have bright T1 and T2 signals. White epidermoid cysts, a rare subtype, appear bright on T1. Schwannoma may have a bright T1 signal related to hemorrhage.

49. Posterior fossa tumors.
   Imaging findings in CP angle tumors. The FALSE answer is:
   A. Arachnoid cyst follows CSF on all pulse sequences.
   B. CP angle meningioma commonly extends into the IAC.
   C. Epidermoid cysts show diffusion restriction.
   D. Hemangioblastoma can present as a CP angle mass.
   E. Vestibular schwannoma shows intense contrast enhancement.

Answer B
— Cerebellopontine angle meningiomas rarely extend into the IAC. Extension into the IAC favors vestibular schwannoma.

3

? 50. **Posterior fossa tumors.**
Differentiating points between CP angle meningioma and schwannoma. The FALSE answer is:
A. Calcification is more likely in meningioma.
B. Dural tail is classically described in meningioma.
C. Hemorrhage is seen in schwannoma.
D. A heterogeneous appearance favors meningioma.
E. Widening of the porus acusticus favors vestibular schwannoma.

✓ **Answer D**
— Schwannomas are more likely to show hemorrhage and cystic changes and hence are more likely to appear heterogeneous on imaging.

? 51. **Posterior fossa tumors.**
Imaging findings in rosette-forming glioneuronal tumor (RGNT). The FALSE answer is:
A. Associated hydrocephalus may be seen.
B. Calcification may be present.
C. Can be solid or cystic.
D. Characteristic location around the fourth ventricle.
E. Intense enhancement is typical.

✓ **Answer E**
— Enhancement of these rare tumors is variable. The most frequently described enhancement pattern is focal, while some masses exhibit heterogeneous enhancement, and a few even display nodular or ring enhancement. Cases with no enhancement in the lesion have also been reported.

? 52. **Diffuse leptomeningeal glioneuronal tumor. The FALSE answer is:**
A. Dominant parenchymal mass.
B. Involvement of the brain.
C. Involvement of the spinal cord.
D. Small subpial cysts.
E. Thick nodular leptomeningeal enhancement.

✓ **Answer A**
— No dominant parenchymal mass is usually seen; however, multiple small discrete enhancing parenchymal masses can be seen especially in the spinal cord. This is a rare newly recognized tumor entity addressed in the WHO 2016 classification of CNS tumors. Radiologically, it presents as

thick nodular leptomeningeal enhancement of the brain and spinal cord affecting the basal cisterns, posterior fossa, and inferior surface of the brain. Small subpial cysts can be seen.

? 53. **Sellar/suprasellar tumors.**
Macroadenoma. The FALSE answer is:
A. Cavernous sinus invasion may be seen.
B. Hemorrhage is a recognized feature.
C. Macroadenomas may have a cystic component.
D. Postcontrast enhancement is minimal.
E. Typically defined as tumors >1 cm.

✓ Answer D
▬ As the pituitary gland is beyond the blood-brain barrier, pituitary tumors generally enhance vividly with intravenous contrast.

? 54. **Sellar/suprasellar tumors.**
Microadenomas. The FALSE answer is:
A. Contrast administration is a must for their detection.
B. May cause bulging of the gland.
C. May cause depression of the sellar floor.
D. A negative MR scan does not exclude microadenoma.
E. They are <10 mm by definition.

✓ Answer A
▬ The sensitivity of nonenhanced MRI scans for microadenoma detection is approximately 70%. Contrast administration increases the sensitivity to 85% but is not always required as the management would not be altered.

? 55. **Sellar/suprasellar tumors.**
Rathke's cleft cyst. The FALSE answer is:
A. Calcification is a recognized finding.
B. Intracystic nodule is pathognomonic.
C. Hemorrhage is common.
D. Located in or above the sella.
E. Variable signal on T1 and T2 images.

✓ Answer C
▬ Rathke's cleft cysts almost never bleed.

3

? 56. Sellar/suprasellar tumors.
   Craniopharyngioma (adamantinomatous type). The FALSE answer is:
   A. Calcification is common.
   B. Cysts are small and not a significant feature.
   C. May have a bright T1 component.
   D. Solid components enhance avidly.
   E. Is typically lobulated and heterogeneous.

✓ Answer B
   — In adamantinomatous craniopharyngiomas, cysts are usually large and a dominant feature present in 90% of cases. They appear as CSF density on CT and have variable MRI signals, appearing iso- to hyperintense on T1, and variable but partly or mostly hyperintense on T2 in 80% of cases.

? 57. Sellar/suprasellar tumors.
   Craniopharyngioma (papillary type). The FALSE answer is:
   A. Calcification is rare.
   B. Causes displacement of adjacent structures.
   C. Cysts are a dominant feature.
   D. Cysts are typically T1 hypointense if present.
   E. Solid components enhance avidly.

✓ Answer C
   — In papillary craniopharyngiomas, cysts are not a dominant feature and if present are usually small.

? 58. Sellar/suprasellar tumors.
   Meningioma. The FALSE answer is:
   A. Calcification is common.
   B. Can invade the cavernous sinus.
   C. Enhances avidly.
   D. May have a small cystic component.
   E. Typically enlarges the sella.

✓ Answer E
   — Although suprasellar meningiomas may extend inferiorly and have a small intrasellar component, they do not typically enlarge the sella turcica.

❓ 59. **Sellar/suprasellar tumors.**
Meningioma versus macroadenoma. The FALSE answer is:
A. A cystic component favors macroadenoma.
B. Hemorrhage favors meningioma.
C. Narrowing of the cavernous ICA is seen in meningioma.
D. Dural tail is described in meningioma.
E. Snowman appearance is typical for macroadenoma.

✅ **Answer B**
— Hemorrhage in a sellar/suprasellar mass favors macroadenoma over meningioma.

❓ 60. **Sellar/suprasellar tumors.**
Masses typically presenting as solid-enhancing lesions.
The FALSE answer is:
A. Adamantinomatous craniopharyngioma.
B. Germinoma.
C. Macroadenoma.
D. Meningioma.
E. Metastasis.

✅ **Answer A**
— Adamantinomatous craniopharyngiomas typically present as cystic and solid tumors.

❓ 61. **Sellar/suprasellar tumors.**
Cystic lesions. The FALSE answer is:
A. Craniopharyngioma.
B. Epidermoid cyst.
C. Macroadenoma.
D. Meningioma.
E. Rathke's cleft cyst.

✅ **Answer D**
— Meningiomas are typical solid-enhancing tumors. If a cystic component is present, it is usually small and not a dominant feature.

3

❓ 62. Sellar/suprasellar tumors.
Pituitary masses that may present as an entirely intrasellar lesion.
The FALSE answer is:
A. Craniopharyngioma.
B. Meningioma.
C. Microadenoma.
D. Pituicytoma.
E. Rathke's cleft cyst.

✅ Answer B
— Meningiomas can have intrasellar components. However, the epicenter of the lesion is always outside the sella turcica.

❓ 63. Sellar/suprasellar tumors.
Hypothalamic hamartoma imaging features. The FALSE answer is:
A. Avid contrast enhancement.
B. Isodense on CT.
C. Iso- to hyperintense to gray matter on T2.
D. Isointense on T1.
E. Solid homogeneous.

✅ Answer A
— Hypothalamic hamartomas do not typically show contrast enhancement.

❓ 64. Pineal region tumors.
Pineal parenchymal tumors: pineocytoma imaging features. The FALSE answer is:
A. Hyperintense on T2.
B. Iso- to hypointense on T1.
C. No enhancement.
D. Peripheral calcification.
E. Well-demarcated.

✅ Answer C
— Pineocytomas typically demonstrate avid homogeneous enhancement.

❓ 65. Pineal region tumors.
Parenchymal versus germ cell tumors. The FALSE answer is:
A. Cystic change excludes pineal parenchymal tumors.
B. Germinomas typically have central calcification.

C. Invasion of adjacent structures favors germinoma.

D. Pineal parenchymal tumors are more likely to spread through CSF.

E. Significant overlap in imaging findings is present.

✅ **Answer A**

▬ Cystic changes are commonly encountered in pineal parenchymal tumors. Germ cell tumors may also have cystic spaces.

❓ 66. **Intraventricular tumor. The FALSE answer is:**

A. Supratentorial ependymomas are more common in young adults.

B. Supratentorial ependymomas have a predilection for the third ventricle.

C. 60% of subependymomas arise in the fourth ventricle

D. Supratentorial subependymomas have a predilection for the atrium of lateral ventricle.

E. Intraventricular meningiomas usually arise in the trigone of the lateral ventricles.

✅ **Answer D**

▬ Supratentorial subependymomas have a predilection for the frontal horn of the lateral ventricle.

❓ 67. **Intraventricular tumor.**

Regarding the most common tumor location. The FALSE answer is:

A. Central neurocytoma at the septum pellucidum.

B. Subependymal giant cell astrocytoma in the foramen of Monro.

C. Chordoid glioma in the frontal horn.

D. Rosette-forming glioneuronal tumor in the fourth ventricle.

E. Metastasis in the lateral ventricle.

✅ **Answer C**

▬ Chordoid glioma is most commonly located in the anterior third ventricle/hypothalamus.

❓ 68. **Intraventricular tumors.**

Tumors located in the body of the lateral ventricle. The FALSE answer is:

A. CPP.

B. Teratoma.

C. PNET.
D. Pilocytic astrocytoma.
E. Meningioma.

✅ **Answer E**
— Intraventricular meningiomas are located within the trigone of the lateral ventricles.

❓ 69. **Intraventricular tumors.**
Choroid plexus tumors. The FALSE answer is:
A. Choroid plexus carcinoma (CPC) is found only in pediatric patients.
B. Choroid plexus papilloma (CPP) arises in the atrium of the lateral ventricle in 50% of cases.
C. CPP arises in the fourth ventricle in 40% of cases.
D. Lateral ventricle lesions are more common in children.
E. Fourth ventricle lesions are more common in adults.

✅ **Answer E**
— Fourth ventricle lesions are evenly distributed among all age groups.

❓ 70. **Intraventricular tumors.**
Tumors commonly associated with calcifications. The FALSE answer is:
A. Ependymoma.
B. Subependymoma.
C. Meningioma.
D. Choroid plexus tumors.
E. Chordoid glioma.

✅ **Answer E**
— Chordoid glioma does not calcify.

❓ 71. **Intraventricular tumors.**
Hyperdense tumors on CT. The FALSE answer is:
A. Central neurocytoma.
B. CPP.
C. Meningioma.
D. Chordoid glioma.
E. Ependymoma.

✅ **Answer E**
— Ependymomas are usually hypodense on CT.

❓ 72. **Intraventricular tumors.**
   Tumors showing avid enhancement. The FALSE answer is:
   A. Ependymoma.
   B. Subependymoma.
   C. Central neurocytoma.
   D. Subependymal giant cell astrocytoma.
   E. Meningioma.

✅ **Answer B**
— Subependymomas show minimal to no enhancement.

❓ 73. **Intraventricular tumors.**
   Pattern of enhancement in intraventricular tumors. The FALSE answer is:
   A. Mild enhancement in CPP.
   B. Avid enhancement in CPC.
   C. Avid enhancement in chordoid glioma.
   D. Heterogeneous enhancement in RGNT.
   E. Avid enhancement in metastasis.

✅ **Answer A**
— Enhancement is avid in all benign, atypical, and malignant choroid plexus tumors.

❓ 74. **Intraventricular tumors.**
   Common features for most intraventricular tumors. The FALSE answer is:
   A. Calcification.
   B. Hemorrhage.
   C. Cystic changes.
   D. Circumscribed borders.
   E. Lobulated margins.

✅ **Answer E**
— While all the other features are seen with most tumor types, lobulated margins are relatively specific for choroid plexus tumors.

? 75. Intraventricular tumors.

Perilesional edema is seen in all the following tumors. The FALSE answer is:

A. Ependymoma.
B. Subependymoma.
C. Central neurocytoma.
D. CPP.
E. Meningioma.

✓ Answer B

— Subependymomas are not associated with perilesional edema.

? 76. Intraventricular tumors.

Tumors showing CSF seeding. The FALSE answer is:

A. Ependymoma.
B. Supependymoma.
C. CPP.
D. CPC.
E. Central neurocytoma.

✓ Answer B

— Subependymomas are not associated with CSF seeding.

? 77. Advanced neuroimaging.

MR spectroscopy: typical imaging spectra of primary neoplasms. The FALSE answer is:

A. Elevated peak of lipid.
B. Elevated peak of lactate.
C. Elevated peak of choline.
D. Elevated peak of myoinositol.
E. Elevated peak of NAA.

✓ Answer E

— Primary brain tumors are associated with reduced peaks of NAA, which is a metabolite seen in normal neurons.

? 78. Advanced neuroimaging.

Role of MR spectroscopy in tumor imaging. The FALSE answer is:

A. No cutoff ratios to distinguish neoplastic from nonneoplastic conditions.

B. Can separate high-grade from low-grade neoplasms and nonneo-plastic conditions.
C. Lipid signal is absent in low-grade neoplasms.
D. A high myoinositol peak is characteristic of low-grade neoplasms.
E. Gliomatosis cerebri have advanced MR imaging features of high-grade neoplasms.

✅ **Answer E**
– Gliomatosis cerebri have advanced MR imaging features of low-grade neoplasms.

❓ 79. **Advanced neuroimaging.**
Typical MR spectroscopic features for secondary neoplasms. The FALSE answer is:
A. Similar to the metabolic profile of primary tumors.
B. Elevated peaks of amino acids.
C. Evaluation of the lesion itself is unreliable to distinguish from primary tumors.
D. Presence of peritumoral edema is helpful in distinguishing from primary tumors.
E. Choline/NAA ratio of greater than 1 in peritumoral edema has 100% accuracy.

✅ **Answer B**
– Elevated peaks of amino acids are associated with cerebral abscesses.

❓ 80. **Advanced neuroimaging.**
MRS: lesions with overlapping metabolic profiles. The FALSE answer is:
A. Gliomas.
B. Lymphoma.
C. Encephalitis.
D. Abscess.
E. Tumefactive demyelination.

✅ **Answer D**
– Abscesses have a distinct spectroscopic pattern that allows differentiation from other entities.

3

? 81. **Advanced neuroimaging.**
   MRS: lesions with overlapping metabolic profiles. The FALSE answer is:
   A. Can distinguish high-grade from low-grade gliomas.
   B. Can distinguish recurrence from treatment changes.
   C. Superior to PET CT in detecting posttreatment recurrence.
   D. Can aid in the planning of targeted biopsy.
   E. Can aid in the planning of radiation target volume.

✓ Answer C
▬ PET CT is superior to MRS in detecting posttreatment recurrence.

? 82. **Advanced neuroimaging.**
   Diffusion-weighted imaging in brain tumors. The FALSE answer is:
   A. Tumefactive demyelination is reliably distinguished from neoplasms.
   B. High-grade gliomas show more restriction than low-grade lesions.
   C. Not accurate in predicting tumor grade in adult tumors.
   D. Useful for distinguishing lymphoma from glioma.
   E. Of great value in distinguishing abscesses from necrotic tumors.

✓ Answer A
▬ The appearance of tumefactive demyelination may overlap with that of tumors on diffusion imaging.

? 83. **Advanced neuroimaging.**
   Diffusion-weighted imaging in pediatric posterior fossa tumors. The FALSE answer is:
   A. Accurate distinction of juvenile pilocytic astrocytoma (JPA) from ependymomas and medulloblastomas.
   B. Maximum diffusion restriction is noted in JPA.
   C. Significant overlap between medulloblastoma and ependymoma.
   D. Best correlated with conventional imaging features.
   E. Atypical teratoid rhabdoid tumor overlaps with medulloblastoma.

✓ Answer B
▬ Minimum restriction is seen with JPA.

❓ 84. Advanced neuroimaging.
Perfusion imaging. The FALSE answer is:
A. Helpful adjunct in differentiating low-grade tumors from high-grade tumors.
B. Improved target selection with stereotactic biopsy.
C. Identify and localize the higher-grade component of the tumor.
D. Useful for differentiating recurrent tumors from radiation necrosis.
E. Tumors tend to have reduced cerebral blood volume.

✅ Answer E
— Tumors tend to have high cerebral blood volume.

❓ 85. Advanced neuroimaging.
Perfusion imaging feature for primary neoplasms. The FALSE answer is:
A. Similar information can be obtained by CT and MR perfusion.
B. Neoplasms show increased permeability parameters.
C. Percentage signal recovery (PSRmax) is the quantitative permeability parameter.
D. Relative tumor blood volume (rTBV) is a valuable perfusion parameter.
E. Arterial spin labeling (ASL) is an MRI technique that requires contrast administration.

✅ Answer E
— Arterial spin labeling (ASL) is a perfusion MRI technique that is noninvasive and does not require contrast administration.

❓ 86. Advanced neuroimaging.
Perfusion imaging: features for intracranial neoplasms. The FALSE answer is:
A. Peritumoral perfusion may distinguish primary from secondary tumors.
B. Lymphoma is readily distinguished from primary tumors.
C. Lymphoma has low relative total blood volume (rTBV) compared to other tumors.
D. Tumefactive demyelination cannot be distinguished from tumors.
E. Abscesses can be distinguished from neoplasms.

✅ **Answer D**

— Tumefactive demyelination can be distinguished by perfusion imaging as it shows low rTBV compared to the surrounding brain tissue.

❓ 87. **Advanced neuroimaging.**
Perfusion imaging features for grading intracranial neoplasms. The FALSE answer is:
  A. A combination of PSR and rTBV gives higher accuracy.
  B. The rTBV increases with the neoplasm grade.
  C. Reliable classification into low-grade and high-grade.
  D. Can separate high-grade tumors into grades III and IV.
  E. Oligodendroglioma grade can be accurately predicted.

✅ **Answer E**

— Oligodendrogliomas are exceptions to the perfusion rules, as high TBV is also seen in low-grade oligodendrogliomas.

❓ 88. **Radiation necrosis versus recurrent tumor. The FALSE answer is:**
  A. Periventricular enhancement within the radiation port suggests radiation necrosis.
  B. New enhancement in a previously nonenhancing lesion suggests tumor recurrence.
  C. The soap bubble pattern of enhancement suggests radiation necrosis.
  D. Involvement of the corpus callosum favors recurrent tumor.
  E. Conventional imaging features show great overlap.

✅ **Answer B**

— New enhancement in a previously nonenhancing lesion suggests radiation necrosis.

❓ 89. **Radiation necrosis versus tumor recurrence: advanced neuroimaging.**
The FALSE answer is:
  A. Recurrent tumors have lower ADC values.
  B. The ADC ratio is more reliable than the ADC value.
  C. Fractional anisotropy is lower in radiation necrosis.
  D. Relative cerebral blood volume is higher in recurrent tumors.
  E. Radiation necrosis has a lower PSR than recurrent tumors.

✅ **Answer E**

– PSR is a measure of lesion permeability; the lower the PSR the higher the lesion permeability. Tumors generally have leaky capillaries and show a lower PSR than radiation necrosis.

❓ 90. **Radiation necrosis versus tumor recurrence, advanced neuroimaging. The FALSE answer is:**

A. PET scan can aid in distinguishing.
B. PET has 100% specificity.
C. Overlapping spectra in spectroscopy.
D. PSR is more reliable than CBV.
E. Tumors are often mixed with radiation necrosis.

✅ **Answer B**

– Overlap exists in PET scans of the two pathologies.

❓ 91. **Radiation necrosis versus tumor recurrence, MRS. The FALSE answer is:**

A. The combination of spectroscopy and perfusion data enhances specificity.
B. Recurrent tumor has a higher choline/creatinine ratio.
C. Recurrent tumor has a higher choline/NAA ratio.
D. A high lipid lactate peak with lower levels of other metabolites is more suggestive of tumor recurrence.
E. Necrosis may have a high choline peak.

✅ **Answer D**

– High lipid lactate peaks are seen with both radiation necrosis and tumor recurrence. However, high lipid lactate with lower levels of other metabolites is more suggestive of radiation necrosis.

❓ 92. **Spinal cord tumors.**
Intramedullary tumors: general imaging features. The FALSE answer is:

A. Are almost always circumscribed.
B. Cause cord expansion.
C. Enhancement is common.
D. Hemorrhage can be seen.
E. Tumoral cysts can be seen.

✅ Answer A

— Intramedullary tumors can be circumscribed as in ependymoma or infiltrative as in astrocytoma.

❓ 93. Spinal cord tumors.

The following spinal tumors are typically intramedullary. The FALSE answer is:

A. Astrocytoma.
B. Ependymoma.
C. Ganglioglioma.
D. Hemangioblastoma.
E. Schwannoma.

✅ Answer E

— Spinal schwannomas are typically extramedullary in location.

❓ 94. Spinal cord tumors.

Intramedullary tumors: ependymoma imaging features. The FALSE answer is:

A. Avid enhancement.
B. Circumscribed outline.
C. Cysts are seen.
D. Eccentric in location.
E. Hemorrhage is present.

✅ Answer D

— Ependymomas are more central than eccentrically located in relation to the cross-sectional area of the cord. Hemorrhage can be seen sometimes and results in the formation of the classic hemosiderin cap at the superior or inferior margins of the mass.

❓ 95. Spinal cord tumors.

Intramedullary tumors: ependymoma versus astrocytoma. The FALSE answer is:

A. Avid homogeneous enhancement excludes astrocytoma.
B. Central location favors ependymoma.
C. Holocord involvement is classically seen in astrocytoma.
D. Infiltrative appearance favors astrocytoma.
E. Location at the conus medullaris favors ependymoma.

✅ **Answer A**

▬ Spinal cord astrocytoma exhibits variable enhancement. They can show minimal enhancement. Avid enhancement can also be seen, and can be homogeneous or heterogeneous. Astrocytomas are eccentrically located in the cord, unlike ependymomas. Holocord involvement is common in children but rare in adults. Although astrocytoma can be located at the conus, it is a rare location.

❓ 96. **Spinal cord tumors.**
Intradural extramedullary tumors: general imaging features. The FALSE answer is:
A. Cord compression.
B. Cord deviation.
C. Cord infiltration.
D. Enhancement.
E. Widened ipsilateral CSF space.

✅ **Answer C**

▬ The cord is compressed and deviated by the tumor but infiltration is classically not seen. Most intradural extramedullary tumors show enhancement. The CSF space ipsilateral to the tumor is widened with narrowing of the contralateral CSF space.

❓ 97. **Spinal cord tumors.**
Tumors that can present as intradural extramedullary masses. The FALSE answer is:
A. Astrocytoma.
B. Meningioma.
C. Metastasis.
D. Neurofibroma.
E. Schwannoma.

✅ **Answer A**

▬ Astrocytoma is an intramedullary tumor. The most common intradural extramedullary masses are meningiomas and schwannomas. Other less common types of intradural masses include benign fibrous histiocytoma (hemangiopericytoma).

❓ 98. **Spinal cord tumors.**
Intradural extramedullary masses: meningioma imaging findings.
The FALSE answer is:
A. Avid enhancement.
B. Dural tail.
C. Calcification.
D. Location in the thoracic region is favored.
E. Hemorrhage.

✅ **Answer E**
— Hemorrhage is rare in meningioma.

❓ 99. **Spinal cord tumors.**
Intradural extramedullary tumors: schwannomas imaging findings.
The FALSE answer is:
A. Bony remodeling.
B. Cystic changes.
C. Hemorrhage is present.
D. Minimal enhancement.
E. Widened intervertebral foramen.

✅ **Answer D**
— Schwannomas usually show avid enhancement, although they can be heterogeneous due to the presence of cystic changes or hemorrhage.

❓ 100. **Spinal cord tumors.**
Intradural extramedullary masses: signs differentiating schwannoma from meningioma. The FALSE answer is:
A. Arachnoid isolation sign: meningioma.
B. Calcification: meningioma.
C. Dumb-bell sign: schwannoma.
D. Dural tail sign: meningioma.
E. Ginkgo leaf sign: schwannoma.

✅ **Answer E**
— The Ginkgo leaf sign is typical for spinal meningioma. It is described on axial contrast-enhanced T1 images with the leaf representing the compressed distorted cord and the stem mostly representing the nonenhanced denticulate ligament.

Bibliography

1. Rapalino O, Smirniotopoulos JG. Extra-axial brain tumors. Handb Clin Neurol. 2016;135:275–91.
2. Mühl-Benninghaus R. Extraaxiale Tumoren des zentralen Nervensystems [Extra-axial tumors of the central nervous system]. Radiologe. 2017;57(9):715–27. German.
3. Papanagiotou P. Intra-axial brain tumors. Radiologe. 2012;52(6):567–81.
4. Aronica E, Crino PB. Epilepsy related to developmental tumors and malformations of cortical development. Neurotherapeutics. 2014;11(2):251–68.
5. Barkley AS, Kuo CH, Leary SES, Ojemann JG, Susarla SM. Unusual radiographic presentation of intracranial mature teratoma and resection via supraorbital approach. World Neurosurg. 2019;122:81–4.
6. Bruzzone MG, D'Incerti L, Farina LL, Cuccarini V, Finocchiaro G. CT and MRI of brain tumors. Q J Nucl Med Mol Imaging. 2012;56(2):26.
7. Berberat J, Grobholz R, Boxheimer L, Rogers S, Remonda L, Roelcke U. Differentiation between calcification and hemorrhage in brain tumors using susceptibility-weighted imaging: a pilot study. Am J Roentgenol. 2014;202(4):847–50.
8. Rauscher A, Sedlacik J, Barth M, et al. Magnetic susceptibility weighted MR phase imaging of the human brain. AJNR Am J Neuroradiol. 2005;26:736–42.
9. Leung D, Han X, Mikkelsen T, Nabors LB. Role of MRI in primary brain tumor evaluation. J Natl Compr Cancer Netw. 2014;12(11):1561–8.
10. Cha S. Update on brain tumor imaging: from anatomy to physiology. AJNR Am J Neuroradiol. 2006;27:475–87.
11. Badve C, Yu A, Dastmalchian S, Rogers M, Ma D, Jiang Y, et al. MR fingerprinting of adult brain tumors: initial experience. Am J Neuroradiol. 2017;38(3):492–9.
12. Jiang Y, Ma D, Seiberlich N, et al. MR fingerprinting using fast imaging with steady state precession (FISP) with spiral readout. Magn Reson Med. 2015;74:1621–31. https://doi.org/10.1002/mrm.25559.
13. Thomas RP, Xu LW, Lober RM, et al. The incidence and significance of multiple lesions in glioblastoma. J Neurooncol. 2013;112:91–7. https://doi.org/10.1007/s11060-012-1030-1.
14. Smirniotopoulos JG, Murphy FM, Rushing EJ, Rees JH, Schroeder JW. Patterns of contrast enhancement in the brain and meninges. Radiographics. 2007;27(2):525–51 [cited 2020 Dec 22]. Available from: https://pubs.rsna.org/doi/10.1148/rg.272065155.
15. Provenzale JM, Mukundan S, Dewhirst M. The role of blood-brain barrier permeability in brain tumor imaging and therapeutics. AJR Am J Roentgenol. 2005;185:763–7.
16. Phillips ME, Ryals TJ, Kambhu SA, Yuh WT. Neoplastic vs inflammatory meningeal enhancement with Gd-DTPA. J Comput Assist Tomogr. 1990;14:536–41.
17. Gupta S, Gupta RK, Banerjee D, Gujral RB. Problems with the dural tail sign. Neuroradiology. 1993;35:541–2.
18. Takano S, Kamiyama H, Tsuboi K, Matsumura A. Angiogenesis and antiangiogenic therapy for malignant gliomas. Brain Tumor Pathol. 2004;21:69–73.
19. Takeuchi H, Kubota T, Sato K, Arishima H. Ultrastructure of capillary endothelium in pilocytic astrocytomas. Brain Tumor Pathol. 2004;21:23–6.
20. Beni-Adani L, Gomori M, Spektor S, Constantini S. Cyst wall enhancement in pilocytic astrocytoma: neoplastic or reactive phenomena. Pediatr Neurosurg. 2000;32:234–9. https://doi.org/10.1159/000028944.

21. Masdeu JC, Moreira J, Trasi S, Visintainer P, Cavaliere R, Grundman M. The open ring: a new imaging sign in demyelinating disease. J Neuroimaging. 1996;6:104–7.
22. Schwartz KM, Erickson BJ, Lucchinetti C. Pattern of T2 hypointensity associated with ring-enhancing brain lesions can help to differentiate pathology. Neuroradiology. 2006;48:143–9.
23. Hartmann M, Jansen O, Heiland S, Sommer C, Munkel K, Sartor K. Restricted diffusion within ring enhancement is not pathognomonic for brain abscess. AJNR Am J Neuroradiol. 2001;22:1738.
24. Cha S, Knopp EA, Johnson G, Wetzel SG, Litt AW, Zagzag D. Intracranial mass lesions: dynamic contrast-enhanced susceptibility-weighted echo-planar perfusion MR imaging. Radiology. 2002;223:11–29.
25. Raz E, Zagzag D, Saba L, Mannelli L, Di Paolo PL, D'Ambrosio F, Knopp E. Cyst with a mural nodule tumor of the brain. Cancer Imaging. 2012;12(1):237–44.
26. Shin JH, Lee HK, Khang SK, et al. Neuronal tumors of the central nervous system: radiologic findings and pathologic correlation. Radiographics. 2002;22:1177–89.
27. Pierallini A, Bonamini M, Di Stefano D, Siciliano P, Bozzao L. Pleomorphic xanthoastrocytoma with CT and MRI appearance of meningioma. Neuroradiology. 1999;41:30–4.
28. Erdogan C, Hakyemez B, Yildirim N, Parlak M. Brain abscess and cystic brain tumor: discrimination with dynamic susceptibility contrast perfusion-weighted MRI. J Comput Assist Tomogr. 2005;29(5):663–7.
29. Provenzale JM, Wang GR, Brenner T, Petrella JR, Sorensen AG. Comparison of permeability in high-grade and low-grade brain tumors using dynamic susceptibility contrast MR imaging. Am J Roentgenol. 2002;178(3):711–6.
30. AlRayahi J, Zapotocky M, Ramaswamy V, Hanagandi P, Branson H, Mubarak W, et al. Pediatric brain tumor genetics: what radiologists need to know? Radiographics. 2018;38(7):2102–22.
31. Belden CJ, Valdes PA, Ran C, Pastel DA, Harris BT, Fadul CE, et al. Genetics of glioblastoma: a window into its imaging and histopathologic variability. Radiographics. 2011;31(6):1717–40.
32. Altman DA, Atkinson DS, Brat DJ. Glioblastoma multiforme. Radiographics. 2007;27(3):883–8.
33. Koeller KK, Rushing EJ. Oligodendroglioma and its variants: radiologic-pathologic correlation. Radiographics. 2005;25(6):1669–88.
34. Zulfiqar M, Yousem DM, Lai H. ADC values and prognosis of malignant astrocytomas: does lower ADC predict a worse prognosis independent of grade of tumor—a meta-analysis. Am J Roentgenol. 2013;200(3):624–9.
35. Provenzale JM, York G, Moya MG, Parks L, Choma M, Kealey S, et al. Correlation of relative permeability and relative cerebral blood volume in high-grade cerebral neoplasms. Am J Roentgenol. 2006;187(4):1036–42.
36. Gempt J, Soehngen E, Förster S, et al. Multimodal imaging in cerebral gliomas and its neuropathological correlation. Eur J Radiol. 2014;83:829–34. https://doi.org/10.1016/j.ejrad.2014.02.006.
37. Perkins A, Liu G. Primary brain tumors in adults: diagnosis and treatment. Am Fam Physician. 2016;93(3):211–7.
38. Chalal RA, Kessaci F, Mansouri B. Posterior fossa tumors in adults: MR imaging. In: EPOS. European Congress of Radiology—ECR 2017; 2017.

39. Arslanoglu A, Aygun N, Tekhtani D, Aronson L, Cohen K, Burger PC, et al. Imaging findings of CNS atypical teratoid/rhabdoid tumors. Am J Neuroradiol. 2004;25(3):476–80.
40. Kerleroux B, Cottier JP, Janot K, Listrat A, Sirinelli D, Morel B. Posterior fossa tumors in children: radiological tips & tricks in the age of genomic tumor classification and advance MR technology. J Neuroradiol. 2020;47(1):46–53.
41. Poretti A, Meoded A, Huisman TAGM. Neuroimaging of pediatric posterior fossa tumors including review of the literature. J Magn Reson Imaging. 2012;35(1):32–47.
42. Koeller KK, Rushing EJ. From the archives of the AFIP: medulloblastoma: a comprehensive review with radiologic-pathologic correlation. Radiographics. 2003;23(6):1613–37.
43. Helton KJ, Phillips NS, Khan RB, et al. Diffusion tensor imaging of tract involvement in children with pontine tumors. AJNR Am J Neuroradiol. 2006;27(4):786–93.
44. Koeller KK, Rushing EJ. From the archives of the AFIP: pilocytic astrocytoma: radiologic-pathologic correlation. Radiographics. 2004;24(6):1693–708.
45. Yuh EL, Barkovich AJ, Gupta N. Imaging of ependymomas: MRI and CT. Childs Nerv Syst. 2009;25(10):1203–13.
46. Fink JR. Imaging of cerebellopontine angle masses: self-assessment module. AJR Am J Roentgenol. 2010;195(3):S15–21.
47. Silk PS, Lane JI, Driscoll CL. Surgical approaches to vestibular schwannomas: what the radiologist needs to know. Radiographics. 2009;29(7):1955–70.
48. Fink JR. Imaging of cerebellopontine angle masses: self-assessment module. Am J Roentgenol. 2010;195(3_Suppl):S15–21.
49. Venkatasamy A, Le Foll D, Karol A, Lhermitte B, Charpiot A, Debry C, et al. Differentiation of vestibular schwannomas from meningiomas of the internal auditory canal using perilymphatic signal evaluation on T2-weighted gradient-echo fast imaging employing steady state acquisition at 3T. Eur Radiol Exp. 2017;1(1):8.
50. Hsu C, Kwan G, Lau Q, Bhuta S. Rosette-forming glioneuronal tumour: imaging features, histopathological correlation and a comprehensive review of literature. Br J Neurosurg. 2012;26(5):668–73.
51. Gardiman MP, Fassan M, Orvieto E, D'Avella D, Denaro L, Calderone M, et al. Diffuse leptomeningeal glioneuronal tumors: a new entity? Brain Pathol. 2010;20(2):361–6.
52. Boxerman JL, Rogg JM, Donahue JE, et al. Preoperative MRI evaluation of pituitary macroadenoma: imaging features predictive of successful transsphenoidal surgery. AJR Am J Roentgenol. 2010;195(3):720–8.
53. Friedman TC, Zuckerbraun E, Lee ML, et al. Dynamic pituitary MRI has high sensitivity and specificity for the diagnosis of mild Cushing's syndrome and should be part of the initial workup. Horm Metab Res. 2007;39(6):451–6.
54. Byun WM, Kim OL, Kim D. MR imaging findings of Rathke's cleft cysts: significance of intracystic nodules. AJNR Am J Neuroradiol. 2000;21(3):485–8.
55. Bonneville F, Cattin F, Marsot-Dupuch K, Dormont D, Bonneville J-F, Chiras J. T1 signal hyperintensity in the sellar region: spectrum of findings. Radiographics. 2006;26(1):93–113.
56. Sartoretti-Schefer S, Wichmann W, Aguzzi A, Valavanis A. MR differentiation of adamantinomatous and squamous-papillary craniopharyngiomas. AJNR Am J Neuroradiol. 1997;18(1):77–87.

57. Smith AB, Horkanyne-Szakaly I, Schroeder JW, et al. From the radiologic pathology archives: mass lesions of the dura: beyond meningioma-radiologic-pathologic correlation. Radiographics. 2014;34(2):295–312.

58. Pisaneschi M, Kapoor G. Imaging the sella and parasellar region. Neuroimaging Clin N Am. 2005;15(1):203–19.

59. Connor SE, Penney CC. MRI in the differential diagnosis of a sellar mass. Clin Radiol. 2003;58(1):20–31.

60. Shin JL, Asa SL, Woodhouse LJ, et al. Cystic lesions of the pituitary: clinicopathological features distinguishing craniopharyngioma, Rathke's cleft cyst, and arachnoid cyst. J Clin Endocrinol Metab. 1999;84(11):3972–82.

61. Rao VJ, James RA, Mitra D. Imaging characteristics of common suprasellar lesions with emphasis on MRI findings. Clin Radiol. 2008;63(8):939–47.

62. Amstutz DR, Coons SW, Kerrigan JF, et al. Hypothalamic hamartomas: correlation of MR imaging and spectroscopic findings with tumor glial content. AJNR Am J Neuroradiol. 2006;27(4):794–8.

63. Smith AB, Rushing EJ, Smirniotopoulos JG. From the archives of the AFIP: lesions of the pineal region: radiologic-pathologic correlation. Radiographics. 2010;30(7):2001–20.

64. Dumrongpisutikul N, Intrapiromkul J, Yousem DM. Distinguishing between germinomas and pineal cell tumors on MR imaging. Am J Neuroradiol. 2012;33(3):550–5.

65. Shogan P, Banks KP, Brown S. AJR teaching file: intraventricular mass. Am J Roentgenol. 2007;189(6_Suppl):S55–7.

66. Glastonbury CM, Osborn AG, Salzman KL. Masses and malformations of the third ventricle: normal anatomic relationships and differential diagnoses. Radiographics. 2011;31(7):1889–905.

67. Houle V, Bélair M, Allaire GS. AIRP best cases in radiologic-pathologic correlation: choroidal melanoma. Radiographics. 2011;31(5):1231–6.

68. Grygotis LA, Chew FS. Choroid plexus carcinoma of the lateral ventricle. Am J Roentgenol. 1997;169(5):1400.

69. Zarghouni M, Vandergriff C, Layton KF, et al. Chordoid glioma of the third ventricle. Proc (Bayl Univ Med Cent). 2012;25(3):285–6.

70. Mermuys K, Jeuris W, Vanhoenacker PK, Van Hoe L, D'Haenens P. Supratentorial ependymoma. Radiographics. 2005;25(2):486–90.

71. Koeller KK, Sandberg GD, Armed Forces Institute of Pathology. From the archives of the AFIP. Cerebral intraventricular neoplasms: radiologic-pathologic correlation. Radiographics. 2002;22(6):1473–505.

72. Smith AB, Smirniotopoulos JG, Horkanyne-Szakaly I. From the radiologic pathology archives: intraventricular neoplasms: radiologic-pathologic correlation. Radiographics. 2013;33(1):21–43.

73. Zhang TJ, Yue Q, Lui S, et al. MRI findings of choroid plexus tumors in the cerebellum. Clin Imaging. 2011;35(1):64–7.

74. Ragel BT, Osborn AG, Whang K, et al. Subependymomas: an analysis of clinical and imaging features. Neurosurgery. 2006;58(5):881–90.

75. Koral K, Kedzierski RM, Gimi B, et al. Subependymoma of the cerebellopontine angle and prepontine cistern in a 15-year-old adolescent boy. AJNR Am J Neuroradiol. 2008;29(1):190–1.

76. Vallée A, Guillevin C, Wager M, Delwail V, Guillevin R, Vallée J-N. Added value of spectroscopy to perfusion MRI in the differential diagnostic performance of common malignant brain tumors. Am J Neuroradiol. 2018;39(8):1423–31.

77. Huang W, Alexander GE, Daly EM, et al. High brain myo-inositol levels in the predementia phase of Alzheimer's disease in adults with Down's syndrome: a 1H MRS study. Am J Psychiatry. 1999;156(12):1879–86.

78. Sharma A, Kumar R. Metabolic imaging of brain tumor recurrence. Am J Roentgenol. 2020;215(5):1199–207.

79. Stoffey RD, Clinical MR. Spectroscopy: techniques and applications. Am J Roentgenol. 2011;196(5):W662.

80. Tien RD, Lai PH, Smith JS, Lazeyras F. Single-voxel proton brain spectroscopy exam (PROBE/SV) in patients with primary brain tumors. Am J Roentgenol. 1996;167(1):201–9.

81. Kono K, Inoue Y, Nakayama K, Shakudo M, Morino M, Ohata K, et al. The role of diffusion-weighted imaging in patients with brain tumors. Am J Neuroradiol. 2001;22(6):1081–8.

82. Jaremko JL, Jans LBO, Coleman LT, Ditchfield MR. Value and limitations of diffusion-weighted imaging in grading and diagnosis of pediatric posterior fossa tumors. Am J Neuroradiol. 2010;31(9):1613–6.

83. Feldman SC, Chu D, Schulder M, Barry M, Cho E-S, Liu W-C. The blood oxygen level–dependent functional MR imaging signal can be used to identify brain tumors and distinguish them from normal tissue. Am J Neuroradiol. 2009;30(2):389–95.

84. Geer CP, Simonds J, Anvery A, Chen MY, Burdette JH, Zapadka ME, et al. Does MR perfusion imaging impact management decisions for patients with brain tumors? A prospective study. Am J Neuroradiol. 2012;33(3):556–62.

85. Bulakbasi N, Kocaoglu M, Farzaliyev A, Tayfun C, Ucoz T, Somuncu I. Assessment of diagnostic accuracy of perfusion MR imaging in primary and metastatic solitary malignant brain tumors. Am J Neuroradiol. 2005;26(9):2187–99.

86. Halshtok Neiman O, Sadetzki S, Chetrit A, et al. Perfusion-weighted imaging of peritumoral edema can aid in the differential diagnosis of glioblastoma mulltiforme versus brain metastasis. Isr Med Assoc J. 2013;15:103–5.

87. Shah R, Vattoth S, Jacob R, Manzil FFP, O'Malley JP, Borghei P, et al. Radiation necrosis in the brain: imaging features and differentiation from tumor recurrence. Radiographics. 2012;32(5):1343–59.

88. Mullins ME, Barest GD, Schaefer PW, et al. Radiation necrosis versus glioma recurrence: conventional MR imaging clues to diagnosis. AJNR Am J Neuroradiol. 2005;26(8):1967–72.

89. Clarke JL, Chang S. Pseudoprogression and pseudoresponse: challenges in brain tumor imaging. Curr Neurol Neurosci Rep. 2009;9:241–6. https://doi.org/10.1007/s11910-009-0035-4.

90. Brandes AA, Tosoni A, Spagnolli F, et al. Disease progression or pseudoprogression after concomitant radiochemotherapy treatment: pitfalls in neurooncology. Neuro Oncol. 2008;10(3):361–7.

91. Shih RY, Koeller KK. Intramedullary masses of the spinal cord: radiologic-pathologic correlation. Radiographics. 2020;40(4):1125–45.

92. Buch K. Invited commentary: a framework for the differential diagnosis of benign and malignant intramedullary tumors. Radiographics. 2020;40(4):1146–7.

93. Botelho RV, de Oliveira MF, Kuntz C. Differential diagnosis of spinal disease. In: Winn HR, editor. Youmans and Winn neurological surgery. 7th ed. Amsterdam: Elsevier; 2017. p. 2322–36.

94. Herbrecht A, Messerer M, Parker F. Development of a lateralization index for intramedullary astrocytomas and ependymomas. Neurochirurgie. 2017;63(5):410–2.
95. Koeller KK, Shih RY. Intradural extramedullary spinal neoplasms: radiologic-pathologic correlation. Radiographics. 2019;39(2):468–90.
96. Koeller KK, Rosenblum RS, Morrison AL. Neoplasms of the spinal cord and filum terminale: radiologic-pathologic correlation. Radiographics. 2000;20(6):1721–49.
97. Zhai X, Zhou M, Chen H, Tang Q, Cui Z, Yao Y, Yin Q. Differentiation between intraspinal schwannoma and meningioma by MR characteristics and clinic features. Radiol Med. 2019;124(6):510–21.
98. Abul-kasim K, Thurnher MM, Mckeever P, et al. Intradural spinal tumors: current classification and MRI features. Neuroradiology. 2008;50(4):301–14.
99. Yamaguchi S, Takeda M, Takahashi T, et al. Ginkgo leaf sign: a highly predictive imaging feature of spinal meningioma. J Neurosurg Spine. 2015;23(5):1–5.

3

Management of CNS Tumors (General Principles)

*Mohamed J. Mubarak, Mohammed A. Al-Dhahir,
Hayder R. Salih, Mustafa Ismail,
Mohamed M. Arnaout, and Samer S. Hoz*

© The Author(s), under exclusive license to Springer Nature Switzerland AG 2024
S. S. Hoz et al. (eds.), *Surgical Neuro-Oncology*,
https://doi.org/10.1007/978-3-031-53642-7_4

❓ 1. Pregnancy and brain tumors.
General considerations. The FALSE answer is:
A. Should immediately carry out an abortion.
B. Should proceed with full radiological investigations if needed.
C. Dexamethasone is beneficial.
D. Should be careful with the antiepileptics.
E. To delay chemotherapy until postnatal.

4

✓ Answer A
- MRI is the preferred modality for diagnosis and follow-up in pregnancy due to the lack of ionizing radiation, greater resolution, and better sensitivity.
- If the mother's life or function is in jeopardy, surgery must be done under special anesthesia consideration.
- The use of steroids is of great help in postponing surgery until the third trimester or even after full-term delivery.

❓ 2. Pregnancy and brain tumors.
Anesthesia. The FALSE answer is:
A. Can cause developmental abnormalities in the third trimester.
B. The risk of spontaneous abortion is increased.
C. Aspiration is significant at induction.
D. Supine hypotension syndrome should be avoided.
E. Hypotension can cause premature contraction.

✓ Answer A
- Anesthesia drugs during craniotomy can cause developmental abnormalities in the first trimester.
- Hypotension should be avoided throughout the procedure which has a negative impact on oxygen delivery to the fetus.
- Avoid the supine position which causes mechanical compression on the vena cava.

❓ 3. Pregnancy and brain tumors.
Delivery. The FALSE answer is:
A. Can be achieved safely at 32 weeks.
B. Can be planned before craniotomy.
C. A cesarean section is preferred.
D. Should administer general anesthesia.
E. Can use regional anesthesia.

✅ **Answer E**
- An epidural block is contraindicated in the presence of an intracranial mass.
- When delivery and craniotomy are planned to be done simultaneously, delivery of the fetus by cesarean section is done first, followed by craniotomy.

❓ 4. **Pregnancy and brain tumors.**
Pituitary tumors. The FALSE answer is:
   A. Increase in size physiologically during pregnancy.
   B. Increase in size of adenoma during pregnancy.
   C. More pronounced in the second and third trimesters.
   D. Adenoma is usually of the micro type.
   E. The risk of hemorrhage is increased.

✅ **Answer D**
- The pituitary gland increases in size physiologically in pregnancy by 45%.
- A preexisting pituitary macroadenoma is more commonly associated with enlargement during pregnancy compared to a microadenoma.

❓ 5. **Pregnancy and brain tumors.**
Pituitary tumors. The FALSE answer is:
   A. Most can be observed with frequent ophthalmologic evaluations.
   B. Apoplexy necessitates urgent surgery.
   C. The transsphenoidal approach is safe in pregnancy.
   D. Should carry adjuvant radiotherapy after pregnancy only.
   E. Should encourage early breastfeeding in prolactinoma.

✅ **Answer E**
- Breastfeeding increases prolactin secretion, and thus, cessation should be considered in the case of prolactinoma.

❓ 6. **Early postoperative seizure in tumor surgery. The FALSE answer is:**
   A. Seen more in intra-axial tumors.
   B. Incidences increase with preoperative seizure.
   C. Incidence is less in minimally invasive techniques.
   D. Risk increases after 48 hours.
   E. AEDs are given for no more than 1 week in the low-risk group.

✅ **Answer D**
- Postoperative seizure is attributed to corticotomy of the supratentorial brain compartment typically in intra-axial tumors.
- The incidence is higher in the first 48 hours postsurgery.
- It is recommended to use the antiepileptics medications for no more than a week.

❓ 7. **Tumor embolization. The FALSE answer is:**
   A. Facilitates tumor resection.
   B. It does not change the mortality.
   C. May increase morbidity.
   D. Can be an alternative to surgery.
   E. Complete devascularization is not always possible.

✅ **Answer D**
- Tumor embolization is an adjunctive tool in the management of central nervous system tumors.
- Attention must be paid to the dangerous anastomotic connections to avoid the risk of unintended embolization of critical structures.
- Anatomy of the vascular supply and drainage of the tumor must be well understood as inadvertent embolization of the vasa nervosa of the cranial nerve or a territory supplied by the main artery can have deleterious effects.
- Cerebral edema and stroke are the main morbidities of embolization.

❓ 8. **Postoperative worsening of neurological deficit. The FALSE answer is:**
   A. Higher incidence with benign tumors.
   B. Early prophylaxis measures reduce the rate of incidence.
   C. Can be reduced by using navigation.
   D. Can be reduced by using intraoperative MRI.
   E. Fluorescence-guided surgery reduces the incidence.

✅ **Answer A**
- The incidence of new or worsened neurological deficits postoperatively has been observed to be higher in surgeries for malignant intra-axial brain tumors.
- The advancement of diagnostic and intraoperative techniques has helped increase the free margin of tumor resection.
- The maximization of resection in brain tumors leads to better postoperative neurological outcomes and hence overall survival.

9. **The advantage of 5-ALA intraoperative fluorescence. The FALSE answer is:**
   A. Real-time information.
   B. Information is provided through the microscope directly.
   C. Information is provided from tissue directly and not from images.
   D. Provides three-dimensional information.
   E. Can be repeated as often as necessary.

✅ **Answer D**
- 5-ALA fluorescence technique provides real-time information.
- Extended resection can be made only depending on the area of fluorescence.
- Reduces reliability on imaging which may be inaccurate with intraoperative brain shift.
- Drawbacks: two-dimensional, visibility can be changed by overhanging brain tissue, blood, and hemostatic agents.

10. **Intraoperative MRI (iMRI) in tumor surgery. The FALSE answer is:**
   A. Typically for intra-axial tumors.
   B. Expensive.
   C. Need for training.
   D. Maximizes the resection and reduces reoperating on gliomas.
   E. No change in survival rate in high-grade glioma.

✅ **Answer E**
- Intraoperative MRI allows the surgeon to discover the residual and remove it in the same setting.
- Can incorporate other new diagnostic and mapping techniques like DTI.
- Drawbacks: expensive technology, need for training, and inability to control lost surgical plane due to brain shift.

11. **Intraoperative CT scan (iCT). The FALSE answer is:**
   A. Allows real-time tumor identification.
   B. Helps in navigation resetting.
   C. Better used for skull base lesions.
   D. Helps in maximizing the resection.
   E. Improves postoperative general outcome.

✅ **Answer C**
- Intraoperative CT scans and other imaging techniques are better for intra-axial tumor resection.

❓ 12. Postoperative peritumoral edema. The FALSE answer is:
A. Rarely encountered in intra-axial tumors.
B. Reduced by using steroids.
C. Can result from suboptimal head positioning intraoperatively.
D. Can result from suboptimal head positioning postoperatively.
E. Can result from a brain vessel injury.

✓ Answer A

4

- It is important that the surgeon predicts and avoids this complication as the consequences are devastating.
- It adversely affects the local and overall surgical outcome.
- It is important to pay attention to the head positioning before surgery and in the postoperative observation period.
- The use of steroids, unobstructed venous drainage, CSF drainage, maintaining low-normal carbon dioxide perioperatively, and elevation of the head help alleviate postoperative edema.

❓ 13. Postoperative peritumoral edema.
Controlled hyperventilation. The FALSE answer is:
A. Can be done during surgery.
B. Decrease $PaCO_2$ causes an increase in rCBF.
C. Can reduce the ICP.
D. The physiological mechanism is respiratory alkalosis.
E. Target $PaCO_2$ level is 30–35 mmHg.

✓ Answer B

- Controlled hypertension is a rescue measure to reduce edema and raised ICP.
- Can be done temporarily during surgery when the brain is bulging.
- The reduced $PaCO_2$ causes a decrease in rCBF. This can be helpful immediately but harmful when sustained.
- The recommended target level of $PaCO_2$ is 30–35 mmHg for no longer than a few hours.

❓ 14. Postoperative peritumoral edema.
Osmotherapy. The FALSE answer is:
A. The level of osmolality is solely determined by plasma urea.
B. The goal of treatment is euvolemia or slight hypervolemia.
C. Target osmolality in brain edema ranges from 300 to 320 mOsm/L.

D. The osmotic agent should be chemically inert, nontoxic, and excluded by the blood-brain barrier.

E. Mannitol has an issue of causing hypotension, renal insufficiency, and pulmonary edema.

✅ **Answer A**
— Osmolality is determined by the level of urea, sodium, and glucose.

❓ 15. **Advantages of reoperating on high-grade glioma. The FALSE answer is:**
A. Cytoreduction of a residual/recurrence.
B. Upgrading or augmenting the original diagnosis.
C. To relieve symptoms.
D. To exclude radiation necrosis.
E. Allows to stop adjuvant therapy.

✅ **Answer E**
— Reoperation can facilitate adjuvant chemoradiotherapy and allows for the implantation of chemotherapy and radiotherapy delivery devices in the cavity.
— Reducing the tumor mass is the key to successful adjuvant therapy.
— Age, symptoms, performance score, and fitness for future therapy are factors to consider before redo surgery.

❓ 16. **Meningioma.**
Surgical management. The FALSE answer is:
A. Indicated if the patient is symptomatic.
B. Indicated if the growth is more than 3 cm/year.
C. Surgery can be done to prevent future symptoms in asymptomatic patients.
D. Can wait and watch in some cases upon the patient's wishes.
E. Simpson grade predicts the recurrence rate after surgery.

✅ **Answer B**
— Surgery should always aim for total excision, as the recurrence rate is lowest with lower Simpson grades.
— In symptomatic patients, surgery is mandatory. In asymptomatic patients, surgery is easier and has fewer complications with small tumors (<3 cm) when the ICP is normal and tumor infiltration between structures is less.
— Patients can choose to wait and watch, provided serial neuroimaging shows no growth faster than 1 cm/year.

? 17. **Meningioma.**
   Radiation therapy. The FALSE answer is:
   A. Improves local control.
   B. Depends on the extent of resection.
   C. The risk of radiation should be weighed against the risk of recurrence.
   D. Stereotactic radiosurgery is considered for tumors <4 cm.
   E. Stereotactic radiosurgery can be considered for multiple meningiomas.

4

✅ **Answer D**
- Stereotactic radiosurgery is a continuously evolving treatment of residual and recurrent small meningiomas less than 3.5 cm in size and even in cases with multiple lesions. The best outcome is seen in tumors less than 1 cm with minimized radiation injury.
- The risk of radiation injury should be weighed against watching the lesion before starting radiotherapy.

? 18. **DVT in craniotomy patient.**
   Prophylaxis. The FALSE answer is:
   A. More effective with pharmacological agents.
   B. Heparin increases the risk of hemorrhage.
   C. Mechanical and pharmacological prophylaxes are equally effective.
   D. Mechanical and pharmacological can be both used simultaneously.
   E. Need not be started for all pediatric patients.

✅ **Answer B**
- Heparin does not increase the risk of hemorrhage.

? 19. **DVT in craniotomy patient.**
   Risk factors. The FALSE answer is:
   A. Obesity.
   B. Short duration surgery.
   C. Malignancy
   D. Smoking.
   E. Higher age group.

✅ **Answer B**
- The longer the surgery duration under general anesthesia, the higher the risk for DVT.
- Other risk factors are failing heart, use of contraceptives, smoking, previous thromboembolic events, sepsis, and stroke.

❓ 20. **Management of intraoperative DIC. The FALSE answer is:**
   A. Needs platelet transfusion.
   B. Needs cryoprecipitate.
   C. PCC corrects the INR.
   D. Activated PCC contains three factors.
   E. The use of local hemostats can help for some time.

✅ **Answer D**
- Intraoperative DIC is an emergency intraoperative situation.
- Needs to replenish the coagulation system precursors.
- Activated PCC contains four factors (II, VII, IX, and X).

❓ 21. **Incidental low-grade gliomas. The FALSE answer is:**
   A. WHO II.
   B. MR spectroscopy is helpful.
   C. PET scan improves the accuracy of biopsy.
   D. Functional mapping is necessary.
   E. The survival rate is 24 months.

✅ **Answer E**
- Incidental gliomas are usually discovered early in the course of the disease.
- Need to use novel diagnostic technology for better biopsy and maximal safe resection, especially in the eloquent brain areas.
- Survival is up to 10 years depending on the histology and extent of resection.

❓ 22. **Low-grade glioma.**
   Preoperative functional mapping. The FALSE answer is:
   A. Allows understanding of the surgical risk.
   B. Functional MRI is reliable.
   C. EEG to localize the seizure.
   D. DTI is helpful.
   E. Does not change the extent of resection.

Answer E

- LGG can infiltrate the normal functional tissues surrounding the glioma. Utilizing functional planning techniques allows for a more precise extent of tumor resection while avoiding damage to eloquent areas.

23. Brachytherapy. The FALSE answer is:
   A. External beam radiation.
   B. Has some concerns regarding radiation to the surgeon.
   C. Is an option in treating craniopharyngioma.
   D. Weak against solid tumors due to lack of homogeneity.
   E. The site of treatment must be either surgically accessible or an existing body cavity.

Answer A

- Brachytherapy is a type of radiation therapy delivered internally by placing a radioactive source usually placed by a surgeon.

24. Stereotactic radiosurgery. The FALSE answer is:
   A. Currently uses X-ray.
   B. Considered a minimally invasive technique.
   C. Should fix the head on a frame.
   D. Single session procedure.
   E. The dose of radiation depends on the pathology.

Answer A

- The project of stereotactic radiosurgery started with X-ray radiation. Currently, Gamma and other types of radiation are used.
- It is a minimally invasive technique that delivers large doses to the target with low doses of radiation to the surrounding normal brain parenchyma.

25. Stereotactic radiosurgery (SRS).
   Indications. The FALSE answer is:
   A. Large meningioma in the skull base.
   B. Some traditionally radioresistant lesions.
   C. Multiple brain metastases.
   D. Brain stem neoplasia.
   E. Postoperative residuals.

✓ **Answer A**
- SRS is suitable for small skull base lesions including meningiomas.
- Has been shown to be effective in melanoma, sarcoma, and renal carcinoma which are traditionally radioresistant.

? 26. **Stereotactic radiosurgery (SRS).**
Brain metastatic disease. The FALSE answer is:
A. Class I evidence is available.
B. Can be given to multiple metastases.
C. Can be used as a stand-alone or combined with other modalities.
D. Effective in increasing overall patient survival.
E. Local control of the disease cannot be achieved.

✓ **Answer E**
- Local control of metastatic lesions can be achieved with SRS.

? 27. **Radiation necrosis. The FALSE answer is:**
A. Occurs typically after 6 weeks.
B. May need surgery.
C. May need biopsy.
D. Depends on the dose.
E. Steroids can help.

✓ **Answer A**
- Radiation necrosis is typically seen after more than 6 months from radiotherapy.
- Can mimic local tumor recurrence and form a diagnostic dilemma especially when symptomatic.
- May necessitate surgery for biopsy or relief of mass effect.

? 28. **Brain metastatic disease.**
Favorable outcome factors in stereotactic radiosurgery (SRS). The FALSE answer is:
A. Controlled primary disease.
B. High Karnofsky performance score.
C. Elder age group.
D. Singularity of the metastasis.
E. Small spherical lesions.

✅ **Answer C**
- A favorable outcome is seen in younger age groups.

❓ 29. **Brain metastatic disease.**
   Factors favoring surgery. The FALSE answer is:
   A. Mass effect exerted by the lesion.
   B. Lesion less than 2 cm.
   C. Brain edema.
   D. Uncertainty of the diagnosis.
   E. Tumors are known to be radioresistant.

✅ **Answer B**
- Metastasis less than 3 cm in size is typically suitable for less invasive procedures, i.e., SRS.
- Surgery is useful for obtaining tissue biopsy which gives a clear roadmap regarding tumor management.

❓ 30. **Brain metastatic disease.**
   Whole brain radiotherapy (WBRT) treatment. The FALSE answer is:
   A. The total dose is <20 Gy.
   B. Reserved for diffuse disease.
   C. Used in leptomeningeal involvement.
   D. Useful in occult metastatic lesions.
   E. Not advisable in oligometastasis.

✅ **Answer A**
- The total dose is 25–40 Gy.
- WBRT is associated with significant cognitive decline. Therefore, the aim is to reserve WBRT for cases with multiple metastases, primarily for palliative purposes.

❓ 31. **Brain metastatic disease.**
   Indications of surgical intervention. The FALSE answer is:
   A. Polymetastasis.
   B. Dominant lesion.
   C. Controlled extracranial disease.
   D. Karnofsky Performance Scale (KPS) should be more than 70.
   E. Age less than 65.

✅ **Answer A**

– Surgery for brain metastatic disease is relatively contraindicated except for the dominant large lesion in the case of oligometastasis.

❓ 32. **Brain metastatic disease.**
   Technical issues of surgery. The FALSE answer is:
   A. Brain metastasis can be surrounded by gliotic tissue.
   B. Piecemeal resection is favorable for deep-seated tumors.
   C. Supratotal resection offers extra safe margins.
   D. Supratotal resection improves outcome.
   E. En-bloc resection is associated with higher complication rates.

✅ **Answer E**

– En-bloc resection is associated with lower complication rates.

❓ 33. **Resection with tubular retractor for intra-axial tumors. The FALSE answer is:**
   A. Used in superficial tumors.
   B. Can lead to vascular injuries.
   C. Better if combined with DTI.
   D. Has interoperator technical differences.
   E. Better to be combined with a microscope.

✅ **Answer A**

– The tubular retractor allows the removal of deep-seated tumors with a minimally destructive trajectory.

❓ 34. **Neuronavigation system. The FALSE answer is:**
   A. Is a replacement for the frame-based stereotaxy.
   B. Useful for skin incision planning.
   C. The surgical trajectory can be planned.
   D. Can calculate and hence accommodate the intraoperative brain shift.
   E. Does not increase the surgical time.

✅ **Answer D**

– The main drawback of neuronavigation in tumor resection surgery is brain shift, which necessitates resetting of the neuronavigation system data.

❓ 35. **Primary spinal tumors.**

Spinal radiation therapy. The FALSE answer is:

A. A surgical adjunct in primary malignant tumors.

B. First-line treatment in primary benign tumors.

C. Carry concern of radiation toxicity to the spinal cord.

D. Carry concern of radiation-induced sarcoma.

E. Stereotactic radiosurgery is helpful.

4

✓ **Answer B**

— Radiation has no role in the treatment of benign primary tumors of the spinal column.

— SRS reduces the rate and intensity of radiation injury to the surrounding tissue, particularly the spinal cord.

❓ 36. **Primary spinal tumors.**

Surgical management. The FALSE answer is:

A. Indicated if symptomatic.

B. The cure rate is high.

C. Need neoadjuvant and adjuvant therapy in malignant tumors.

D. Spinal tumors with epidural involvement are good candidates for en-bloc resection.

E. Piecemeal resection is a choice in some cases.

✓ **Answer D**

— Spinal tumors with epidural involvement are not good candidates for en-bloc resection because the risk of neurological injury is high. In these cases, en-bloc resection is substituted with piecemeal resection or subtotal tumor removal.

❓ 37. **Intramedullary tumors surgical management. The FALSE answer is:**

A. Surgery is the preferred option.

B. Preserving postoperative neurological function is paramount.

C. Benign tumors should be totally excised.

D. Malignant tumors should be totally excised.

E. The absence of malignant features indicate the end of surgical excision.

✅ **Answer D**
- The single determinant factor of postoperative outcome in intramedullary tumor surgery is the presence of a tumor-cord interface.
- Malignant tumors are infiltrative and complete removal results often in neurological damage.

❓ 38. **Intradural craniocervical junction tumors surgical intervention. The FALSE answer is:**
   A. Minimal bone removal is preferred.
   B. Neurophysiological monitoring is preferred.
   C. Requires preoperative tracheostomy.
   D. Severe neurological injury results from traction.
   E. Severe neurological injury results from flexion.

✅ **Answer C**
- Cardiopulmonary evaluation is necessary to assess the need for postoperative tracheostomy. Tracheostomy is rarely required preoperatively.
- Some tumors cause instability of the craniovertebral junction and if missed, can cause severe neurological deficits while positioning the patient in excessive flexion.
- Minimal bone removal preserves the stability of the joint.
- Neurophysiological monitoring intraoperatively can help avoid traction injury to the upper cord and brain stem.

❓ 39. **Delivery of therapeutics to the brain. The FALSE answer is:**
   A. Biochemical disruption of the blood-brain barrier.
   B. Intracavitary delivery systems.
   C. Third ventricular endoscopy.
   D. Lipophilic analogs.
   E. Catheter with direct delivery of drugs.

✅ **Answer C**
- Intrathecal chemotherapeutics can be beneficial in the treatment of leptomeningeal tumors as diffusion of the drug from the CSF space into the parenchyma is limited.
- Third ventricular endoscopy has no role in the delivery of therapeutics to the brain.

Bibliography

1. Bonfield CM, Engh JA. Pregnancy and brain tumors. Neurol Clin. 2012;30(3):937–46.
2. Chapter 123: Brain tumors during pregnancy. In: Youmans neurological surgery. 7th ed.
3. Joiner EF, Youngerman BE, Hudson TS, Yang J, Welch MR, McKhann GM, et al. Effectiveness of perioperative antiepileptic drug prophylaxis for early and late seizures following oncologic neurosurgery: a meta-analysis. J Neurosurg. 2019;130(4):1274–82.
4. Brandel MG, Rennert RC, Wali AR, Santiago-Dieppa DR, Steinberg JA, Ramos CL, et al. Impact of preoperative endovascular embolization on immediate meningioma resection outcomes. Neurosurg Focus. 2018;44(4):1–7.
5. Wong JM, Panchmatia JR, Ziewacz JE, Bader AM, Dunn IF, Laws ER, et al. Patterns in neurosurgical adverse events: intracranial neoplasm surgery. Neurosurg Focus. 2012;33(5):1–3.
6. Stummer W, Suero ME. Fluorescence imaging/agents in tumor resection. Neurosurg Clin N Am. 2017;28(4):569–83.
7. Rao G. Intraoperative MRI and maximizing extent of resection. Neurosurg Clin N Am. 2017;28(4):477–85.
8. Wang JL, Elder JB. Techniques for open surgical resection of brain metastases. Neurosurg Clin N Am. 2020;31(4):527–36.
9. Raslan A, Bhardwaj A. Medical management of cerebral edema. Neurosurg Focus. 2007;22(5):1–2.
10. Robin AM, Lee I, Kalkanis SN. Reoperation for recurrent glioblastoma Multiforme. Neurosurg Clin N Am. 2017;28(3):407–28.
11. Rockhill J, Mrugala M, Chamberlain MC. Intracranial meningiomas: an overview of diagnosis and treatment. Neurosurg Focus. 2007;23(4):1–7.
12. Shaikhouni A, Baum J, Lonser RR. Deep vein thrombosis prophylaxis in the neurosurgical patient. Neurosurg Clin N Am. 2018;29(4):567–74.
13. Bar-Natan M, Hymes KB. Management of intraoperative coagulopathy. Neurosurg Clin N Am. 2018;29(4):557–65.
14. Noorani I, Sanai N. Surgical management of incidental gliomas. Neurosurg Clin N Am. 2017;28(3):397–406.
15. Kekhia H, Rigolo L, Norton I, Golby AJ. Special surgical considerations for functional brain mapping. Neurosurg Clin N Am. 2011;22(2):111–32.
16. Chapter 262. In: Youmans neurological surgery. 6th ed.
17. Chapter 264. In: Youmans neurological surgery. 7th ed.
18. Chapter 265. In: Youmans neurological surgery. 7th ed.
19. Chapter 267. In: Youmans neurological surgery. 7th ed.
20. Lee D, Riestenberg RA, Haskell-Mendoza A, Bloch O. Brain metastasis recurrence versus radiation necrosis: evaluation and treatment. Neurosurg Clin N Am. 2020;31(4):575–87.
21. Starkweather CK, Choi BD, Alvarez-Breckenridge C, Brastianos PK, Oh K, Wang N, et al. Initial approach to the patient with multiple newly diagnosed brain metastases. Neurosurg Clin N Am. 2020;31(4):505–13.
22. Chapters 292 and 293. In: Youmans neurological surgery. 7th ed.
23. Chapter 308. In: Youmans neurological surgery. 6th ed.
24. Chapter 125. In: Youmans neurological surgery. 7th ed.

Specific CNS Tumors

Contents

WHO Classification of CNS Tumors (General Principles)

Oday Atallah, Abdulaziz Y. Alahmed,
Mostafa H. Algabri, Saleh A. Saleh,
Younus M. Al-Khazaali, Arwa S. Alabedi,
and Maliya Delawan

? 1. **WHO classification: general features. The FALSE answer is:**
A. The latest version of the WHO classification is the 2021 edition.
B. The initial edition of the WHO classification was published in 1979.
C. The current WHO classification is the fourth edition.
D. The present WHO classification utilizes Arabic numerals.
E. The new classification utilizes terms such as "types" and "sub-types."

✓ Answer C
— The most recent classification corresponds to the fifth edition.

5

? 2. **WHO classification: major groups. The FALSE answer is:**
A. Schwannomas.
B. Gliomas, glioneuronal, and neuronal tumors.
C. Embryonal tumors.
D. Melanocytic tumors.
E. Germ cell tumors.

✓ Answer A
— Schwannomas are not a major group in the WHO 2021 classification of CNS tumors. They are categorized as a subtype under the major group of cranial and paraspinal nerve tumors.

? 3. **Gliomas, glioneuronal, and neuronal tumors: types. The FALSE answer is:**
A. Adult-type diffuse gliomas.
B. Pediatric-type diffuse high-grade gliomas.
C. Adult-type low-grade gliomas.
D. Circumscribed astrocytic gliomas.
E. Glioneuronal and neuronal tumors.

✓ Answer C
— There is no adult-type low-grade glioma, in contrast to pediatric-type diffuse low-grade gliomas.

? 4. **Pineal tumors: types. The FALSE answer is:**
A. Pineocytoma.
B. Pineal parenchymal tumor of intermediate differentiation.
C. Pineoblastoma.
D. Medullary tumor of the pineal region.
E. Desmoplastic myxoid tumor of the pineal region.

✅ **Answer D**
- Medullary tumors are not well known to affect the pineal region. Another type of pineal tumor is papillary tumor of the pineal region.

❓ 5. **Astroblastoma: general information. The FALSE answer is:**
  A. This tumor is categorized as a circumscribed astrocytic glioma.
  B. 20% of individuals express MN-1 mutations.
  C. The majority of astroblastomas are located in the cerebral hemispheres.
  D. In the fifth edition, astroblastoma is not assigned a formal grade.
  E. It may exhibit a multicystic or "bubbly" appearance.

✅ **Answer B**
- MN-1 mutations account for 70% of astroblastoma cases.

❓ 6. **Medulloblastoma (MB), the proportion of subtypes. The FALSE answer is:**
  A. *WNT*-activated: 40%.
  B. *SHH*-activated/*TP53* wild-type: 30%.
  C. Non-*WNT*/non-*SHH* is the most common MB subtype: 50–60%.
  D. Group 3: 25%.
  E. Group 4: 35%.

✅ **Answer A**
- The *WNT*-activated subtype accounts for approximately 10% of all medulloblastomas.

❓ 7. **Tumors of the sellar region: types. The FALSE answer is:**
  A. Papillary craniopharyngioma.
  B. Lymphomatoid craniopharyngioma.
  C. Pituitary adenoma.
  D. Pituicytoma.
  E. Pituitary blastoma.

✅ **Answer B**
- There are only two types of craniopharyngioma: papillary and adamantinomatous craniopharyngiomas.

? 8. Distribution of primary CNS tumors among children between 0 and 14 years of age: the more prevalent tumor is the following. The FALSE answer is:

A. Malignant glioma > craniopharyngioma.
B. Embryonal neoplasms > meningioma.
C. Embryonal neoplasms > meningioma.
D. Craniopharyngioma > malignant glioma.
E. Malignant glioma > meningioma.

✅ Answer B

— Malignant gliomas are more common in children than craniopharyngioma. The distribution of primary CNS tumors among children 0–14 years of age is as follows:
  – Malignant glioma: 30%.
  – Pilocytic astrocytoma: 18%.
  – Embryonal neoplasms: 15%.
  – Meningioma: 2%.
  – Craniopharyngioma: 4%.

? 9. Distribution of primary CNS tumors among adolescents between 15 and 19 years of age: the more prevalent tumor is the following. The FALSE answer is:

A. Pituitary adenoma > glioneuronal tumors.
B. Pituitary adenoma > pilocytic astrocytoma.
C. Lymphoma > pilocytic astrocytoma.
D. Pilocytic astrocytoma > lymphoma.
E. Glioneuronal tumors > lymphoma.

✅ Answer C

— Pilocytic astrocytoma is more common than lymphoma among adolescents between 15 and 19 years of age. The distribution of primary CNS tumors in this group is as follows:
  – Pituitary adenoma: 27%.
  – Pilocytic astrocytoma: 10%.
  – Glioneuronal tumors: 8%.
  – Glioblastoma 3%.
  – Lymphoma: 1%.

② 10. **Distribution of brain tumors among adults: the more prevalent tumor is the following. The FALSE answer is:**
   A. Metastases > meningioma.
   B. Glioblastoma > metastases.
   C. Meningioma > glioblastoma.
   D. Glioblastoma > lymphoma.
   E. Glioblastoma > oligodendroglioma.

✅ Answer B

— Metastases are more common than glioblastoma in adults. The distribution of brain tumors in this group is as follows:
   – Metastases: 50%.
   – Meningioma: 18%.
   – Glioblastoma: 7%.
   – Lymphoma: 2%.
   – Oligodendroglioma: 2%.

② 11. **Extra-axial intracranial cysts: types. The FALSE answer is:**
   A. Arachnoid cyst.
   B. Epidermoid cyst.
   C. Dermoid cyst.
   D. Pineal cyst.
   E. Neuroglial cyst.

✅ Answer E

— Neuroglial cysts are intra-axial cysts.

② 12. **Diffuse midline glioma: genes/molecular profiles. The FALSE answer is:**
   A. H3 K27.
   B. TSC1.
   C. ACVR1.
   D. EGFR.
   E. PDGFRA.

✅ Answer B

— TSC1 has been expressed in cases of subependymal giant cell astrocytoma.

❓ 13. Pituitary blastoma: general information. The FALSE answer is:
   A. It has been added to the WHO's most current classification.
   B. It is a rare embryonal tumor.
   C. The median age is 8 months.
   D. Pituitary blastomas are WHO grade II.
   E. Pituitary blastomas are linked to either somatic or germline *DICER1* mutations.

✓ Answer D
— Pituitary blastomas are WHO grade IV.

❓ 14. CNS neuroblastoma: general information. The FALSE answer is:
   A. It reaches its peak at age 25.
   B. High vascularity and necrosis are prominent features.
   C. It is associated with a mutation in the FOXR2 gene.
   D. The majority are sporadic.
   E. Imaging reveals a massive heterogeneous supratentorial mass.

✓ Answer A
— It has a peak at 5 years of age.

Bibliography

1. Louis DN, Perry A, Wesseling P, Brat DJ, Cree IA, Figarella-Branger D, Hawkins C, Ng HK, Pfister SM, Reifenberger G, Soffietti R, von Deimling A, Ellison DW. The 2021 WHO classification of tumors of the central nervous system: a summary. Neuro Oncol. 2021;23(8):1231–51.
2. Chen W, Soon YY, Pratiseyo PD, et al. Central nervous system neuroepithelial tumors with MN1-alteration: an individual patient data meta-analysis of 73 cases. Brain Tumor Pathol. 2020;37:145–53.
3. Louis DN, Wesseling P, Aldape K, et al. cIMPACT-NOW update 6: new entity and diagnostic principle recommendations of the cIMPACT-UTRECHT meeting on future CNS tumor classification and grading. Brain Pathol. 2020;30:844–56.
4. Hirose T, Nobusawa S, Sugiyama K, et al. Astroblastoma: a distinct tumor entity characterized by alterations of the X chromosome and MN1 rearrangement. Brain Pathol. 2018;28:684–94.
5. Mhatre R, Sugur HS, Nandeesh BN, et al. MN1 rearrangement in astroblastoma: study of eight cases and review of literature. Brain Tumor Pathol. 2019;36:112–20.
6. Osborn AG, Louis DN, Poussaint TY, Linscott LL, Salzman KL. The 2021 World Health Organization classification of tumors of the central nervous system: what neuroradiologists need to know. Am J Neuroradiol. 2022;43:928.

7. Park YW, Vollmuth P, Foltyn-Dumitru M, Sahm F, Choi KS, Park JE, Ahn SS, Chang JH, Kim SH. The 2021 WHO classification for gliomas and implications on imaging diagnosis: part 3-summary of imaging findings on glioneuronal and neuronal tumors. J Magn Reson Imaging. 2023;58:1680.

8. Chen W, Guo S, Wang Y, Shi Y, Guo X, Liu D, Li Y, Wang Y, Xing H, Xia Y, Li J, Wu J, Liang T, Wang H, Liu Q, Jin S, Qu T, Li H, Yang T, Zhang K, Wang Y, Ma W. Novel insight into histological and molecular astrocytoma, IDH-mutant, grade 4 by the updated WHO classification of central nervous system tumors. Cancer Med. 2023;12:18666.

9. Fernandes RT, Teixeira GR, Mamere EC, Bandeira GA, Mamere AE. The 2021 World Health Organization classification of gliomas: an imaging approach. Radiol Bras. 2023;56(3):157–61.

10. Guo X, Gu L, Li Y, Zheng Z, Chen W, Wang Y, Wang Y, Xing H, Shi Y, Liu D, Yang T, Xia Y, Li J, Wu J, Zhang K, Liang T, Wang H, Liu Q, Jin S, Qu T, Guo S, Li H, Wang Y, Ma W. Histological and molecular glioblastoma, IDH-wildtype: a real-world landscape using the 2021 WHO classification of central nervous system tumors. Front Oncol. 2023;13:1200815.

11. Malta TM, Snyder J, Noushmehr H, Castro AV. Advances in central nervous system tumor classification. Adv Exp Med Biol. 2023;1416:121–35.

12. Miller DC. The World Health Organization classification of tumors of the central nervous system, fifth edition, 2021: a critical analysis. Adv Tech Stand Neurosurg. 2023;46:1–21.

13. Villa C, Baussart B, Assié G, Raverot G, Roncaroli F. The World Health Organization classifications of pituitary neuroendocrine tumours: a clinico-pathological appraisal. Endocr Relat Cancer. 2023;30(8):e230021.

14. Bagchi A, Dhanda SK, Dunphy P, Sioson E, Robinson GW. Molecular classification improves therapeutic options for infants and young children with medulloblastoma. J Natl Compr Cancer Netw. 2023;1–9:1097.

15. Bondy ML, Scheurer ME, Malmer B, Barnholtz-Sloan JS, Davis FG, Il'yasova D, Kruchko C, BJ MC, Rajaraman P, Schwartzbaum JA, Sadetzki S, Schlehofer B, Tihan T, Wiemels JL, Wrensch M, Buffler PA, Brain Tumor Epidemiology Consortium. Brain tumor epidemiology: consensus from the Brain Tumor Epidemiology Consortium. Cancer. 2008;113(7 Suppl):1953–68.

Meningeal Tumors (General Principles)

Usama AlDallal, Leen Azzam, Sami Al-Horani, Ebtesam Abdulla, Saad Mallah, Sanad M. A. Kamal, and Samer S. Hoz

© The Author(s), under exclusive license to Springer Nature Switzerland AG 2024
S. S. Hoz et al. (eds.), *Surgical Neuro-Oncology*,
https://doi.org/10.1007/978-3-031-53642-7_6

? 1. **Meningioma.**

   Definition. The FALSE answer is:

   A. Most common primary central nervous system tumor.
   B. Is usually benign.
   C. Is located superficially.
   D. Affects males more than females.
   E. Is an extra-axial tumor.

✓ Answer D

— Meningiomas affect females more than males.

? 2. **Meningioma.**

   Definition. The FALSE answer is:

   A. Is most commonly located along the falx, convexity, or sphenoid bone.
   B. Arises from the dura mater.
   C. Psammoma bodies are a classic histological finding.
   D. Slow-growing and noninfiltrating.
   E. They form a diffuse sheet of tumor cells.

✓ Answer B

— Meningioma arises from arachnoid cap cells of the arachnoid layer.

? 3. **Meningioma.**

   Definition. The FALSE answer is:

   A. Often occurs along intracranial venous sinuses.
   B. Can cause symptoms such as headaches, seizures, and changes in vision.
   C. Can be treated via surgical removal, radiation therapy, or observation.
   D. They are more common in children than they are in adults.
   E. EMA is one of the most expressed immunohistochemical markers in meningioma.

✓ Answer D

— They are more common in adults than children, especially in adults above the age of 40.

? 4. **Meningioma.**
Epidemiology: prevalence. The FALSE answer is:
A. In the US, around 5% of primary brain tumors are meningiomas.
B. Meningiomas occur in 8 out of every 100,000 people each year.
C. Most meningiomas (80–85%) are benign tumors (grade 1).
D. The second most common (~15%) grade of meningioma is atypical (grade 2).
E. Only 1–3% of meningiomas are malignant (grade 3).

✓ **Answer A**
▬ In the US, around 39% of primary brain tumors are meningiomas. This number, as per autopsy results, is expected to be even higher.

? 5. **Meningioma.**
Epidemiology: risk factors. The FALSE answer is:
A. The primary environmental risk factor is exposure to ionizing radiation.
B. An association between hormones and meningioma risk has been suggested, especially considering the increased incidence in females during peak reproductive years.
C. A positive family history of meningioma is the main overall risk factor for the development of meningiomas.
D. Attempts to link specific chemical exposure, cellphone use, and head trauma with meningioma risk have proved inconclusive.
E. There is a well-studied association between breast cancer and meningioma.

✓ **Answer C**
▬ While it is true that a few studies have revealed an increased risk of meningioma with increasing numbers of affected first-degree relatives, the total number of families with multiple members diagnosed with meningioma are relatively rare, and most such families are currently attributed to inherited *NF2* mutations. At present, no family-based linkage or segregation analyses studies of meningioma have been reported.

? 6. **Meningioma.**
Epidemiology: molecular etiology. The FALSE answer is:
A. Deletion and inactivation of NF2 on chromosome 22 is a predominant feature in sporadic meningiomas.
B. Other regions include 14q, 1p, 6q, and 18q.

C. Meningiomas are reported in families of several cancer predisposition syndromes including NF1, PTCH, CREBBP, VHL, PTEN, and CDKN2A.
D. The complexity of genetic variations decreases with tumor grade.
E. Epigenetically, DNA methylation events may impact meningioma biology more significantly than DNA copy number mutations.

✅ **Answer D**
— Only a small number of mutations may be necessary for most meningiomas. Additionally, the complexity of genetic aberrations increases with tumor grade, not decreases. Furthermore, the slow growth of meningiomas makes long latency an issue; this makes it difficult to identify the source and timing of the initiating mutations, presenting a further complication for epidemiology studies.

6

❓ 7. **Meningioma.**
   Pathology: WHO grade 2. The FALSE answer is:
   A. Only perivascular spread or indentation of the brain without pial breach.
   B. Has an uninterrupted patternless appearance.
   C. At least three features such as increased cellularity, small cells with a high N:C ratio, and prominent nucleoli.
   D. WHO grade 2 for meningioma is atypical meningioma.
   E. Has a foci of spontaneous necrosis.

✅ **Answer A**
— Unequivocal brain invasion may also occur.

❓ 8. **Meningioma.**
   Pathology: WHO grade 3. The FALSE answer is:
   A. TERT promoter mutation.
   B. Homozygous deletion of CDKN2A.
   C. Heterozygous deletion of CDKN2B.
   D. Frank anaplasia, sarcoma, carcinoma, or melanoma-like appearance.
   E. WHO grade 3 for meningioma is anaplastic meningioma.

✅ **Answer C**
— Homozygous deletion of CDKN2B.

? 9. **Meningioma.**
Pathology: subtypes with a higher risk of recurrence. The FALSE answer is:
A. Atypical meningioma.
B. Clear cell meningioma.
C. Chordoid meningioma.
D. Papillary meningioma.
E. Transitional meningioma.

✓ Answer E
▬ Transitional meningiomas (WHO grade I) have a better prognosis and lower risk of recurrence than other subtypes.

? 10. **Meningioma.**
Subtypes and characteristics. The FALSE answer is:
A. The WHO classification scheme recognizes 15 variations of meningiomas according to their cell type as seen under a microscope.
B. WHO grade 1 meningiomas are classified into 13 subtypes.
C. WHO grade I (benign) subtypes include fibrous (fibroblastic), psammomatous, angiomatous, microcytic, and secretory.
D. WHO grade II (atypical) subtypes include choroid, clear cell, and atypical.
E. WHO grade III (malignant) subtypes include papillary, rhabdoid, anaplastic, and meningothelial.

✓ Answer D
▬ Malignant (grade III) subtypes of meningioma include papillary, rhabdoid, and anaplastic only. Meningothelial is another example of a benign (grade I) subtype.
▬ B—Other benign subtypes include meningothelial, fibrous (fibroblastic), psammomatous, angiomatous, microcystic, secretory, transitional (mixed), lymphoplasmacyte-rich, and metaplastic meningioma[5].

? 11. **Meningioma.**
Subtypes and characteristics: anatomical classification. The FALSE answer is:
A. Cerebellopontine angle meningiomas are located near the margin of the cerebellum.
B. Intraorbital meningiomas are located in or around the eye sockets.

C. Suprasellar meningiomas are located near the portion of the temporal bone that contains parts of the auditory apparatus.
D. Tentorium meningiomas are located near where the cerebral hemispheres connect with the cerebellum and brain stem.
E. Parasagittal/falx meningiomas are located adjacent to the dural fold that separates the two brain hemispheres.

✅ **Answer C**

— Suprasellar meningiomas are located near the area of the skull where the pituitary gland is found. The meningioma located near the portion of the temporal bone that contains parts of the auditory apparatus is the petrous ridge meningioma.
— Other anatomic meningiomas include cavernous sinus meningioma, cerebral convexity meningioma, foramen magnum meningioma, intraventricular meningioma, olfactory groove meningioma, posterior fossa meningioma, sphenoid meningioma, and spinal meningioma.

❓ 12. **Meningioma.**
   Subtypes and characteristics: anatomic-based symptoms. The FALSE answer is:
   A. Falx and parasagittal meningiomas may lead to impaired levels of brain functioning (e.g., reasoning and memory), leg weakness/numbness, and seizures.
   B. Suprasellar meningiomas may cause vision problems due to compression of the optic nerves/chiasm.
   C. Posterior fossa meningiomas may cause facial symptoms or loss of hearing due to compression of cranial nerves, unsteady gait, and problems with coordination.
   D. Sphenoid meningiomas may cause vision problems, loss of sensation in the face, or facial numbness and seizures.
   E. Intraventricular meningiomas may lead to a buildup of pressure in the eyes, leading to a bulging appearance and potential loss of vision.

✅ **Answer E**

— Intraventricular meningiomas may block the flow of cerebrospinal fluid, resulting in obstructive hydrocephalus. This may lead to headaches, lightheadedness, and changes in mental function. The meningioma that may lead to a buildup of pressure in the eyes, a bulging appearance, and potential loss of vision is the intraorbital meningioma.

- Other anatomic-based symptoms include the following:
  - Spinal meningiomas may cause back pain or pain in the limbs caused by compression of the nerves that run into the spinal cord.
  - Olfactory groove meningiomas may lead to loss of smell due to compression of the nerves that run between the brain and the nose. If the tumor grows large enough, vision problems may occur due to compression of the optic nerve.
  - Convexity meningiomas may cause seizures, headaches, and neurological deficits.

❓ 13. **Meningioma.**
Molecular genetics. The FALSE answer is:
A. Skull Base lesions can carry an AKT1 mutation.
B. Skull Base lesions can carry a TRAF7 mutation.
C. Skull Base lesions can carry an SMO mutation.
D. Skull Base lesions can carry a TERT promoter mutation.
E. Skull Base lesions can carry a PIK3CA mutation.

✅ **Answer D**
- Skull base lesions do not carry TERT promoter mutations.

❓ 14. **Meningioma.**
Molecular genetics. The FALSE answer is:
A. Loss of 1p, 6, 10q, 14q, and/or 18 in higher-grade meningiomas.
B. Monosomy 22/22q.
C. Strong and diffuse SSTR2A immunoreactivity.
D. Presence of TRAF7, AKT1, KLF4, SMO, PIK3CA.
E. Monoallelic inactivation of NF2.

✅ **Answer E**
- WHO diagnostic criteria for meningioma specify suggestive histopathological features combined with biallelic inactivation of NF2, not monoallelic.

❓ 15. **Meningioma.**
Molecular genetics: WHO grade III. The FALSE answer is:
A. TERT promoter mutation.
B. Homozygous deletion of CDKN2A and/or CDKN2B.
C. Loss of H3p.K27me3.
D. SMARCB1 mutation.
E. Loss of H3p.K28me3 in anaplastic malignant meningioma.

✅ **Answer D**

— SMARCB1 mutations occur in desmoplastic myxoid tumors of the pineal region.

❓ 16. **Meningioma.**
   Etiology: risk factors. The FALSE answer is:
   A. Female gender.
   B. Family history of meningioma.
   C. Age over 60 years.
   D. Obesity.
   E. Exposure to high levels of mobile phone radiation.

6

✅ **Answer E**

— Current studies have not provided evidence of increased risk.

❓ 17. **Meningioma.**
   Etiology: molecular mechanisms. The FALSE answer is:
   A. Mutation in NF2.
   B. Survivin protein.
   C. Growth factors and growth factor receptors such as HER2 and platelet-derived growth factor.
   D. Mutation in MYC.
   E. Mutation in TERT gene.

✅ **Answer D**

— The most common mutation is NF2. However, studies have shown that MYC is more associated with gliomas.

❓ 18. **Meningioma.**
   Etiology. The FALSE answer is:
   A. Ionizing radiation.
   B. Male gender.
   C. Chronic viral infection.
   D. Exposure to asbestos.
   E. Tobacco smoking.

✅ **Answer B**

— Meningioma is associated with the female gender more than the male gender.

❓ 19. Meningioma.
  Clinical presentation: atypical. The FALSE answer is:
  A. Atypical meningiomas are more likely to have aggressive growth.
  B. Atypical meningiomas are less likely to cause focal neurological deficits.
  C. Visual disturbances can result from atypical meningiomas.
  D. Surgical resection is the primary treatment for atypical meningiomas.
  E. They often present with headaches and seizures.

✅ Answer B
▬ Atypical meningiomas are associated with more aggressive growth and are more likely to cause focal neurological deficits than typical meningiomas.

❓ 20. Meningioma.
  Clinical presentation: skull base. The FALSE answer is:
  A. Skull base meningiomas are often associated with cranial nerve deficits.
  B. They can cause symptoms related to their specific location.
  C. Skull base meningiomas are exclusively found in the anterior skull base.
  D. They may cause seizures.
  E. Surgical resection of skull base meningiomas can be complex.

✅ Answer C
▬ Skull base meningiomas can occur in various locations along the skull base, including the anterior middle and posterior skull base.

❓ 21. Meningioma.
  Clinical presentation: parasagittal. The FALSE answer is:
  A. Seizures.
  B. Gait disturbance.
  C. Hemiparesis.
  D. Headache.
  E. Vision problems.

✅ Answer B
▬ Gait disturbances are not typically associated with meningiomas in parasagittal locations. These tumors often cause seizures, hemiparesis, headache, and vision problems due to their location near the cerebral hemispheres.

? 22. **Meningioma.**
   Staging and classification: WHO grading system. The FALSE answer is:
   A. Mitotic activity.
   B. Brain invasion.
   C. Presence of nucleoli.
   D. Ki-67 labeling index.
   E. Tumor location within the skull.

✓ **Answer E**
− The WHO grading system primarily relies on histological criteria, such as mitotic activity, nucleoli, and Ki-67 labeling index, rather than tumor location within the skull.

6

? 23. **Meningioma.**
   Staging and classification. The FALSE answer is:
   A. Clear cell meningiomas are characterized by the presence of clear cytoplasm.
   B. Choroid meningiomas often have a papillary architecture.
   C. Psammomatous meningiomas are associated with psammoma bodies.
   D. Secretory meningiomas may contain mucin-filled vacuoles.
   E. Papillary meningiomas are considered benign.

✓ **Answer E**
− Papillary meningiomas, while generally considered a low-grade subtype, are not always considered benign. They may have a more variable clinical course.

? 24. **Meningioma.**
   Staging and classification: NF2 gene mutation. The FALSE answer is:
   A. Meningothelial.
   B. Clear cell.
   C. Fibrous.
   D. Transitional.
   E. Schwannomatosis-associated.

✓ **Answer A**
− Meningothelial meningiomas are not typically associated with NF2 gene mutation.

? 25. **Meningioma.**
Diagnostic procedures. The FALSE answer is:
A. Dural tail sign is pathognomonic for meningioma.
B. 50% of meningiomas present with extraventricular edema.
C. The meningioma base has a direct attachment to the meninges.
D. Hyperostosis is suggestive of meningioma.
E. Meningioma may present with calcification on plain X-ray.

✓ **Answer A**
− The dural tail sign can occur in plasmacytoma, pleomorphic xanthoas-trocytoma, meningioma, and Rosa-Dorfman disease.

? 26. **Meningioma.**
Surgery: NF2 mutant meningiomas. The FALSE answer is:
A. Tend to arise in more surgically inaccessible locations.
B. Have a higher tendency to become atypical and malignant.
C. NF2 mutant meningiomas are more commonly found among males.
D. The surgical approach typically involves wide dural resection and bone removal with cranioplasty.
E. More frequently require postoperative radiotherapy.

✓ **Answer A**
− NF2 mutant meningiomas are more likely to originate in surgically acces-sible locations, such as the convexity.

? 27. **Meningioma.**
Surgery: meningiomas with mutations in SMO and SUFU. The FALSE answer is:
A. Often occur in the midline anterior skull base, along the olfac-tory groove or planum sphenoidale.
B. Are more commonly lower-grade.
C. Are associated with hyperostosis.
D. Are associated with higher rates of recurrence.
E. Bony involvement due to hyperostosis should be completely resected.

✓ **Answer E**
− The complete removal of bony involvement due to hyperostosis is often not pursued as it can risk CSF leak.

❓ 28. Meningioma.
Surgery: meningiomas originating from the tuberculum sellae region. The FALSE answer is:
A. Are associated with *POLR2A* mutations.
B. Are associated with an aggressive clinical course.
C. Extend along the clivus.
D. May extend into the cerebellopontine angle.
E. The extent of resection is often limited due to vascular and cranial nerve involvement.

✅ Answer B
– Meningiomas originating from the tuberculum sellae region are associated with a benign clinical course.

6

❓ 29. Meningioma.
Endoscope-assisted surgery: factors favoring the supraorbital approach over the endonasal approach. The FALSE answer is:
A. Meningiomas with significant lateral extension.
B. Meningiomas encroaching on the supraclinoid ICA.
C. In patients with a subchiasmatic lesion and a prefixed chiasm.
D. Patients with adequate preoperative olfaction.
E. Meningiomas without significant invasion of the lamina cribra and roof of nasal fossae.

✅ Answer C
– For patients with a subchiasmatic lesion and a prefixed chiasm, the preferred route is the endonasal approach. Any transcranial approach would necessitate optic apparatus retraction and could pose a potential risk of visual decline.

❓ 30. Meningioma.
Endoscope-assisted surgery: factors that limit the endoscope endonasal approach. The FALSE answer is:
A. Tumors >3 cm.
B. Tumors with encasement of the carotid arteries and/or ACA complex.
C. Absence of an arachnoid plane between the tumor and the encased blood vessels.
D. Giant olfactory groove meningiomas with significant extension into the nasal cavities and paranasal sinuses.
E. Extensive circumferential invasion of the optic canal.

✅ **Answer D**

━ The endonasal approach allows for staged or combined procedures and is effective for managing giant olfactory groove meningiomas with extensive extension into the nasal cavities and paranasal sinuses.

❓ 31. **Meningioma.**
Stereotactic radiosurgery (SRS). The FALSE answer is:
   A. Approximately 80–90% of meningiomas are radiosensitive.
   B. May be used to treat microscopic or gross residual meningioma after surgery.
   C. May be used as a primary treatment without surgery.
   D. Doses ranging from 12 to 18 Gy are typically used.
   E. Skull base locations away from the convexity are associated with poorer outcomes following SRS.

✅ **Answer E**

━ Skull base locations away from the convexity or parasagittal regions are associated with improved outcomes following SRS. Other factors associated with improved outcomes also include smaller tumor size and imaging-defined tumors.

❓ 32. **Meningioma.**
   Recurrence: Ki-67 proliferation index (PI). The FALSE answer is:
   A. An increase in Ki-67 PI is associated with a higher hazard ratio in recurrence.
   B. Ki-67 PI is a definitive predictor for the likelihood of recurrence in meningioma patients.
   C. Ki-67 PI does not show significant variation between nonrecurrent and recurrent meningiomas.
   D. Lower Ki-67 PI percentages show a lesser incidence of recurrence after the first year compared to higher percentages.
   E. Ki-67 PI is more associated with time to recurrence than actual recurrence likelihood.

✅ **Answer B**

━ While there is an association between higher Ki-67 PI and increased risk of recurrence, the most robust relationship is between the Ki-67 PI and the time it takes for recurrence, not the likelihood of recurrence itself.

? 33. **Meningioma.**
   Recurrence: molecular markers. The FALSE answer is:
   A. SMO mutations are linked to an increased risk of meningioma recurrence.
   B. POLR2A mutations are directly associated with a heightened risk of meningioma recurrence.
   C. TP53 mutations are significant indicators of meningioma recurrence.
   D. NF2 mutations correlate with increased recurrence in meningiomas.
   E. Tumor recurrence is not solely tied to WHO grade; individual mutations can independently elevate recurrence risk.

6

✓ Answer C
— TP53 mutations are not recognized as significant indicators for meningioma recurrence. While TP53 mutations play a critical role in various malignancies, they are not primarily associated with meningioma progression or recurrence. Other mutations, such as NF2, POLR2A, and SMO have a more defined role in meningioma pathogenesis and recurrence risk.

? 34. **Meningioma.**
   Recurrence: Simpson grading. The FALSE answer is:
   A. Grade I removal represents macroscopically complete removal and has a 9% recurrence rate.
   B. Grade II removal specifically aims to leave a small portion of the tumor behind to minimize surgical complications.
   C. Grade III removal does not involve any coagulation or resection of the dural attachment and has a 29% recurrence rate.
   D. Grade IV represents partial removal with a recurrence rate of 44%.
   E. The higher the grade in the Simpson grading system, the higher the recurrence rate.

✓ Answer B
— The grading system is:
   – Grade I: Complete removal with excision of dural attachment; 9% recurrence.
   – Grade II: Complete removal with coagulation of dural attachment; 19% recurrence.

– Grade III: Complete removal without dural coagulation; 29% recurrence.
– Grade IV: Partial removal with some tumor left; 44% recurrence.
– Grade V: Simple decompression, potentially with biopsy; recurrence not specified.

35. **Meningioma.**
    Recurrence: histological features. The FALSE answer is:
    A. A higher recurrence risk is linked with increased mitotic activity.
    B. Psammomatous meningiomas, characterized mainly by psammoma bodies, have a high recurrence risk.
    C. Chordoid meningiomas, categorized as WHO grade 2, possess recurrence rates similar to atypical meningiomas.
    D. Clear cell meningiomas, often found in the CPA and spine, present typically at age 24, and are designated WHO grade 2 due to elevated recurrence and CSF seeding risks.
    E. WHO grade 3 Rhabdoid Meningiomas are marked by high rates of proliferation and recurrence.

Answer B
– Psammomatous meningiomas, while they are characterized by the presence of psammoma bodies, are generally benign and are categorized as WHO grade I, which means they usually have a lower risk of recurrence.
– Some histologic subtypes are more prone to recurrence; atypical meningiomas, a grade II subtype, have a recurrence rate of 29%. This rate is comparable to other grade II meningioma subtypes, including clear cell and chordoid variants.

36. **Meningioma.**
    Follow-up and prognosis. The FALSE answer is:
    A. Ten-year relative survival for nonmalignant was 93.2% in children 0–14, 95% in young adults 15–39, and 82.5% in adults 40+ years old.
    B. Ten-year relative survival for malignant meningioma is 38.5% for the population aged 20–44 years, and 78% for ages 75+ years.
    C. The 5-year relative survival rate for malignant meningioma is 67%.
    D. The 10-year relative survival rate for malignant meningioma is 60%.
    E. Ten-year relative survival for nonmalignant meningiomas was 83.4%.

✅ **Answer B**

– Meningiomas can be broadly categorized into nonmalignant and malignant types, with the nonmalignant variant exhibiting significantly better survival outcomes compared to its malignant counterpart.

– Furthermore, studies underscore the age-dependent prognosis of meningiomas. Younger populations, specifically children and adolescents, tend to exhibit better survival rates when compared to older adults. For instance, 10-year relative survival for malignant meningioma was 78% for the population aged 20–44 years, and 38.5% for ages 75+ years. This suggests that as age advances, the prognosis for meningioma patients tends to worsen.

6

❓ 37. **Meningioma.**

   Follow-up and prognosis. The FALSE answer is:
   A. Ten-year relative survival is 83.2% for nonmalignant tumors in the cerebral meninges.
   B. Ten-year relative survival is 94.8% for nonmalignant tumors in the spinal meninges.
   C. Ten-year relative survival is 71.1% for malignant tumors in the spinal meninges.
   D. Ten-year relative survival is 59.9% for malignant tumors in the cerebral meninges.
   E. Five-year relative survival is 95.4% for malignant tumors in the spinal meninges.

✅ **Answer E**

– Spinal meningiomas generally have a better survival rate than those found in the cerebral meninges, especially when the tumors are nonmalignant. The significantly high 5-year relative survival rate of 95% for malignant tumors in the spinal meninges is inconsistent with general observations about malignant tumors. Typically, malignant tumors have a lower survival rate than their nonmalignant counterparts.

❓ 38. **Meningioma.**

   Follow-up and prognosis. The FALSE answer is:
   A. Follow-up of WHO grade 1 meningiomas should be performed by MRI every 12 months, after 5 years every 2 years.
   B. Follow-up of WHO grade 2 meningiomas should be performed by MRI every 6 months, after 5 years every 12 months.

C. Follow-up of WHO grade 3 meningiomas depends on clinical progression and should be done at least every 3–6 months.

D. MRI is the gold standard for follow-up imaging.

E. T2-weighted MRI is superior to the T1 sequence with gadolinium injection.

✅ **Answer E**

▬ For follow-up imaging, MRI is the preferred method. Typically, the size of a meningioma is assessed using the T1 sequence enhanced with a gadolinium injection. When it comes to measurements, the data from T2-weighted axial MRI is almost equivalent to that from the T1 sequence with gadolinium. Although it is generally recommended to monitor using the gadolinium-enhanced, T1-weighted sequences, using only T2-weighted imaging can be a viable alternative for tracking smaller meningiomas.

Bibliography

1. Buerki RA, Horbinski CM, Kruser T, Horowitz PM, James CD, Lukas RV. An overview of meningiomas. Future Oncol. 2018;14(21):2161–77.
2. Greenberg MS. Greenberg's handbook of neurosurgery. 10th ed. Thieme; 2023.
3. Kumar P, Clark ML. Kumar & Clark's cases in clinical medicine e-book. Elsevier Health Sciences; 2020.
4. Wiemels J, Wrensch M, Claus EB. Epidemiology and etiology of meningioma. J Neurooncol. 2010;99:307–14.
5. Traylor JI, Kuo JS. AANS: meningiomas. American Association of Neurological Surgeons. Accessed 10 Oct 2023. https://www.aans.org/en/Patients/Neurosurgical-Conditions-and-Treatments/Meningiomas.
6. AlSahlawi A, Aljelaify R, Magrashi A, et al. New insights into the genomic landscape of meningiomas identified FGFR3 in a subset of patients with favorable prognoses. Oncotarget. 2019;10(53):5549.
7. Ostrom QT, Price M, Neff C, et al. CBTRUS statistical report: primary brain and other central nervous system tumors diagnosed in the United States in 2015–2019. Neuro Oncol. 2022;24(Suppl_5):v1–v95.
8. Fountain DM, Soon WC, Matys T, Guilfoyle MR, Kirollos R, Santarius T. Volumetric growth rates of meningioma and its correlation with histological diagnosis and clinical outcome: a systematic review. Acta Neurochir. 2017;159:435–45.
9. Di Carlo DT, Capo G, Fava A, et al. Petroclival meningiomas: the risk of post-operative cranial nerve deficits among different surgical approaches—a systematic review and meta-analysis. Acta Neurochir. 2020;162:2135–43.
10. Giordan E, Sorenson TJ, Lanzino G. Optimal surgical strategy for meningiomas involving the superior sagittal sinus: a systematic review. Neurosurg Rev. 2020;43:525–35.

11. WHO. WHO classification of tumors, Head and neck tumours, vol. 5. 5th ed. International Agency for Research on Cancer, WHO Classification of Tumours Editorial Board; 2021.

12. Louis DN, Perry A, Wesseling P, et al. The 2021 WHO classification of tumors of the central nervous system: a summary. Neuro Oncol. 2021;23(8):1231–51.

13. Brastianos PK, Horowitz PM, Santagata S, et al. Genomic sequencing of meningiomas identifies oncogenic SMO and AKT1 mutations. Nat Genet. 2013;45(3):285–9.

14. Mirian C, Skyrman S, Bartek J Jr, et al. The Ki-67 proliferation index as a marker of time to recurrence in intracranial meningioma. Neurosurgery. 2020;87(6):1289–98.

15. Pawloski JA, Fadel HA, Huang Y-W, Lee IY. Genomic biomarkers of meningioma: a focused review. Int J Mol Sci. 2021;22(19):10222.

16. Simpson D. The recurrence of intracranial meningiomas after surgical treatment. J Neurol Neurosurg Psychiatry. 1957;20(1):22.

17. Goldbrunner R, Stavrinou P, Jenkinson MD, et al. EANO guideline on the diagnosis and management of meningiomas. Neuro Oncol. 2021;23(11):1821–34.

18. Dincer A, Morales-Valero SF, Robert SM, Tabor JK, O'Brien J, Yalcin K, et al. Surgical strategies for intracranial meningioma in the molecular era. J Neurooncol. 2023;162(2):253–65.

19. Cappabianca P, d'Avella E, Cavallo LM, Solari D. Meningiomas: criteria for modern surgical indications. Mini-invasive Surg. 2020;4:83. https://doi.org/10.20517/2574-1225.2020.67.

20. Chen WC, Lucas CG, Magill ST, Rogers CL, Raleigh DR. Radiotherapy and radiosurgery for meningiomas. Neurooncol Adv. 2023;5(Suppl 1):i67–83. Published 2023 Jun 3. https://doi.org/10.1093/noajnl/vdac088.

21. Fathi AR, Roelcke U. Meningioma. Curr Neurol Neurosci Rep. 2013;13:1–8.

22. Bulleid LS, James Z, Lammie A, Hayhurst C, Leach PA. The effect of the revised WHO classification on the incidence of grade II meningioma. Br J Neurosurg. 2020;34(5):584–6.

23. Dalle Ore CL, Magill ST, Yen AJ, Shahin MN, Lee DS, Lucas CH, Chen WC, Viner JA, Aghi MK, Theodosopoulos PV, Raleigh DR. Meningioma metastases: incidence and proposed screening paradigm. J Neurosurg. 2019;132(5):1447–55.

24. Varlotto J, Flickinger J, Pavelic MT, Specht CS, Sheehan JM, Timek DT, Glantz MJ, Soggc S, Dimaio C, Moser R, Yunus S. Distinguishing grade I meningioma from higher grade meningiomas without biopsy. Oncotarget. 2015;6(35):38421.

25. Goldbrunner R, Stavrinou P, Jenkinson MD, Sahm F, Mawrin C, Weber DC, Preusser M, Minniti G, Lund-Johansen M, Lefranc F, Houdart E. EANO guideline on the diagnosis and management of meningiomas. Neuro Oncol. 2021;23(11):1821–34.

26. Marosi C, Hassler M, Roessler K, Reni M, Sant M, Mazza E, Vecht C. Meningioma. Crit Rev Oncol Hematol. 2008;67(2):153–71.

27. Dincer A, Morales-Valero SF, Robert SM, Tabor JK, O'Brien J, Yalcin K, Fulbright RK, Erson-Omay Z, Dunn IF, Moliterno J. Surgical strategies for intracranial meningioma in the molecular era. J Neurooncol. 2023;162(2):253–65.

28. Bowers CA, Altay T, Couldwell WT. Surgical decision-making strategies in tuberculum sellae meningioma resection. Neurosurg Focus. 2011;30(5):E1.

29. Schroeder HW, Hickmann AK, Baldauf J. Endoscope-assisted microsurgical resection of skull base meningiomas. Neurosurg Rev. 2011;34:441–55.

6

30. Clark AJ, Jahangiri A, Garcia RM, George JR, Sughrue ME, McDermott MW, El-Sayed IH, Aghi MK. Endoscopic surgery for tuberculum sellae meningiomas: a systematic review and meta-analysis. Neurosurg Rev. 2013;36:349–59.

31. Fatima N, Meola A, Pollom EL, Soltys SG, Chang SD. Stereotactic radiosurgery versus stereotactic radiotherapy in the management of intracranial meningiomas: a systematic review and meta-analysis. Neurosurg Focus. 2019;46(6):E2.

32. Lam Shin Cheung V, Kim A, Sahgal A, Das S. Meningioma recurrence rates following treatment: a systematic analysis. J Neurooncol. 2018;136:351–61.

33. Youngblood MW, Miyagishima DF, Jin L, Gupte T, Li C, Duran D, Montejo JD, Zhao A, Sheth A, Tyrtova E, Özduman K. Associations of meningioma molecular subgroup and tumor recurrence. Neuro Oncol. 2021;23(5):783–94.

34. Nanda A, Bir SC, Maiti TK, Konar SK, Missios S, Guthikonda B. Relevance of Simpson grading system and recurrence-free survival after surgery for World Health Organization Grade I meningioma. J Neurosurg. 2017;126(1):201–11.

35. Spille DC, Sporns PB, Hess K, Stummer W, Brokinkel B. Prediction of high-grade histology and recurrence in meningiomas using routine preoperative magnetic resonance imaging: a systematic review. World Neurosurg. 2019;128:174–81.

36. Islim AI, Mohan M, Moon RD, Srikandarajah N, Mills SJ, Brodbelt AR, Jenkinson MD. Incidental intracranial meningiomas: a systematic review and meta-analysis of prognostic factors and outcomes. J Neurooncol. 2019;142:211–21.

37. de Almeida AN, Pereira BJ, Aguiar PH, Paiva WS, Cabrera HN, da Silva CC, Teixeira MJ, Marie SK. Clinical outcome, tumor recurrence, and causes of death: a long-term follow-up of surgically treated meningiomas. World Neurosurg. 2017;102:139–43.

38. Durand A, Labrousse F, Jouvet A, Bauchet L, Kalamaridès M, Menei P, Deruty R, Moreau JJ, Fèvre-Montange M, Guyotat J. WHO grade II and III meningiomas: a study of prognostic factors. J Neurooncol. 2009;95:367–75.

Mesenchymal Nonmeningothelial Tumors

Oday Atallah, Khalid M. Alshuqayfi,
Younus M. Al-Khazaali, Fatimah O. Ahmed,
Alkawthar M. Abdulsada, Mayur Sharma,
and Samer S. Hoz

© The Author(s), under exclusive license to Springer Nature Switzerland AG 2024
S. S. Hoz et al. (eds.), *Surgical Neuro-Oncology*,
https://doi.org/10.1007/978-3-031-53642-7_7

? 1. **Mesenchymal, nonmeningothelial tumors: types. The FALSE answer is:**
   A. Hemangioblastoma.
   B. Solitary fibrous tumor/hemangiopericytoma.
   C. Angioleiomyoma.
   D. Meningioma.
   E. Rhabdomyosarcoma.

✓ **Answer D**
— Meningioma is a type of meningeal tumor.

? 2. **Solitary fibrous tumor/hemangiopericytoma: epidemiology. The FALSE answer is:**
   A. It tends to affect adults between the ages of 30 and 50.
   B. It has a high incidence in children.
   C. Men are afflicted more frequently than women.
   D. It accounts for less than 1% of CNS malignancies.
   E. It could be located extracranially.

✓ **Answer B**
— Hemangiopericytomas are rare in children.

? 3. **Solitary fibrous tumor/hemangiopericytoma: pathology. The FALSE answer is:**
   A. It originates from the pericytes of Zimmerman.
   B. It is a mesenchymal tumor of the fibroblastic type.
   C. The tumor is usually benign.
   D. There are three WHO grades 1–3.
   E. It is a highly vascular, soft-tissue tumor.

✓ **Answer C**
— Both benign and malignant forms are possible; WHO grades 1–3 apply.

? 4. **Solitary fibrous tumor/hemangiopericytoma: clinical presentation. The FALSE answer is:**
   A. Headache.
   B. Loss of balance and nausea.
   C. Focal neurological deficits.
   D. Metastasis to the liver, lung, and bone is possible.
   E. Gelastic seizure.

✅ **Answer E**

━ Gelastic seizures are associated with hypothalamic hamartomas.

❓ 5. **Solitary fibrous tumor/hemangiopericytoma: diagnosis. The FALSE answer is:**
   A. The diagnosis is validated by the evaluation of STAT6 expression.
   B. The Ki-67 proliferation index is around 10%.
   C. It might erode nearby bone.
   D. It does not enhance significantly with contrast.
   E. Adjacent cerebral edema is often seen.

✅ **Answer D**

━ It enhances significantly with contrast.

❓ 6. **Solitary fibrous tumor/hemangiopericytoma: treatment. The FALSE answer is:**
   A. Preoperative embolization is recommended.
   B. Surgical resection is considered the preferred therapeutic option.
   C. Radiotherapy does not play a significant role in the treatment.
   D. Chemotherapy is employed in the treatment of extracranial metastases.
   E. Stereotactic radiosurgery represents a viable therapy modality.

✅ **Answer C**

━ Radiotherapy has been shown to decrease recurrence.

❓ 7. **Hemangioblastoma: epidemiology. The FALSE answer is:**
   A. It constitutes around 2% of all cerebral tumors.
   B. It appears in the fourth decade.
   C. It constitutes approximately 10% of the tumors located in the posterior fossa.
   D. Men tend to be affected at a higher frequency compared to women.
   E. This tumor does not occur within the spinal cord.

✅ **Answer E**

━ Among spinal cord tumors, 3–13% are sporadic hemangioblastomas.

8. Hemangioblastoma: pathology. The FALSE answer is:
    A. It is associated with von Hippel-Lindau disease.
    B. It is often classified as WHO grade 1.
    C. Histologically, it resembles renal cell carcinoma.
    D. Approximately 10% manifest sporadically.
    E. Polycythemia may be linked to this tumor.

✔ **Answer D**
− Approximately 70% of hemangioblastomas manifest as sporadic cases.

9. Hemangioblastoma: clinical manifestation. The FALSE answer is:
    A. Headache.
    B. Hydrocephalus.
    C. Nausea/vomiting.
    D. Motor aphasia.
    E. Erythrocytosis.

7

✔ **Answer D**
− Since hemangioblastoma is cerebellar, motor aphasia is infrequent.

10. Hemangioblastoma: diagnosis. The FALSE answer is:
    A. CT reveals lesions that are isodense.
    B. Vertebral angiography exhibits a pronounced presence of blood vessels.
    C. The nodule does not exhibit contrast enhancement on MRI.
    D. CT shows strong contrast enhancement.
    E. The cyst wall does not exhibit enhancement.

✔ **Answer C**
− The nodule is very small and greatly enhances with contrast on MRI.

11. Hemangioblastoma: differential diagnosis. The FALSE answer is:
    A. Lhermitte Duclos disease.
    B. Ependymoma.
    C. Medulloblastoma.
    D. Metastasis.
    E. Pilocytic astrocytoma.

✔ **Answer C**
− Lhermitte Duclos disease is distinguished by the tigroid appearance on MRI.

? 12. **Hemangioblastoma: surgical treatment. The FALSE answer is:**
   A. Sporadic instances, in particular, are curable with surgical excision.
   B. Embolization may serve as a viable alternative to surgical resection.
   C. The mural nodule must be removed.
   D. The removal of the cyst wall is often not recommended.
   E. 5-ALA fluorescence might aid in tumor localization.

✅ **Answer B**
▬ Embolization is frequently employed as a preoperative measure to reduce vascularity.

? 13. **Hemangioblastoma: treatment. The FALSE answer is:**
   A. The removal process is more laborious for solid hemangioblastoma.
   B. Bipolar forceps are used to reduce the size of the tumor.
   C. A division may be observed between the tumor and the base of the fourth ventricle.
   D. Following subtotal resection, adjuvant radiation treatment can stop regrowth.
   E. If the nodule cannot be located, the cyst wall should be removed.

✅ **Answer D**
▬ Adjuvant radiation does not prevent regrowth but does reduce recurrence.

? 14. **Cerebral hemangioma: general information. The FALSE answer is:**
   A. Cerebral hemangiomas are benign vascular malformations in the brain.
   B. They are often present at birth or develop within the first or second year of life.
   C. It has a high risk of rupture leading to intracranial hemorrhage.
   D. It can cause seizures, headaches, and developmental delay in children.
   E. Treatment might include observation, medication, or surgery.

✅ **Answer C**
▬ It does not have a high risk of rupture, unlike arteriovenous malformations.

15. Angiosarcoma: general information. The FALSE answer is:
- A. Cerebral angiosarcomas are a very rare tumor.
- B. They most often occur in younger individuals.
- C. Symptoms include headaches, seizures, and neurological deficits.
- D. Treatment involves a combination of surgery, chemotherapy, and radiation.
- E. There is a high 5-year survival rate for individuals with cerebral angiosarcoma.

Answer E
— Cerebral angiosarcomas are aggressive and have a poor prognosis.

16. Ewing sarcoma: general information. The FALSE answer is:
- A. The prevalence of this condition is highest among the pediatric population.
- B. The incidence peaks in the second decade.
- C. An estimated 1% of all Ewing's sarcomas are cranial sarcomas.
- D. The occipital bone is most frequently impacted.
- E. The tumor is characterized by its rarity and aggressive nature.

Answer D
— The most usually impacted bone is the temporal bone.

17. Kaposi sarcoma: general information. The FALSE answer is:
- A. Human Herpesvirus-8 is linked to it.
- B. The frontal lobe is where most cases occur.
- C. The diameter of the observed lesions varies from 2 mm to 2 cm.
- D. It can show up as homogenous, hyperdense lesions on CT.
- E. Kaposi sarcoma is considered to be an incurable condition.

Answer B
— The cerebellum is the most often seen anatomical site.

Bibliography

1. Greenberg MS. Greenberg's handbook of neurosurgery. (10th edition). Thieme publisher. 2023 Apr 19. section 41. P: 716–21.
2. Tauziède-Espariat A, Hasty L, Métais A, Varlet P. Mesenchymal non-meningothelial tumors of the central nervous system: a literature review and diagnostic update of novelties and emerging entities. Acta Neuropathol Commun. 2023;11(1):22.

3. Meredith DM, Alexandrescu S. Embryonal and non-meningothelial mesenchymal tumors of the central nervous system—advances in diagnosis and prognostication. Brain Pathol. 2022;32(4):e13059.

4. Jellinger K, Paulus W. Mesenchymal, non-meningothelial tumors of the central nervous system. Brain Pathol. 1991;1(2):79–87.

5. Vetrano IG, Gioppo A, Faragò G, Pinzi V, Pollo B, Broggi M, Schiariti M, Ferroli P, Acerbi F. Hemangioblastomas and other vascular origating tumors of brain or spinal cord. Adv Exp Med Biol. 2023;1405:377–403.

6. Hamzah A, Bamsallm M, Alshammari KA, Alghamdi AM, Fallatah MA, Babgi M, Lary A. A bibliometric analysis of the top 100 cited articles for hemangioblastoma of the central nervous system. Neurosurg Rev. 2023;46(1):168.

7. Kuharic M, Jankovic D, Splavski B, Boop FA, Arnautovic KI. Hemangioblastomas of the posterior cranial fossa in adults: demographics, clinical, morphologic, pathologic, surgical features, and outcomes. A systematic review. World Neurosurg. 2018;110: e1049–62.

8. Pan J, Jabarkheel R, Huang Y, Ho A, Chang SD. Stereotactic radiosurgery for central nervous system hemangioblastoma: systematic review and meta-analysis. J Neurooncol. 2018;137(1):11–22.

9. Ampie L, Choy W, Lamano JB, Kesavabhotla K, Kaur R, Parsa AT, Bloch O. Safety and outcomes of preoperative embolization of intracranial hemangioblastomas: a systematic review. Clin Neurol Neurosurg. 2016;150:143–51.

10. Kwon SM, Na MK, Choi KS, Lim TH, Shin H, Lee J, Lee H, Kim W, Cho Y, Kim JG, Ahn C, Jang BH. Impact of extent of resection and postoperative radiotherapy on survival outcomes in intracranial solitary fibrous tumors: a systematic review and meta-analysis. Neurosurg Rev. 2023;46(1):138.

11. Tobias S, Jahshan S, Grober Y, Soustiel JF. Skull base hemangiopericytomas. Acta Neurol Belg. 2022;122(6):1537–45.

12. Gopakumar S, Srinivasan VM, Hadley CC, Anand A, Daou M, Karas PJ, Mandel J, Gopinath SP, Patel AJ. Intracranial solitary fibrous tumor of the skull base: 2 cases and systematic review of the literature. World Neurosurg. 2021;149:e345–59.

13. Giordan E, Marton E, Wennberg AM, Guerriero A, Canova G. A review of solitary fibrous tumor/hemangiopericytoma tumor and a comparison of risk factors for recurrence, metastases, and death among patients with spinal and intracranial tumors. Neurosurg Rev. 2021;44(3):1299–312.

14. Ratneswaren T, Hogg FRA, Gallagher MJ, Ashkan K. Surveillance for metastatic hemangiopericytoma-solitary fibrous tumors-systematic literature review on incidence, predictors and diagnosis of extra-cranial disease. J Neurooncol. 2018;138(3):447–67.

15. Pantanowitz L, Dezube BJ. Kaposi sarcoma in unusual locations. BMC Cancer. 2008;8:190.

16. Zare F, Shahbazi N, Faraji N, Goli R, Mostafaei B, Anari S. A cruel invasion of Ewing's sarcoma of the skull: a rare case report. Int J Surg Case Rep. 2023;108:108380.

17. Kuang R, Li S, Wang Y. Primary cerebral epithelioid angiosarcoma: a case report. BMC Neurol. 2023;23:49.

Diffuse Astrocytic and Oligodendroglial Tumors

*Oday Atallah, Sajjad G. Al-Badri, Mays S. Ahmed,
Fatimah O. Ahmed, Mahmood F. Alzaidy,
Alkawthar M. Abdulsada, and Samer S. Hoz*

© The Author(s), under exclusive license to Springer Nature Switzerland AG 2024
S. S. Hoz et al. (eds.), *Surgical Neuro-Oncology*,
https://doi.org/10.1007/978-3-031-53642-7_8

? 1. **Glial cells. The FALSE answer is:**
   A. Oligodendrocytes.
   B. Astrocytes.
   C. Ependymal cells.
   D. Microglia.
   E. Arachnoid cap cells.

✅ **Answer E**
— Arachnoid cap cells are not classified as a type of glial cells.

? 2. **Diffuse astrocytoma: epidemiology. The FALSE answer is:**
   A. The peak age occurs throughout childhood and young adulthood.
   B. It accounts for approximately 25% of primary brain tumors.
   C. It is classified as a subtype of the pediatric-type diffuse low-grade gliomas.
   D. It constitutes around 15% of gliomas.
   E. Astrocytoma, IDH-mutant is a subtype of the adult-type diffuse gliomas.

✅ **Answer B**
— It contributes to about 5% of primary brain tumors.

? 3. **Diffuse astrocytoma: location. The FALSE answer is:**
   A. The most frequent location is the cerebellum.
   B. The frontal lobe is a common site.
   C. In 20% of cases, deep gray nuclei are involved.
   D. Often occurs in the thalamus in pediatric patients.
   E. Around 30% occur in the temporal lobe.

✅ **Answer A**
— The cerebral hemisphere is most frequently observed as the primary location.

? 4. **Diffuse astrocytoma: pathology. The FALSE answer is:**
   A. Mitotic activity is infrequent.
   B. MIB-1 index is high.
   C. Hemorrhage is uncommon.
   D. GFAP positive.
   E. Calcification may potentially be observed.

✅ **Answer B**
— MIB-1 index is low.

❓ 5. **Diffuse astrocytoma: imaging and treatment. The FALSE answer is:**
   A. Typically, it does not enhance contrast.
   B. On T2-weighted images, it appears as a hyperintense mass.
   C. Surgical resection is not recommended.
   D. Brachytherapy constitutes a viable therapeutic alternative.
   E. Radiation therapy represents a viable therapeutic modality.

✅ **Answer C**
— It is suggested to consider surgical resection and/or biopsy.

❓ 6. **Glioblastoma: epidemiology. The FALSE answer is:**
   A. It accounts for 50% of all astrocytomas.
   B. Glioblastoma accounts for approximately 15% of all intracranial neoplasms.
   C. Men are more commonly affected than women.
   D. The highest occurrence rate is observed in individuals aged 50–70 years.
   E. Glioblastoma is the third most common primary intracranial neoplasm in adults.

✅ **Answer E**
— Glioblastoma is the most common primary intracranial neoplasm in adults.

❓ 7. **Glioblastoma: location. The FALSE answer is:**
   A. Frontal lobe: 40%.
   B. Temporal lobe: 29%.
   C. Parietal lobe: 14%.
   D. Occipital lobe: 14%.
   E. Deep structure: 14%.

✅ **Answer D**
— Glioblastoma occurs in the occipital lobe in about 3% of cases.

❓ 8. **Glioblastoma: pathology. The FALSE answer is:**
   A. Astrocytic differentiation.
   B. Nuclear atypia.

C. Cellular pleomorphism.
D. Necrosis.
E. Psammoma bodies.

✅ **Answer E**
▬ The presence of psammoma bodies is a characteristic feature of meningioma.

❓ 9. **Glioblastoma: primary versus secondary GBM. The FALSE answer is:**
   A. Primary GBM results from malignant degeneration of WHO grade 3 astrocytoma.
   B. Patients with secondary GBM tend to be younger.
   C. Secondary GBM exhibits a lower prevalence.
   D. The clinical histories of primary GBM patients are shorter.
   E. IDH-wildtype is the most common type of primary GBM.

✅ **Answer A**
▬ A secondary GBM results from malignant degeneration of WHO grade 2 or 3 astrocytoma.

8

❓ 10. **Glioblastoma: diagnosis. The FALSE answer is:**
   A. Glioblastomas often exhibit enhancement on contrast-enhanced MRI.
   B. The presence of a "ring" of enhancement surrounding a necrotic core is common.
   C. Frequently demonstrates calcifications on CT scans.
   D. Hemorrhage within the tumor can be a feature of glioblastomas.
   E. Glioblastomas can show both hyper- and hypointense areas on T2-weighted MRI.

✅ **Answer C**
▬ Glioblastomas rarely demonstrate calcifications on CT scans.

❓ 11. **Glioblastoma: treatment. The FALSE answer is:**
   A. Surgery is commonly used to remove as much of the glioblastoma as possible.
   B. Drugs to block certain cell growth pathways have proven to be highly effective in improving overall survival rates.
   C. Chemotherapy is often used to slow the growth of new cancer cells.

D. 5-ALA is used to improve the extent of tumor resection.

E. The fluorescence from 5-ALA is visible with a blue light microscope.

✅ **Answer B**
— Research on targeted drugs is still in progress.

❓ 12. **Glioblastoma: factors against surgical debulking. The FALSE answer is:**
A. Younger individuals.
B. Extensive dominant lobe.
C. Massive butterfly gliomas.
D. Karnofsky score <70.
E. Multicentric gliomas.

✅ **Answer A**
— Surgical debulking is not considered a viable option for elderly people.

❓ 13. **Glioblastoma: differential diagnosis. The FALSE answer is:**
A. Metastasis.
B. Toxoplasmosis.
C. Epidermoid.
D. Lymphoma.
E. Abscess.

✅ **Answer C**
— In contrast to glioblastoma, epidermoid is an extra-axial lesion.

❓ 14. **Oligodendroglioma: general information. The FALSE answer is:**
A. Both males and females are equally impacted.
B. The highest occurrence rate is observed during the age range of 30–60 years.
C. The parietal lobe is the most often seen location.
D. Seizures are the most common presenting symptom.
E. It makes up around 1% of all primary brain tumors.

✅ **Answer C**
— The frontal lobe is the most common site (50%).

? 15. **Oligodendroglioma: pathology. The FALSE answer is:**
   A. Fleshy, cortical, pink mass.
   B. Not well-defined and often merges with the surrounding tissues.
   C. Calcification is a common occurrence.
   D. Necrosis is a frequently observed phenomenon.
   E. Intratumoral bleeding occurs with a high frequency.

✓ **Answer D**
— The occurrence of necrosis is infrequent.

? 16. **Oligodendroglioma: diagnosis. The FALSE answer is:**
   A. Calcifications are observed in around 30–60% of instances.
   B. MRI appearances differ based on histology or molecular diagnosis.
   C. 50% of oligodendrogliomas enhance with contrast to varying degrees.
   D. There is no evidence of diffusion restriction on DWI.
   E. Calcification is exclusively central in location.

8

✓ **Answer E**
— Calcification can exhibit three distinct patterns: central, peripheral, or ribbon-like.

? 17. **Oligodendroglioma: treatment and prognosis. The FALSE answer is:**
   A. The initial course of therapy is surgical resection.
   B. Recurrence is infrequent.
   C. The presence or absence of 1p19q gene deletion affects prognosis.
   D. The approximate 10-year survival rate is 50%.
   E. The recommendation is to utilize adjuvant radiation and chemotherapy.

✓ **Answer B**
— Even though they are well-defined macroscopically, they frequently recur locally and exhibit infiltration at their borders.

Bibliography

1. Greenberg MS. Greenberg's handbook of neurosurgery. (10th edition).Thieme publisher. 2023 Apr 19.
2. Louis DN, Perry A, Wesseling P, Brat DJ, Cree IA, Figarella-Branger D, Hawkins C, Ng HK, Pfister SM, Reifenberger G, Soffietti R, von Deimling A, Ellison DW. The 2021 WHO classification of tumors of the central nervous system: a summary. Neuro Oncol. 2021;23(8):1231–51.
3. Mohile NA, Messersmith H, Gatson NT, Hottinger AF, Lassman A, Morton J, Ney D, Nghiemphu PL, Olar A, Olson J, Perry J, Portnow J, Schiff D, Shannon A, Shih HA, Strowd R, van den Bent M, Ziu M, Blakeley J. Therapy for diffuse astrocytic and oligodendroglial tumors in adults: ASCO-SNO guideline. J Clin Oncol. 2022;40(4):403–26.
4. Tork CA, Atkinson C. Oligodendroglioma [updated 2022 Aug 29]. In: StatPearls. Treasure Island, FL: StatPearls Publishing; 2023.
5. Wu W, Klockow JL, Zhang M, Lafortune F, Chang E, Jin L, Wu Y, Daldrup-Link HE. Glioblastoma multiforme (GBM): an overview of current therapies and mechanisms of resistance. Pharmacol Res. 2021;171:105780.
6. Tykocki T, Eltayeb M. Ten-year survival in glioblastoma. A systematic review. J Clin Neurosci. 2018;54:7–13.
7. Wirsching HG, Galanis E, Weller M. Glioblastoma. Handb Clin Neurol. 2016;134:381–97.
8. Ohgaki H, Kleihues P. The definition of primary and secondary glioblastoma. Clin Cancer Res. 2013;19(4):764–72.
9. Ohgaki H, Kleihues P. Genetic pathways to primary and secondary glioblastoma. Am J Pathol. 2007;170(5):1445–53.
10. Wesseling P, van den Bent M, Perry A. Oligodendroglioma: pathology, molecular mechanisms and markers. Acta Neuropathol. 2015;129(6):809–27.
11. Bromberg JE, van den Bent MJ. Oligodendrogliomas: molecular biology and treatment. Oncologist. 2009;14(2):155–63.
12. Carstam L, Latini F, Solheim O, Bartek J Jr, Pedersen LK, Zetterling M, Beniaminov S, Sjåvik K, Ryttlefors M, Jensdottir M, Rydenhag B, Smits A, Jakola AS. Long-term follow up of patients with WHO grade 2 oligodendroglioma. J Neurooncol. 2023;164(1):65–74.
13. Kapoor M, Gupta V. Astrocytoma [updated 2023 Jul 17]. In: StatPearls. Treasure Island, FL: StatPearls Publishing; 2023.
14. Van den Bent MJ, Reni M, Gatta G, Vecht C. Oligodendroglioma. Crit Rev Oncol Hematol. 2008;66(3):262–72.
15. Engelhard HH, Stelea A, Cochran EJ. Oligodendroglioma: pathology and molecular biology. Surg Neurol. 2002;58(2):111–7; discussion 117.
16. Barresi V, Mafficini A, Calicchia M, Piredda ML, Musumeci A, Ghimenton C, Scarpa A. Recurrent oligodendroglioma with changed 1p/19q status. Neuropathology. 2022;42(2):160–6.
17. Paleologos NA, Cairncross JG. Treatment of oligodendroglioma: an update. Neuro Oncol. 1999;1(1):61–8.

Other Astrocytic Tumors and Gliomas

Rasha A. Al-Youzbaki, Farah M. Hameed, Alkawthar M. Abdulsada, Mustafa Ismail, and Samer S. Hoz

© The Author(s), under exclusive license to Springer Nature Switzerland AG 2024
S. S. Hoz et al. (eds.), *Surgical Neuro-Oncology*,
https://doi.org/10.1007/978-3-031-53642-7_9

1. **Pilocytic astrocytoma.**
   Epidemiology. The FALSE answer is:
   A. Age 0–19 years.
   B. 75% occur in ages less than 15 years
   C. Equal in males and females.
   D. Incidence 0.8/100,000.
   E. Incidence declines after 15 years of age.

✅ **Answer C**
— Slight male predilection.

2. **Pilocytic astrocytoma.**
   Location. The FALSE answer is:
   A. Cerebellum: 42%.
   B. Optic nerve: 25%.
   C. Cerebrum: 36%.
   D. Brain stem: 9%.
   E. Spinal cord: 2%.

✅ **Answer B**
— Optic nerve: 9%.

9

3. **Pilocytic astrocytoma.**
   Pathology. The FALSE answer is:
   A. Vascular proliferation is uncommon.
   B. Breaks through the pia and perivascular space.
   C. Multinucleated giant cells are common.
   D. Mitotic figures may be seen.
   E. 64% infiltrate the parenchyma.

✅ **Answer A**
— Vascular proliferation is common.

4. **Pilocytic astrocytoma.**
   Presentation of optic nerve glioma. The FALSE answer is:
   A. Painless proptosis.
   B. Chiasmal involvement causes proptosis.
   C. Gliosis of optic nerve seen by fundoscopy.
   D. Hypothalamic and pituitary dysfunction.
   E. Hydrocephalus.

✅ **Answer B**
➖ Chiasmal involvement causes visual deficit but does not directly cause proptosis.

❓ 5. **Pilocytic astrocytoma.**
Imaging of optic nerve glioma. The FALSE answer is:
A. Dilatation of optic canal by X-ray.
B. CT is better than MRI in assessing orbital structures.
C. Enhanced fusiform dilatation of the involved nerve.
D. Cystic changes are confined to the chiasm in cases associated with NF1.
E. Sometimes cannot be differentiated from hypothalamic glioma.

✅ **Answer D**
➖ Cystic changes are confined to the chiasm in cases not associated with NF1.

❓ 6. **Pilocytic astrocytoma.**
Brain stem glioma management. The FALSE answer is:
A. Shunting for hydrocephalus.
B. Biopsy is not indicated in diffuse pontine glioma.
C. Radiation is given at a dose of 45–55 Gy over 6 weeks.
D. Surgery is indicated only for the exophytic type.
E. Chemotherapy is indicted for nonresectable lesions.

✅ **Answer E**
➖ No chemotherapeutic regimen has been demonstrated to be effective.

❓ 7. **Pilocytic astrocytoma.**
Imaging of cerebellar pilocytic astrocytoma (PCA). The FALSE answer is:
A. Calcification is occasionally present.
B. MRI of the entire neuroaxis should be done.
C. Mass with nonenhancing central area: 46%.
D. Solid mass with no cyst: 17%.
E. Nonenhancing cyst with enhancing nodule: 21%.

✅ **Answer C**
➖ 16% of cases demonstrate a mass with a nonenhancing central area.

? 8. **Pilocytic astrocytoma.**
   Tectal glioma. The FALSE answer is:
   A. A subgroup of brain stem glioma.
   B. CT scan misses 50% of masses.
   C. VP shunt may be the only treatment.
   D. Stereotactic radiosurgery is given at a dose of 25 Gy.
   E. Endoscopic third ventriculostomy with biopsy can be made.

✔ Answer D
— Stereotactic radiosurgery is given at a dose of less than 14 Gy to avoid side effects.

? 9. **Pilomyxoid astrocytoma (PMA).**
   Epidemiology. The FALSE answer is:
   A. It is a variant of pilocytic astrocytoma.
   B. High predilection for the suprasellar area.
   C. Rarely occurs in the cerebellum.
   D. 40% occurs in an atypical location
   E. 20% occurs in the hypothalamus/optic pathway.

9

✔ Answer E
— 60% occurs in the hypothalamus/optic pathway.

? 10. **Pilomyxoid astrocytoma (PMA).**
   Pathology. The FALSE answer is:
   A. Does not have a designated WHO grade.
   B. Expresses H19.
   C. Expresses BRAF.
   D. Piloid cell and myxoid background.
   E. Angiocentric growth.

✔ Answer C
— Does not express BRAF.

? 11. **Pilomyxoid astrocytoma (PMA).**
   Clinical features/course. The FALSE answer is:
   A. CSF dissemination is rare.
   B. Insidious onset.
   C. Common in infants less than 4 years.
   D. More aggressive than PCA.
   E. May differentiate to GBM.

✅ **Answer A**
- CSF dissemination is common.

❓ 12. **Pilomyxoid astrocytoma (PMA).**
   Imaging. The FALSE answer is:
   A. Hypointense in T1 and hyperintense in T2.
   B. 20% have intratumoral hemorrhage
   C. Homogenous enhancement.
   D. Peritumoral edema.
   E. The entire neuroaxis should be imaged.

✅ **Answer D**
- Peritumoral edema is absent.

❓ 13. **Subependymal giant cell astrocytoma (SEGA).**
   Epidemiology. The FALSE answer is:
   A. Associated with tuberous sclerosis.
   B. Arises in 40% of cases with tuberous sclerosis.
   C. Mean age 11 years.
   D. Occurs near the foramen of Monro.
   E. Sporadic cases rare.

✅ **Answer B**
- Arises in 10–20% of cases with tuberous sclerosis.

❓ 14. **Subependymal giant cell astrocytoma (SEGA).**
   Presentation. The FALSE answer is:
   A. Asymptomatic.
   B. Hydrocephalus.
   C. Headache.
   D. Vomiting.
   E. Seizure.

✅ **Answer E**
- Seizure is due to cortical tuber, not SEGA.

❓ 15. **Subependymal giant cell astrocytoma (SEGA).**
   Pathology. The FALSE answer is:
   A. Size is 10–15 mm.
   B. Most are solitary.

C. MIB-1 is high.
D. Multilobulated.
E. Calcification is common.

✅ **Answer C**
— MIB-1 is low.

❓ 16. **Subependymal giant cell astrocytoma (SEGA).**
Natural history. The FALSE answer is:
A. Benign.
B. Slow-growing.
C. Median growth is 2.5–5.6 mm/year.
D. Infiltrates adjacent brain.
E. Prognosis is good.

✅ **Answer D**
— Rarely infiltrates the brain.

❓ 17. **Subependymal giant cell astrocytoma (SEGA).**
Imaging. The FALSE answer is:
A. Isointense on T1 and hyperintense on T2.
B. Hypodense on CT.
C. Calcification is common.
D. Heterogenous enhancement.
E. Hydrocephalus occurs in 40% of cases.

✅ **Answer E**
— Hydrocephalus occurs in 15% of cases.

❓ 18. **Subependymal giant cell astrocytoma (SEGA).**
Treatment. The FALSE answer is:
A. Observation.
B. Serial imaging every 6 months.
C. Surgical resection is the treatment of choice.
D. SEGA can recur in a few months.
E. No role of chemotherapy.

✅ **Answer E**
— Sirolimus and everolimus are safe and efficacious.

❓ 19. Pleomorphic xanthoastrocytoma (PXA).
   Etiology. The FALSE answer is:
   A. Originates from multipotent neuroectodermal cells.
   B. Expresses neuronal marker.
   C. Originates from preexisting hamartomatous lesion.
   D. Lacks IDH mutation.
   E. 30% have BRAF point mutation.

✅ Answer E
➖ More than half have BRAF point mutation.

❓ 20. Pleomorphic xanthoastrocytoma (PXA).
   Epidemiology. The FALSE answer is:
   A. Less than 1% of all astrocytomas.
   B. Typically present in the fourth and fifth decades of life.
   C. No sex predominance.
   D. Is WHO grade 2.
   E. BRAF V600E.

✅ Answer B
➖ Typically present in the first two decades of life.

❓ 21. Pleomorphic xanthoastrocytoma (PXA).
   Location. The FALSE answer is:
   A. The frontal lobe is the most common site.
   B. 95% are supratentorial
   C. Involvement of the adjacent leptomeninges is common.
   D. Parietal involvement occurs in 20% of cases.
   E. Spinal cord involvement is very rare.

✅ Answer A
➖ The temporal lobe is the most common site, accounting for 40–50% of cases.

❓ 22. Pleomorphic xanthoastrocytoma (PXA).
   Pathology. The FALSE answer is:
   A. Partially cystic mass with nodule.
   B. Dural invasion is rare.
   C. Solitary lesion.
   D. Necrosis is rare.
   E. GFAP negative and S-100 positive.

✅ **Answer E**
- GFAP positive and S-100 positive.

❓ 23. **Pleomorphic xanthoastrocytoma (PXA).**
   Natural history. The FALSE answer is:
   A. Recurrence is common.
   B. Seizure is the presenting symptom.
   C. The 5-year survival rate is 80%.
   D. The 10-year survival rate is 70%.
   E. Mitotic activity is a predictor of biological behavior.

✅ **Answer A**
- Recurrence is uncommon.

❓ 24. **Pleomorphic xanthoastrocytoma (PXA).**
   Imaging. The FALSE answer is:
   A. Cyst and nodule are present in 70% of cases.
   B. Solid mass with intratumoral cyst in 30% of cases.
   C. The overlying skull may be thinned.
   D. Calcification in 40% of cases.
   E. Intratumoral hemorrhage is common.

9

✅ **Answer E**
- Intratumoral hemorrhage is uncommon.

❓ 25. **Anaplastic pleomorphic xanthoastrocytoma.**
   Epidemiology. The FALSE answer is:
   A. WHO grade 3.
   B. The presence of BRAF V600E mutation is associated with higher-grade tumors.
   C. Features similar to grade 2.
   D. Worse prognosis than PXA.
   E. Maximal safe resection followed by radiotherapy should be done.

✅ **Answer B**
- The presence of BRAF V600E mutation is associated with lower-grade tumors.

? 26. **Astroblastomas.**
   Pathology. The FALSE answer is:
   A. Cystic hemispheric parenchymal mass.
   B. Exhibits MGMT promotor methylation.
   C. Have features of astrocytoma and ependymoma.
   D. Have pseudorosette.
   E. IDH-mutant positive.

✓ **Answer E**
━ IDH-mutant negative.

? 27. **Astroblastomas.**
   Epidemiology. The FALSE answer is:
   A. Rare glial tumor.
   B. 0.5–3% of gliomas
   C. The male:female ratio is 2:1.
   D. The median age is 14 years.
   E. Low-grade tumor.

✓ **Answer C**
━ The male:female ratio is 1:2.

? 28. **Astroblastomas.**
   Clinical features. The FALSE answer is:
   A. Deeply located.
   B. Supratentorial.
   C. Cystic–solid.
   D. Bubbly appearance.
   E. Edema is minimal or absent.

✓ **Answer A**
━ Is superficially located.

? 29. **Astroblastomas.**
   Imaging. The FALSE answer is:
   A. Hypointense on T1 and hyperintense on T2.
   B. Heterogenous enhancement.
   C. Three quarters of cases have calcification.
   D. Usually hypodense on NECT.
   E. Restricted diffusion.

✅ **Answer D**
– It is hyperdense on NECT in 85% of cases.

❓ 30. **Astroblastomas.**
Differential diagnosis. The FALSE answer is:
A. Astrocytoma.
B. Neurocytoma.
C. Atypical teratoid/rhabdoid.
D. Atypical meningioma.
E. Pleomorphic xanthoastrocytoma.

✅ **Answer B**
– Oligodendroglioma.

❓ 31. **Chordoid glioma.**
Epidemiology. The FALSE answer is:
A. Located in the anterior third ventricle.
B. Arises from organum vasculum.
C. Rare pediatric tumor.
D. The smallest size is around 1.5 cm.
E. No known risk factors.

9

✅ **Answer C**
– Rare adult tumor.

❓ 32. **Chordoid glioma.**
Pathology. The FALSE answer is:
A. Tan gray in color.
B. Encapsulated.
C. GFAP positive.
D. EMA and CD34 negative.
E. MIB-1 index is low.

✅ **Answer D**
– EMA and CD34 positive

❓ 33. **Chordoid glioma.**
Epidemiology. The FALSE answer is:
A. Less than 1% of all gliomas.
B. Age 35–60 years old.

C. F:M ratio 2:1.

D. May be asymptomatic.

E. Endocrine disturbance is the most common feature.

✅ **Answer E**

➖ Visual deficit is the most common feature; endocrine disturbance accounts for 10–15% of cases only.

❓ **34. Chordoid glioma.**
   Natural history. The FALSE answer is:
   A. Slow-growing.
   B. Often subtotal resection is done.
   C. SIADH is a postoperative complication.
   D. Obesity is a postoperative complication.
   E. Attached to the hypothalamus.

✅ **Answer C**

➖ Diabetes insipidus is a postoperative complication.

❓ **35. Chordoid glioma.**
   Imaging. The FALSE answer is:
   A. NECT hyperdense.
   B. Hemorrhage is common.
   C. An intratumoral cyst is present in 25% of cases.
   D. Homogeneous enhancement.
   E. Displaces the pituitary and stalk posteriorly.

✅ **Answer B**

➖ Hemorrhage is rare.

❓ **36. Angiocentric glioma (AG).**
   Clinical issues. The FALSE answer is:
   A. The most common location is the parietal lobe.
   B. Occur in children and young adult.
   C. Present with focal epilepsy.
   D. Surgical excision is curative.
   E. Low-grade glioma.

✅ **Answer A**

➖ The most common locations are the frontal and temporal lobes.

❓ 37. Angiocentric glioma (AG).
Pathology. The FALSE answer is:
A. Located superficially.
B. Cortical-based.
C. MYB-QK1 fusion.
D. WHO grade 1.
E. MIB-1 is present in more than 10% of cases.

✅ Answer E
– MIB-1 is present in less than 1% of cases.

❓ 38. Angiocentric glioma (AG).
Imaging. The FALSE answer is:
A. Calcification may be present.
B. No enhancement.
C. Hyperintense in T2MRI.
D. Well-circumscribed.
E. Necrosis is absent.

✅ Answer D
– It presents as a diffusely infiltrating expansile cortical mass.

9

Bibliography

1. Ostrom QT, Gittelman H, Liao P, et al. CBTRUS statistical report: primary brain and central nervous system tumors diagnosed in the United States in 2007–2011. Neuro Oncol. 2014;16(Suppl 4):iv1–iv63.
2. Burkhard C, Di Pattre PL, Schuller D, et al. A population-based study of the incidence and survival rates in patients with pilocytic astrocytoma. J Neurosurg. 2003;98:1170–4.
3. Collins VP, Jones DT, Giannini C. Pilocytic astrocytoma: pathology, molecular mechanisms and markers. Acta Neuropathol. 2015;129:775–88.
4. Packer RJ, Lange B, Ater J, et al. Carboplatin and vincristine for recurrent and newly diagnosed low-grade gliomas of childhood. J Clin Oncol. 1993;11:850–6.
5. Bonfield CM, et al. Pediatric cerebellar astrocytoma: a review. Childs Nerv Syst. 2015;31(10):1677–85.
6. Epstein F, McCleary EL. Intrinsic brain-stem tumors of childhood: surgical indications. J Neurosurg. 1986;64:11–5.
7. Epstein FJ, Farmaer J-P. Brain-stem glioma growth patterns. J Neurosurg. 1993;78: 408–12.

8. Coakley KJ, Huston J, Scheithauer BW, et al. Pilocytic astrocytomas: well-demarcated magnetic resonance appearance despite frequent infiltration histologically. Mayo Clin Proc. 1995;70:747–51.

9. Austin EJ, Alvord EC. Recurrences of cerebellar astrocytomas: a violation of Collins' law. J Neurosurg. 1988;68:41–7.

10. Oka K, Kin Y, Go Y, et al. Neuroendoscopic approach to tectal tumors: a consecutive series. J Neurosurg. 1999;91:964–70.

11. Rosenfeld A, et al. A case series characterizing pilomyxoid astrocytomas in childhood. J Pediatr Hematol Oncol. 2016;38(2):e63–6.

12. Kleinschmidt-DeMasters BK, et al. Pilomyxoid astrocytoma (PMA)shows significant differences in gene expression vs. pilocytic astrocytoma (PA) and variable tendency toward maturation to PA. Brain Pathol. 2015;25(4):429–40.

13. Arulrajah S, Huisman TA. Pilomyxoid astrocytoma of the spinal cord with cerebrospinal fluid and peritoneal metastasis. Neuropediatrics. 2008;39:243–5.

14. Alkonyi B, et al. Differential imaging characteristics and dissemination potential of pilomyxoid astrocytomas versus pilocytic astrocytomas. Neuroradiology. 2015;57(6):625–38.

15. Arroyo MS, et al. Acute management of symptomatic subependymal giant cell astrocytoma with everolimus. Pediatr Neurol. 2017;72:81–5.

16. Appalla D, et al. Mammalian target of rapamycin inhibitor induced complete remission of a recurrent subependymal giant cell astrocytoma in a patient without features of tuberous sclerosis complex. Pediatr Blood Cancer. 2016;63(7):1276–8.

17. Pachow D, et al. The mTOR signaling pathway as a treatment target for intracranial neoplasms. Neuro Oncol. 2015;17(2):189–99.

18. Chow CW, Klug GL, Lewis EA. Subependymal giant-cell astrocytoma in children: an unusual discrepancy between histological and clinical features. J Neurosurg. 1988;68:880–3.

19. Ouyang T, et al. Subependymal giant cell astrocytoma: current concepts, management, and future directions. Childs Nerv Syst. 2014;30(4):561–70.

20. Krishnan A, et al. Cross-sectional imaging review of tuberous sclerosis. Radiol Clin North Am. 2016;54(3):423–40.

21. Lohkamp LN, et al. MGMT promoter methylation and BRAF V600E mutations are helpful markers to discriminate pleomorphic xanthoastrocytoma from giant cell glioblastoma. PLoS One. 2016;11(6):e0156422.

22. Ida CM, et al. Pleomorphic xanthoastrocytoma: natural history and long-term follow-up. Brain Pathol. 2015;25(5):575–86.

23. Kumar S, Retnam TM, Menon G, et al. Cerebellar hemisphere, an uncommon location for pleomorphic xanthoastrocytoma and lipidized glioblastoma multiformis. Neurol India. 2003;51:246–7.

24. Weldon-Linne CM, Victor TA, Groothuis DR, et al. Pleomorphic xanthoastrocytoma: ultrastructural and immunohistochemical study of a case with a rapidly fatal outcome following surgery. Cancer. 1983;52:2055–63.

25. Fouladi M, Jenkins J, Burger P, et al. Pleomorphic xanthoastrocytoma: favorable outcome after complete surgical resection. Neuro Oncol. 2001;3:184–92.

26. Jiménez-Heffernan JA, et al. Cytologic features of pleomorphic xanthoastrocytoma, WHO grade II. A comparative study with glioblastoma. Diagn Cytopathol. 2017;45(4):339–44.

27. Pahapill PA, Ramsay DA, Del Maestro RF. Pleomorphic xanthoastrocytoma: case report and analysis of the literature concerning the efficacy of resection and the significance of necrosis. Neurosurgery. 1996;38:822–8; discussion 828–9.

28. Lehman NL, et al. Morphological and molecular features of astroblastoma, including BRAFV600E mutations, suggest an ontological relationship to other cortical-based gliomas of children and young adults. Neuro Oncol. 2017;19(1):31–42.

29. Mallick S, et al. Patterns of care and survival outcomes in patients with astroblastoma: an individual patient data analysis of 152 cases. Childs Nerv Syst. 2017;33:1295.

30. Aldape KD, et al. Astroblastoma. In: Louis DN, et al., editors. WHO classification of tumours of the central nervous system. Lyon: International Agency for Research on Cancer; 2016. p. 121–2.

31. Cunningham DA, et al. Neuroradiologic characteristics of astroblastoma and systematic review of the literature: 2 new cases and 125 cases reported in 59 publications. Pediatr Radiol. 2016;46(9):1301–8.

32. Erwood AA, et al. Chordoid glioma of the third ventricle: report of a rapidly progressive case. J Neurooncol. 2017;132(3):487–95.

33. Morais BA, et al. Chordoid glioma: case report and review of the literature. Int J Surg Case Rep. 2015;7C:168–71.

34. Brat DJ, Fuller GN. Chordoid glioma of the third ventricle. In: Louis DN, et al., editors. WHO classification of tumours of the central nervous system. Lyon: International Agency for Research on Cancer; 2016. p. 116–8.

9

Embryonal Tumors

*Ahmed M. N. ElGhamry, Younus M. Al-Khazaali,
Zinah A. Alaraji, and Samer S. Hoz*

© The Author(s), under exclusive license to Springer Nature Switzerland AG 2024
S. S. Hoz et al. (eds.), *Surgical Neuro-Oncology*,
https://doi.org/10.1007/978-3-031-53642-7_10

? 1. Embryonal tumors: WHO 2016 classification. The FALSE answer is:
A. Medulloblastomas, genetically defined.
B. Medulloblastomas, histologically defined.
C. Medulloblastoma, NOS.
D. CNS neuroblastoma.
E. Central neurocytoma.

✓ Answer E
— Central neurocytoma is a type of neuronal and mixed neuronal-glial tumor.

? 2. Embryonal tumors: WHO 2016 classification. The FALSE answer is:
A. Medulloepithelioma.
B. CNS ganglioneuroblastoma.
C. Gangliocytoma.
D. Embryonal tumors with multilayered rosettes.
E. Atypical teratoid/rhabdoid tumor.

✓ Answer C
— Gangliocytoma is a type of neuronal and mixed neuronal-glial tumor.

? 3. Medulloblastomas (MDBs). The FALSE answer is:
A. Are all WHO grade IV.
B. Small cell embryonal tumor.
C. Peak in the first decade of life.
D. The second most common pediatric brain malignancy.
E. Common in the posterior fossa in children.

✓ Answer D
— Medulloblastoma is the most common pediatric brain malignancy.

? 4. Medulloblastoma: histologic types. The FALSE answer is:
A. Desmoplastic.
B. Extensive nodularity.
C. Classic.
D. Large cell.
E. Reticular.

✓ Answer E
— There are four histologic types of medulloblastoma: classic, desmoplastic/nodular, extensive nodular, and large cell/anaplastic.

10

❓ 5. **Medulloblastoma: genetic categories. The FALSE answer is:**
   A. WNT-activated.
   B. SHH-activated.
   C. IDH wildtype.
   D. Non-WNT/non-SHH, group 3.
   E. Non-WNT/non-SHH, group 4.

✅ **Answer C**
- IDH wildtype is a type of glioma.
- The four genetic types of medulloblastoma
   - WNT-activated.
   - SHH-activated (TP53-mutant, wildtype).
   - Non-WNT/non-SHH, group 3.
   - Non-WNT/non-SHH, group 4.

❓ 6. **Medulloblastoma: clinical presentation. The FALSE answer is:**
   A. High ICP.
   B. Seizure is the most common presentation.
   C. Cerebellar signs.
   D. Early obstructive hydrocephalus.
   E. Associated spinal drop mets.

✅ **Answer B**
- Seizure is not the most common clinical presentation of medulloblastoma. Common signs are papilledema, truncal and appendicular ataxia, nystagmus, EOM palsies, and macrocrania in infants and young children.

❓ 7. **Medulloblastoma: radiological features. The FALSE answer is:**
   A. Arises from the floor of the fourth ventricle.
   B. Mostly in the posterior fossa midline in children.
   C. Typically hyperdense on CT.
   D. 20% have calcification.
   E. Mostly enhances with contrast.

✅ **Answer A**
- Medulloblastoma arises from the roof of the fourth ventricle and tends to protrude into it while ependymoma arises from the floor of the fourth ventricle.

8. Medulloblastoma, classic type. The FALSE answer is:
   A. Densely packed undifferentiated small round cells.
   B. Mild-to-moderate nuclear pleomorphism.
   C. Predominant in children.
   D. The least common histologic type of MDBs.
   E. Found in all four molecular MDB clusters.

Answer D
— Classic medulloblastoma is the most common histologic type of MDBs, accounting for about 75% of MDBs.

9. Desmoplastic/nodular MDB. The FALSE answer is:
   A. Accounts for around 20% of all MDBs.
   B. Occurs only in the cerebellar midline.
   C. Bimodal age distribution.
   D. Associated with Gorlin syndrome in early childhood.
   E. Reticulin-free zones (pale islands).

Answer B
— Desmoplastic MDBs occur in the cerebellar hemispheres and midline. Classic MDBs are restricted to the cerebellar midline.

10. MDB with extensive nodularity. The FALSE answer is:
   A. Predominant in infants.
   B. Mostly in the cerebellar hemispheres.
   C. Reticulin-free nodules rich in neuropil matrix.
   D. Cells arranged in parallel rows.
   E. Favorable outcome.

Answer B
— More than 80% occur in the cerebellar vermis.

11. Medulloblastoma, large cell anaplastic type. The FALSE answer is:
   A. 10–25% of medulloblastomas.
   B. Male predominance.
   C. Most involve the cerebellar vermis.
   D. Common in metastatic cases.
   E. Low risk with SHH-activated TP53-mutant type.

✅ **Answer E**

━ It is considered high risk with SHH-activated TP53-mutant and group 3 types.

❓ 12. **Medulloblastoma, WNT-activated. The FALSE answer is:**
   A. Accounts for about 10% of all MDBs.
   B. Male:female ratio is 1:2.
   C. The predominant histologic variant is of the anaplastic morphology.
   D. The putative cell of origin: lower rhombic lip progenitor cells.
   E. Frequent genetic mutations: CTNNB1, DDX3X, TP53.

✅ **Answer C**

━ The predominant histologic variant is of the classic morphology. It is a low-risk tumor that typically occurs in older children.

❓ 13. **Medulloblastoma, SHH-activated, TP53-mutant. The FALSE answer is:**
   A. Male:female ratio is 1:1.
   B. Predominant histologic variant: large cell/anaplastic.
   C. The putative cell of origin: cerebellar granule neuron cell precursors of the external granule cell layer and cochlear nucleus.
   D. Frequent genetic mutations: TP53.
   E. Large cell/anaplastic morphology is low-risk.

✅ **Answer E**

━ Large cell/anaplastic morphology is high-risk.

❓ 14. **Medulloblastoma, SHH-activated, TP53-wildtype. The FALSE answer is:**
   A. Male:female ratio is 1:1.
   B. WHO grade III.
   C. Predominant histologic variant: desmoplastic/nodular.
   D. The putative cell of origin: cerebellar granule neuron cell precursors of the external granule cell layer and cochlear nucleus.
   E. Frequent genetic mutations: PTCH1, SUFU.

✅ **Answer B**

━ Medulloblastoma is WHO grade IV. Desmoplastic/nodular morphology is low-risk. It is prevalent in infants and adults.

❓ 15. **Medulloblastoma, non-WNT/non-SHH, group 3. The FALSE answer is:**

A. Typically presents in infancy and childhood.

B. Male:female ratio is 2:1.

C. Predominant histologic variants: desmoplastic/nodular.

D. Putative cell of origin: cerebellar granule neuron cell precursors of the external granule cell layer.

E. Genetic mutations: PVT1-MYC, GFI1/GFI1B.

✅ **Answer C**

— Predominant histologic variants: classic and large cell/anaplastic morphology. With regard to prognosis, classic morphology typically corresponds to a standard-risk tumor, while large cell/anaplastic morphology is associated with a high-risk tumor.

❓ 16. **Medulloblastoma: poor prognosticators. The FALSE answer is:**

A. Younger age (especially if <3 years).

B. Disseminated (metastatic) disease.

C. Not to perform gross-total removal.

D. Poor Karnofsky performance score.

E. SHH-activated with desmoplastic histology.

✅ **Answer E**

— Medulloblastoma, SHH-activated with desmoplastic histology is considered low-risk.

10

■ **Postoperative Risk Stratification in Medulloblastoma**
Standard-Risk Patients

— Total or near total surgical resection.[1]

— No CNS metastases on MRI of brain and spine.

— No tumor cells on cytospin of lumbar CSF.

— No clinical evidence of extra-CNS metastases.

— MDB classification

– SHH-activated, TP53-wildtype with classic histology.

– Non-WNT/non-SHH, group 3 or 4, with classic histology.

---

1   Near total resection: <1.5 cm² on axial-plane early postop MRI. This criterion is controversial as much of the data is from the CT era.

Low-Risk Patients

— MDB classification
  – WNT-activated group
    – β-catenin mutation (mandatory testing).
    – β-catenin nuclear immunopositivity by immunohistochemistry and monosomy 6 (optional testing).
  – SHH-activated, TP53-wildtype group
    – Desmoplastic/nodular histology.
    – Extensive nodularity histology.
— Total or near total surgical resection.[1]

High-Risk Patients

— Large cell/anaplastic histology with
  – SHH-activated, TP53-mutant.
  – Non-WNT/non-SHH, group 3.
— Unresectable tumor or residual tumor >1.5 cm^2 on axial-plane early postop MRI.
— Extra-CNS metastases.

❓ 17. **Medulloblastoma: treatment options. The FALSE answer is:**
  A. Maximal surgical resection.
  B. VP shunt for hydrocephalus.
  C. Gliadel wafers.
  D. Adjuvant conventional radiotherapy.
  E. Adjuvant chemotherapy.

✅ **Answer C**
— Gliadel wafers are used in the treatment of high-grade gliomas.

❓ 18. **Embryonal tumors with multilayered rosettes. The FALSE answer is:**
  A. Mostly in children under 2 years.
  B. It is more common in girls.
  C. Most are supratentorial in location.
  D. Includes CNS PNET only.
  E. Amplification of C19MC on chromosome 19.

✅ **Answer D**
— It includes ETANTR, ependymoblastoma, and CNS PNET.
— Amplification of C19MC on chromosome 19 is present in both CNS PNET and ETANTR.

? 19. **Embryonal tumors with multi-layered rosettes (ETMR), pathology. The FALSE answer is:**
A. Amplification of C17MC.
B. Undifferentiated neuroepithelial cells.
C. Well-differentiated neuropil.
D. Ependymoblastic rosettes.
E. Has no epithelial-like formation.

✓ **Answer A**
− ETMR is associated with the amplification of C19MC. Unlike medulloblastoma, ETMR has no epithelial-like formation.

? 20. **Atypical Teratoid/Rhabdoid Tumors (AT/RTs). The FALSE answer is:**
A. Highly aggressive embryonal tumors of the CNS.
B. Primarily in children under 3 years.
C. Consist of only one cell type.
D. Most have biallelic inactivation of SMARCB1 (or INI1) on chromosome 22.
E. Leptomeningeal dissemination in 15–20% of cases.

✓ **Answer C**
− ATRTs have widely divergent cell populations, including mesenchymal, epithelial, glial, and neuronal cell lines accounting for the "teratoid" descriptor.

10

Bibliography

1. Louis DN, Perry A, Reifenberger G, et al. The 2016 World Health Organization classification of tumors of the central nervous system: a summary. Acta Neuropathol (Berl). 2016;131(6):803–20.
2. Greenberg MS, MD. Handbook of neurosurgery. 9th ed. Thieme Medical Publishers; 2020.
3. Shih RY, Koeller KK. Embryonal tumors of the central nervous system: from the radiologic pathology archives. Radiographics. 2018;38(2):525–41.
4. https://www.cancer.gov/types/brain/hp/child-cns-embryonal-treatment-pdq.
5. McGovern SL, Grosshans D, Mahajan A. Embryonal brain tumors. Cancer J. 2014;20(6):397–402. https://doi.org/10.1097/PPO.0000000000000081.
6. Kristensen BW, Priesterbach-Ackley LP, Petersen JK, Wesseling P. Molecular pathology of tumors of the central nervous system. Ann Oncol. 2019;30(8):1265–78. https://doi.org/10.1093/annonc/mdz164.

7. Singh N. Desmoplastic/nodular medulloblastoma. PathologyOutlines.com. http://www. pathologyoutlines.com/topic/cnstumormedulloblastomadesmo.html. Accessed 19 Nov 2020.

8. Pei YC, Huang GH, Yao XH, Bian XW, Li F, Xiang Y, Yang L, Lv SQ, Liu J. Embryonal tumor with multilayered rosettes, C19MC-altered (ETMR): a newly defined pediatric brain tumor. Int J Clin Exp Pathol. 2019;12(8):3156–63.

9. Rieken S, Gaiser T, Mohr A, Welzel T, Witt O, Kulozik AE, Wick W, Debus J, Combs SE. Outcome and prognostic factors of desmoplastic medulloblastoma treated within a multidisciplinary treatment concept. BMC Cancer. 2010;10(1):1.

10. Yeh-Nayre LA, Malicki DM, Vinocur DN, Crawford JR. Medulloblastoma with excessive nodularity: radiographic features and pathologic correlate. Case Rep Radiol. 2012;2012:1.

11. Huang PI, Lin SC, Lee YY, Ho DM, Guo WY, Chang KP, Chang FC, Liang ML, Chen HH, Liu YM, Yen SH. Large cell/anaplastic medulloblastoma is associated with poor prognosis—a retrospective analysis at a single institute. Childs Nerv Syst. 2017;33: 1285–94.

12. Cambruzzi E. Medulloblastoma, WNT-activated/SHH-activated: clinical impact of molecular analysis and histogenetic evaluation. Childs Nerv Syst. 2018;34:809–15.

13. Menyhárt O, Győrffy B. Principles of tumorigenesis and emerging molecular drivers of SHH-activated medulloblastomas. Ann Clin Transl Neurol. 2019;6(5):990–1005.

14. Bartek J. Elucidating the role of DNA damage and human cytomegalovirus in medulloblastoma and glioblastoma, Doctoral dissertation. Karolinska Institutet, Sweden.

15. Ellison DW, Dalton J, Kocak M, Nicholson SL, Fraga C, Neale G, Kenney AM, Brat DJ, Perry A, Yong WH, Taylor RE. Medulloblastoma: clinicopathological correlates of SHH, WNT, and non-SHH/WNT molecular subgroups. Acta Neuropathol. 2011;121:381–96.

16. Wong GC, Li KK, Wang WW, Liu AP, Huang QJ, Chan AK, Poon MF, Chung NY, Wong QH, Chen H, Chan DT. Clinical and mutational profiles of adult medulloblastoma groups. Acta Neuropathol Commun. 2020;8:1–4.

17. Brandes AA, Franceschi E, Tosoni A, Blatt V, Ermani M. Long-term results of a prospective study on the treatment of medulloblastoma in adults. Cancer. 2007;110(9): 2035–41.

18. Raghuram N, Khan S, Mumal I, Bouffet E, Huang A. Embryonal tumors with multilayered rosettes: a disease of dysregulated miRNAs. J Neurooncol. 2020;150:63–73.

19. Horwitz M, Dufour C, Leblond P, Bourdeaut F, Faure-Conter C, Bertozzi AI, Delisle MB, Palenzuela G, Jouvet A, Scavarda D, Vinchon M. Embryonal tumors with multilayered rosettes in children: the SFCE experience. Childs Nerv Syst. 2016;32:299–305.

20. Biegel JA. Molecular genetics of atypical teratoid/rhabdoid tumors. Neurosurg Focus. 2006;20(1):1–7.

Ependymal and Choroid Plexus Tumors

*Khalil Al-Qadasi, Sara Benchekroun,
Khalid M. Alshuqayfi, Ahmed Muthana,
and Samer S. Hoz*

© The Author(s), under exclusive license to Springer Nature Switzerland AG 2024
S. S. Hoz et al. (eds.), *Surgical Neuro-Oncology*,
https://doi.org/10.1007/978-3-031-53642-7_11

? 1. **Ependymomas: definition. The FALSE answer is:**
   A. It arises from the ependymal cell lining in the ventricles and central canal of the spinal cord.
   B. It tends to occur in cranial locations in adults.
   C. They may occur anywhere along the neuraxis.
   D. Can arise within the brain parenchyma.
   E. Posterior fossa is the typical location for pediatrics.

✓ Answer B

— Ependymomas most commonly occur in the spinal cord in adults. They comprise 5–6% of intracranial gliomas, 9% of pediatric brain tumors, and 60% of spinal cord gliomas. They are more common in the pediatric population (69%) and occur mainly in the posterior fossa. The incidence of pediatric intracranial ependymomas in the US is around 200 cases per year.

? 2. **Ependymomas: epidemiology. The FALSE answer is:**
   A. Systemic spread is rare.
   B. Are the most common primary spinal glioma below the mid-thoracic region.
   C. Are likely to have drop metastasis via CSF.
   D. There is a higher incidence in patients with NF1.
   E. It is an intramedullary spinal cord tumor.

✓ Answer D

— The incidence is higher in patients with NF type 2.

? 3. **Ependymomas: pathology. The FALSE answer is:**
   A. Papillary type is considered the classic lesion of ependymomas and is classified as WHO grade II.
   B. The tanycytic type is a rare WHO grade I tumor characterized by the presence of true rosettes.
   C. Subependymomas are WHO I and typically located in the lateral and fourth ventricles.
   D. Ependymomas are usually well-circumscribed lesions.
   E. The myxopapillary type is WHO I and is typically located at the filum terminale.

✅ **Answer B**

▬ WHO classification of ependymomas:

- WHO I: myxopapillary (occurs only in filum terminale), and subependymomas
- WHO II: cellular, papillary (classic lesion, can metastasize in up to 30% of cases), clear cell, tanycytic (rare, cells appear similar to ependymoglial cells, and true rosette are absent)
- WHO III: anaplastic ependymomas

❓ 4. **Subependymomas. The FALSE answer is:**
   A. WHO grade II.
   B. Typically occur in the fifth and sixth decades.
   C. Most common location is the fourth ventricle.
   D. Histologically, they occasionally appear with loose pseudorosettes.
   E. They usually enhance in the contrast studies.

✅ **Answer E**

▬ Subependymomas are benign slow-growing tumors WHO I of ependymal origin that account for less than 10% of ependymal neoplasms.

▬ Most commonly occur in the fifth and sixth decades of life where they appear attached to the ventricular wall by a narrow pedicle usually in the posterior fourth and anterior lateral ventricles.

▬ On MRI studies, they are circumscribed, nodular nonenhancing mass lesions attached to the ventricular wall.

▬ Histologically they appear hypovascular with low cellularity and occasional loose pseudorosette.

❓ 5. **Ependymomas: radiology. The FALSE answer is:**
   A. Imaging of the whole craniospinal axis must be done.
   B. Often show obstructive hydrocephalus.
   C. Can be easily distinguished from medulloblastomas by MRI with contrast.
   D. Commonly appear on CT as a calcified lesion and often have a cystic component.
   E. On MRI, they are typically hypointense on T1 and hyperintense on T2.

✅ **Answer C**
- MRI is the study of choice.
- Imaging must be done for the entire craniospinal axis with and without contrast due to the possibility of drop mets.
- Usually appear in the floor of the fourth ventricle, often with HCP.
- Usually it is difficult to distinguish it from medulloblastomas by radiological studies.
- CT is not as detailed for the posterior fossa but commonly demonstrates a calcified lesion, often with a cystic component.
- On MRI, they demonstrate heterogenous contrast enhancement and are typically hypointense on T1 and hyperintense on T2.

❓ 6. **Ependymomas: radiotherapy (XRT). The FALSE answer is:**
    A. They are radiosensitive tumors.
    B. For cranial XRT, traditional therapy involves 45 Gy to the tumor bed.
    C. Spinal XRT is required, even if there are no drop mets.
    D. XRT is undesirable under the age of 3 years.
    E. The survival time is 2 years longer for 50% of patients receiving XRT compared to those without it.

✅ **Answer C**
- Ependymomas rank second only to medulloblastomas in radiosensitivity.
- Traditional therapy involves 45–48 Gy to the cranial tumor bed (recurrence is treated with an additional 15–20 Gy).
- XRT is undesirable in patients younger than 3 years old due to side effects.
- Spinal XRT is mostly administered in cases of drop metastases or positive CSF cytology. Prophylactic XRT is a topic of controversy.
- The 5-year survival rate increases from 20–40% without XRT to 40–80% with XRT, and the survival time is 2 years longer for 50% of patients receiving XRT compared to those without it.

❓ 7. **Choroid plexus tumors: definition. The FALSE answer is:**
    A. Are rare neuroepithelial tumors.
    B. Are mostly choroid plexus papillomas (CPP), WHO I.
    C. There is an association with Von Hippel-Lindau disease.
    D. Rarely produce drop mets.
    E. Atypical CPP have more mitotic figures than CPP.

11

✅ **Answer D**
- They are rare neuroepithelial tumors, most are histologically benign.
  WHO classification:
  - Choroid plexus papilloma (WHO I)
  - Atypical choroid plexus papilloma (WHO II)
  - Choroid plexus carcinoma (WHO III)
- They are usually slow-growing, but may sometimes grow rapidly.
- There is an association with Von Hippel-Lindau disease.
- All may produce drop mets in the CSF, but WHO III tumors do so more commonly.
- Atypical CPP have more mitotic figures than CPP without frank signs of malignancy seen in CPC.
- Resection is the mainstay of treatment in grade I and grade II tumors and adjuvant treatment is usually reserved for the less frequently occurring choroid plexus carcinoma (CPC).

❓ 8. **Choroid plexus papilloma (CPP): definition. The FALSE answer is:**
   A. Most frequently found in the third ventricles.
   B. Usually enhances with contrast on MRI.
   C. Typically causes hydrocephalus.
   D. Can spread to other parts of the CNS through CSF.
   E. After resection, the rate of recurrence is low.

✅ **Answer A**
- In children, they most commonly occur at a median age of 3.5 years and the lateral ventricles are the most frequent site of growth.
- When present in the lateral ventricles, it is mostly found in the atrium.
- When they occur in adults, the fourth ventricle is the most frequent site of growth.

❓ 9. **Choroid plexus tumors: epidemiology. The FALSE answer is:**
   A. Prevalence is 0.4–1%.
   B. 70% of patients are <2 years.
   C. The main clinical presentation is signs and symptoms of increased ICP.
   D. Total removal will lead to cure of the hydrocephalus.
   E. They usually enhance on CT and MRI.

✅ **Answer D**

- Prevalence: 0.4–1% of all intracranial tumors.
- It might occur at any age, but 70% of patients are <2 years of age.
- The most frequent locations are the lateral or fourth ventricles and the CPA. In adults, these lesions are usually infratentorial whereas in children they tend to be supratentorial.
- HCP results from overproduction of CSF and complete removal of these tumors does not always cure the HCP.
- Brain CT or MRI with/without contrast usually demonstrates a densely enhancing multilobulated intraventricular mass (fronds), and HCP is common.

❓ 10. **Choroid plexus: anatomy. The FALSE answer is:**
   A. It is located in the pia mater.
   B. It is formed by ependymal cells located in the ventricles and central canal of the spinal cord.
   C. It can be found everywhere in the ventricular system except in the third ventricle and the cerebral aqueduct.
   D. It secretes up to 500 mL of CSF per day in the adult brain.
   E. The ependymal cells participate in the formation of the blood-brain barrier and regulate the exchange between CSF and the blood.

✅ **Answer C**

11

- The choroid plexus is found in all the ventricles of the brain except the frontal/occipital horn of the lateral ventricles and the cerebral aqueduct.
- Secretes about 500 mL of CSF per day. High CSF production can lead to hydrocephalus and can be associated with tumors of the choroid plexus while insufficient CSF production can affect brain development.

❓ 11. **Choroid plexus carcinoma (CPC): characteristics. The FALSE answer is:**
   A. CPC can be differentiated from CPP based on their histological features such as increased necrosis, increased mitotic activity, and changes in growth.
   B. CPC most commonly occurs in the lateral ventricles followed by the fourth ventricle.
   C. CPC is the most common choroid plexus tumor found in the pediatric population.
   D. CPC can lead to excess production of CSF.
   E. Frequently, adjacent invasion of the parenchymal brain is present with CPC.

✅ **Answer C**

- 20–40% of choroid plexus tumors are CPC in children but the most common choroid plexus tumor found in the pediatric population is CPP.
- CPC represents between 0.4% and 0.6% of all brain tumors but is much higher in the pediatric population making up between 1% and 4% of all brain tumors.
- 80% of CPCs occur in the pediatric population.

❓ 12. **Chordoid gliomas (CG): definition. The FALSE answer is:**
   A. Usually emerge from the anterior portion of the third ventricle.
   B. The cells are commonly found in a stroma characterized by mucinous vacuolation.
   C. When symptomatic, patients present with headache, ataxia, and nausea/vomiting.
   D. Considered a high-grade tumor by WHO classification.
   E. It can be associated with hydrocephalus and hypothalamic dysfunction.

✅ **Answer D**

- CGs are WHO grade II neuroepithelial tumors. They are composed of clusters and cords of cells that are found in a mucinous matrix and test positive for GFAP staining, a marker for glial origin.
- They are rare tumors that are slow-growing and are mostly seen in the anterior portion of the third ventricle and suprasellar region.

❓ 13. **Chordoid meningioma: pathology. The FALSE answer is:**
   A. Chordoid meningioma rarely occurs in the ventricular system, with a preference for the lateral ventricles when it does occur.
   B. Meningiomas are usually benign.
   C. There is a low rate of recurrence after resection of this tumor.
   D. They are most frequently found in the inner part of the cranial dura near the falx cerebri.
   E. Meningioma accounts for approximately 50% of primary intracranial tumors.

✅ **Answer E**

- Meningioma accounts for 25% of primary intracranial tumors. They mostly occur in adults between 50 and 60 years old.
- Chordoid meningiomas are rare and can be hard to diagnose.
- When they arise from the intraventricular system, they originate from stromal arachnoid cells of the choroid plexus.

❓ 14. **Colloid cyst: pathology. The FALSE answer is:**
A. Benign lesion of epithelial cells containing gelatinous material.
B. Mostly found in the third ventricle.
C. Mostly found in the pediatric population.
D. The cyst can lead to hydrocephaly and ventriculomegaly.
E. Most colloid cysts are asymptomatic and found incidentally on imaging.

✅ **Answer C**
- Most patients presenting with a colloid cyst are between 30 and 70 years old.
- 99% of colloid cysts are found in the third ventricle or near the foramen of Monro.
- Most of the time, colloid cysts do not grow large enough to cause issues.

❓ 15. **Tuberous sclerosis complex (TSC): brain manifestations. The FALSE answer is:**
A. Lesions found in the brain appear in adulthood.
B. TSC involves subependymal nodules (SENs) found in the lateral ventricle.
C. SENs are hamartomas that do not usually cause any neurological deficits.
D. SENs growing in the foramen of Monro have the potential to transform into subependymal giant cell tumors.
E. TSC lesions in the brain are best seen with MRI.

11

✅ **Answer A**
- Tuberous sclerosis is an autosomal dominant disease but most of them are new mutations.
- Lesions appear in childhood but can also continue to be present throughout adulthood.
- The second most commonly found condition in childhood tuberous sclerosis is subependymal nodules.

❓ 16. **Choroid plexus papilloma (CPP): diagnosis. The FALSE answer is:**
A. CT scan is diagnostic for CPP.
B. On MRI, T1-weighted images, the lesion is hypo or isointense in comparison to the brain.
C. On MRI, T2-weighted images, the lesion is hyperintense relative to the brain.

D. On CT scan, it reveals an intraventricular mass characterized by hyperdensity and lobulated contour.

E. Histopathologically, it has similar features to bilateral villous hypertrophy of the choroid plexus.

✅ **Answer D**

– CT scan is diagnostic for CPP and demonstrates an intraventricular hypodense mass with lobulated contour.

– On histopathological examination, CPP and bilateral villous hypertrophy of the choroid plexus have similar features, but they can be differentiated on CT and MRI which show a lesion characterized by homogenous enhancement and heightened density.

❓ 17. **Colloid cyst: diagnosis. The FALSE answer is:**

A. In symptomatic patients, usually presents with headache, nausea, and vomiting.

B. CT commonly reveals a hyperdense spheric lesion in the third ventricle, posterior to the foramen of Monro.

C. MRI is the standard for diagnosis of colloid cysts.

D. It is hyperintense on T2-weighted images and hypointense on T1-weighted images.

E. In adults, it is the most common third ventricular lesion encountered.

✅ **Answer D**

– On MRI, T2-weighted images often show a hypointense lesion while 50% of cases have hyperintense lesions seen in T1-weighted images but they can also be iso or hypointense depending on the composition of the cyst.

– They are mostly found incidentally.

– A colloid cyst wall can be seen around it and is formed with an outer thin layer of fibrous connective tissue and an inner layer of columnar epithelium.

❓ 18. **Intraventricular meningiomas: management. The FALSE answer is:**

A. Resection appears to result in a reduction of presurgical symptoms.

B. Visual deficits are rarely seen postresection of intraventricular meningiomas.

C. Interhemispheric approach of intraventricular meningiomas is favored when located in the superior region of the lateral ventricles.

D. The most common location is in the lateral ventricles.

E. They rarely occur in the fourth ventricle.

✅ **Answer B**

— The morbidity and mortality rates are low following the resection of intraventricular meningiomas. However, visual deficits are frequently observed after surgery for lesions within the lateral ventricles.

— Recurrence is rarely seen postresection.

❓ 19. **Choroid plexus papilloma: treatment. The FALSE answer is:**

A. Tumors are usually fragile and have a high tendency for bleeding during surgery.

B. There is no role for chemotherapy or radiation for CPP treatment.

C. The 5-year survival rate postsurgical removal of CPP is 30–40%.

D. Postoperative subdural collection is not uncommon.

E. On MRI, lesions are typically hypointense on T1 and hyperintense on T2.

✅ **Answer C**

— While benign lesions may be curable through surgery, the procedure can be challenging due to the tumor's fragility and the risk of bleeding from choroidal arteries.

— CPP is classified as WHO I and is considered a benign tumor. Surgical resection is curative, and adjuvant treatment is typically reserved for the less common choroid plexus carcinoma (CPC).

— Following transcortical tumor excision, a subdural collection may develop, requiring subdural-peritoneal shunting.

— A 5-year survival rate of 84% can be achieved following surgical removal of CPP.

— On MRI, they typically appear hypointense on T1, hyperintense on T2, and may show multiple flow voids.

11

Bibliography

1. Greenberg MS. Handbook of neurosurgery. 8th ed. Thieme Medical Publishers; 2016.
2. Ramkissoon S. Surgical pathology of neoplasms of the central nervous system. In: Pathobiology of human disease. Academic Press; 2014.

3. Hosmann A, Hinker F, Dorfer C, et al. Management of choroid plexus tumors—an institutional experience. Acta Neurochir. 2019;161:745–54. https://doi.org/10.1007/s00701-019-03832-5.

4. Harbaugh RE, Shaffrey C, Couldwell WT, Berger MS. Neurosurgery knowledge update. A comprehensive review. Thieme; 2015.

5. Elsharkawy AE, Abuamona R, Bergmann M, Salem S, Gafumbegete E, Röttger E. Cortical anaplastic ependymoma with significant desmoplasia: a case report and literature review. Case Rep Oncol Med. 2013;2013:354873, 6 p. https://doi.org/10.1155/2013/354873.

6. Gerstner ER. Seminars in neurology ependymoma. Thieme Medical Publishers; 2018.

7. Joseph JJ, Das JM. Choroid plexus papilloma. In: StatPearls. Treasure Island, FL: StatPearls Publishing; 2023.

8. NCI. Choroid plexus tumors diagnosis and treatment. NIH; Aug 2023. https://www.cancer.gov/rare-brain-spine-tumor/tumors/choroid-plexus-tumors.

9. Johnson GW, Mian AY, Dahiya S, Rich KM, Chicoine MR, Limbrick DD. Cystic dissemination of choroid plexus papilloma: illustrative cases. J Neurosurg Case Lessons. 2022;4 https://doi.org/10.3171/case22360.

10. Sethi D, Arora R, Garg K, Tanwar P. Choroid plexus papilloma. Asian J Neurosurg. 2017;12:139–41. https://doi.org/10.4103/1793-5482.153501.

11. Javed K, Reddy V, Lui F. Neuroanatomy, choroid plexus [updated 2023 Jul 24]. In: StatPearls. Treasure Island, FL: StatPearls Publishing; 2023. https://www.ncbi-nlm-nih-gov.acces.bibl.ulaval.ca/books/NBK538156/.

12. Gopal P, Parker JR, Debski R, Parker JC Jr. Choroid plexus carcinoma. Arch Pathol Lab Med. 2008;132:1350–4. https://doi.org/10.5858/2008-132-1350-cpc.

13. Ampie L, Choy W, Lamano JB, Kesavabhotla K, Mao Q, Parsa AT, Bloch O. Prognostic factors for recurrence and complications in the surgical management of primary chordoid gliomas: a systematic review of literature. Clin Neurol Neurosurg. 2015;138:129–36. https://doi.org/10.1016/j.clineuro.2015.08.011.

14. Wilson JL, Ellis TL, Mott RT. Chordoid meningioma of the third ventricle: a case report and review of the literature. Clin Neuropathol. 2011;30(2):70–4. https://doi.org/10.5414/npp30070.

15. Tenny S, Thorell W. Colloid brain cyst [updated 2022 Sep 20]. In: StatPearls. Treasure Island, FL: StatPearls Publishing; 2023. https://www.ncbi-nlm-nih-gov.acces.bibl.ulaval.ca/books/NBK470314/.

16. Moncef B. Management of subependymal giant cell tumors in tuberous sclerosis complex: the neurosurgeon's perspective. World J Pediatr. 2010;6:103–10. https://doi.org/10.1007/s12519-010-0025-2.

17. Sayah A, Berkowitz F, Thakkar RS. The black rim susceptibility sign in the MRI evaluation of intracranial colloid cysts. J Neuroimaging. 2021;31:1028–34. https://doi.org/10.1111/jon.12870.

18. Lagman C, et al. Fatal colloid cyst: a systematic review. World Neurosurg. 2017;107:409–15. https://doi.org/10.1016/j.wneu.2017.07.183.

Neuronal and Mixed Neuronal-Glial Tumors

Dominic E. Mahoney, Giulio Anichini, Kevin O'Neill, Maliya Delawan, and Li Ma

? 1. **Gangliocytomas. The FALSE answer is:**
   A. Account for between 0.1% and 0.5% of all brain tumors.
   B. Seizure and headache are the most common presenting features.
   C. Most commonly occur in the frontal lobe.
   D. Typically present within the first three decades of life.
   E. There is a slight male predilection in the incidence.

✅ **Answer C**
- The majority of gangliocytomas occur in the temporal lobe, either in isolation or in combination with the frontal or parietal lobe.
- This is possibly due to the division of granular neurons in the subgranular layer of the dentate gyrus that continues postnatally.

? 2. **Gangliocytomas. The FALSE answer is:**
   A. Frequently stain positively for synaptophysin and neurofilament epitopes.
   B. Are WHO grade I lesions.
   C. May be challenging to distinguish from ganglioma.
   D. The average relative incidence is around 10%.
   E. Stroma consists of nonneoplastic glia.

✅ **Answer D**
- Relative incidence in a case series of epilepsy ranged from 0% to 3.2%.
- Stroma of gangliocytoma is typically comprised of nonneoplastic glial features; however, this may be challenging to distinguish from the glial component of a ganglioglioma.

12

? 3. **Ganglioglioma. The FALSE answer is:**
   A. Can occur at any location along the neuraxis—including the optic nerve.
   B. Is among the rarest tumors found.
   C. Typically WHO grade I.
   D. Recurrence-free survival at 7.5 years is >90%.
   E. The rate of anaplastic transformation from grade I is between 0.6% and 2.6%.

✅ **Answer B**
- Gangliogliomas are among the commonest tumors found in pathological specimens from the epilepsy surgical case series.
- Higher rates of anaplastic transformation of ganglioma are seen in pediatric patients.

4. Ganglioglioma. The FALSE answer is:
A. IDH mutation or 1p19q codeletion excludes this diagnosis.
B. BRAF V600E mutations are seen in 25% of cases.
C. Calcification and perivascular lymphocytic infiltration are recognized features.
D. Chromogranin A expression is typically weak or absent.
E. Occasional mitoses and small necrotic foci may be found.

✅ **Answer D**
- Chromogranin A expression is weak or absent in normal neurons and is typically extensively expressed in dysplastic neuronal populations such as those making up gangliogliomas.
- Mitoses and necrosis are typically high-grade features but may still be seen in gangliogliomas.

5. Dysplastic gangliocytoma of the cerebellum (aka Lhermitte-Duclos disease). The FALSE answer is:
A. Typically only arises in one cerebellar hemisphere but may extend into the vermis.
B. Found almost exclusively in children.
C. Is a recognized feature of Cowden's syndrome.
D. Has no clear gender-based predilection.
E. Typically appears as areas of T2 hyperintensity with thickened folia.

✅ **Answer B**
- Dysplastic gangliocytoma of the cerebellum has been identified in patients of various ages, from neonates to septuagenarians—most cases have been identified in adults.

6. Dysplastic gangliocytoma of the cerebellum (aka Lhermitte-Duclos disease). The FALSE answer is:
A. The commonest presenting features include dysmetria and hydrocephalus.
B. May present with seizures.
C. Cerebellar cytoarchitecture is often distorted by the lesion.
D. Associated with breast cancer.
E. Lesions typically do not enhance radiologically.

✅ **Answer C**
- Cerebellar architecture is relatively preserved, though the affected folia is enlarged and distorted.
- Lhermitte-Duclos disease is a feature of Cowden syndrome, an autosomal-dominant condition also associated with an increased risk of breast and endometrial cancer, and colonic polyps.

❓ 7. **Dysembryoplastic neuroepithelial tumor (DNET). The FALSE answer is:**
   A. Typically located in the temporal lobe.
   B. IDH mutation or 1p/19q codeletion excludes the diagnosis.
   C. Is associated with dysplastic cortex in approximately 80% of cases.
   D. Do not contain neurons resembling dysplastic ganglion cells.
   E. Axons running parallel to the cortex are a pathognomic feature.

✅ **Answer E**
- DNETs contain a "specific glioneuronal element" which consists of bundles of axons running perpendicular to the cortical surface, lined by oligodendrocyte-like cells suspended in a mucoid matrix.
- Although neurons in the tumor and dysplastic cortex show cytological abnormalities, they do not resemble dysplastic ganglion cells as in gangliogliomas.

❓ 8. **Dysembryoplastic neuroepithelial tumor (DNET). The FALSE answer is:**
   A. Typically present with drug-resistant, complex partial seizures.
   B. Often cystic and may contain microcalcifications.
   C. Ki-67 index of approximately 5% is typical.
   D. *BRAF V600E* mutations may be identified in over 50%.
   E. Simple, complex, and nonspecific/diffuse forms exist.

12

✅ **Answer C**
- High mitotic indices are rarely seen in DNETs—the typical Ki-67 index ranges from 0% to 1.6%.

❓ 9. **Dysembryoplastic neuroepithelial tumor (DNET). The FALSE answer is:**
   A. Demonstrates high T2 signal with partial FLAIR suppression.
   B. Two subtypes exist.
   C. Perilesional hyperintensity on FLAIR is characteristic.
   D. Do not demonstrate restricted diffusion.
   E. Multinodular and vacuolating neuronal tumor (MVNT) is a differential.

✅ **Answer B**

- Three subtypes exist: simple, complex, and nonspecific. However, non-specific DNETs are a controversial entity and currently lack specific pathological criteria.
- The high FLAIR signal seen around these lesions results in the characteristic "bright ring sign"—this should not be confused with the T2-FLAIR mismatch often seen in low-grade gliomas.
- MVNT appears similar to DNET, although the former is juxtacortical rather than intracortical.

❓ 10. **Desmoplastic infantile ganglioglioma (DIG) and astrocytoma (DIA). The FALSE answer is:**
   A. Microscopy depicts pleomorphic neuroepithelium with neoangiogenesis.
   B. Present as cystic masses with hyperdense and enhancing peripheries on CT.
   C. Leptomeningeal fibrosis is a typical pathological feature.
   D. Underlying Virchow-Robin spaces are often occupied by tumor cells.
   E. GFAP is profusely expressed in the desmoplastic meningeal component.

✅ **Answer A**

- Neoangiogenesis is not seen in either DIG or DIA.
- A component containing poorly differentiated neuroepithelial cells with densely basophilic nuclei is often seen.

❓ 11. **Desmoplastic infantile ganglioglioma (DIG) and astrocytoma (DIA). The FALSE answer is:**
   A. Present with signs of increased ICP, seizures, and focal neurology.
   B. Gross total resection is associated with long-term survival.
   C. Recurrence is rare.
   D. Demonstrate low mitoses and no necrosis.
   E. Tumors may regress following subtotal resection.

✅ **Answer D**

- DIG and DIA may show high mitotic rates and areas of intralesional necrosis.

- Reports have been published describing radiological regression following subtotal resection.
- Recurrence is rare but has been reported. Progression with histological features of GBM has been reported in residual tumors following subtotal resection.

? 12. **Central neurocytoma. The FALSE answer is:**
  A. Consists of a homogenous tumor population within an irregular stroma.
  B. May contain 1p/19q codeletion.
  C. *EGFR* amplification may be present.
  D. Choline and GABA have both been found in high levels in these tumors.
  E. Are thought to arise from subventricular zone progenitor cells.

✓ Answer C
- p53 and *EGFR* amplification are absent.
- Central neurocytomas are considered WHO grade II tumors, and contain both immature and differentiating neuronal lineages.
- 1p/19q codeletion may be present but isolated 1p deletion is more common.
- Chromosomal gains in 2p, 7, 10q, 13q, and 18q have been reported in up to a fifth of central neurocytomas.

? 13. **Central neurocytoma. The FALSE answer is:**
  A. Typically present with raised ICP, visual, memory, or hormonal disturbances.
  B. Surgery is the mainstay of treatment.
  C. Recurrence may be as high as 22% in >12 years.
  D. There is no role for adjuvant radiotherapy following total resection.
  E. Radiosurgery may result in superior tumor control with lower morbidity.

✓ Answer D
- Irradiation following incomplete resection or in cases of atypical neurocytoma may yield some prognostic benefit.
- Tumors with an MIB index <2 with total resection are unlikely to benefit significantly from irradiation.

12

❓ 14. Central neurocytoma. The FALSE answer is:

A. The extent of surgical resection is the most important prognostic factor.

B. Radiotherapy may be advisable after resection.

C. The prognostic influence of the Ki-67 index is unclear.

D. Anaplastic features are generally not associated with poorer prognosis.

E. Risk factors for recurrence include younger age, short preoperative history, and lack of cortical dysplasia.

✔ Answer E

- Older age, longer preoperative course, and presence of cortical dysplasia are associated with an increased risk of recurrence or resistant seizures.
- Some authors recommend the application of radiotherapy following gross total resection to mitigate the risk of recurrence.
- There is a disparity in the literature concerning the relevance of MIB-1 findings, with some authors reporting an association between higher Ki-67 indices and poorer prognoses, while others finding no clear correlation.
- More than three mitoses per ten high-power fields have been associated with increased recurrence risk.
- Interestingly, anaplasia is not a poor prognostic indicator in these tumors.

❓ 15. Anaplastic ganglioglioma. The FALSE answer is:

A. *CDKN2A* and *BRAF* V600E mutations are diagnostic.

B. These are WHO grade III.

C. Malignant changes are typically seen in the glial component.

D. Features include increased cellularity, pleomorphism, and necrosis.

E. Histology of these lesions may not simply be related to prognosis.

✔ Answer A

- Although *CDKN2A* and *BRAF* V600E mutations have been observed in some anaplastic gangliogliomata in published case series, these mutations are not essential for the diagnosis.
- There is conflicting evidence in published case series with respect to the prognostic importance of histopathology in anaplastic gangliocytomas.
- Two case series demonstrate poorer prognosis with high-grade features, another study found no relationship, whilst a fourth study found anaplastic features to confer favorable event-free survival among pediatric patients.

? 16. **Anaplastic ganglioglioma. The FALSE answer is:**
   A. Typically has elevated Ki-67 indices.
   B. Often shows suppression in *PDGFRA* and *CDK4*.
   C. May present de novo or from the transformation of irradiated ganglioglioma.
   D. Surgical resection plays a crucial role in the management.
   E. May be mimicked by diffuse midline gliomata H3 K27M.

✓ **Answer B**
 ▪ *PDGFRA* and *CDK4* are both oncogenes, the upregulation of which has been observed in anaplastic ganglioglioma.
 ▪ H3 K27M midline gliomata represent a phenotypically diverse group of tumors that can mimic anaplastic ganglioglioma among others.

? 17. **Papillary glioneuronal tumor. The FALSE answer is:**
   A. More common in males.
   B. Most commonly peri−/intraventricular.
   C. Typically possesses a significant cystic component.
   D. Generally carries a good prognosis but may exhibit dissemination.
   E. *KIAA1549-BRAF* fusion oncogene is typically seen.

✓ **Answer E**
 ▪ The translocation t(9;17)(q31;q24) resulting in the fusion oncogene *SLC44A1-PRKCA* is often seen in papillary glioneuronal tumors—the *KIAA1549-BRAF* fusion gene is associated with diffuse leptomeningeal glioneuronal tumors.

12

? 18. **Rosette-forming glioneuronal tumor. The FALSE answer is:**
   A. Contains neurocytes-forming rosettes or perivascular pseudorosettes.
   B. Contains cell populations resembling pilocytic astrocytoma.
   C. Most frequently occurs in the posterior fossa.
   D. Predominantly a tumor of childhood.
   E. Is thought to arise from subependymal pluripotent progenitor cells.

✓ **Answer D**
 ▪ The average age at the time of presentation is 32 years (range: 8–70 years).

19. **Rosette-forming glioneuronal tumor. The FALSE answer is:**
   A. Gross total surgical resection generally forms the mainstay of treatment.
   B. Often T2 hyperintense with variable contrast enhancement.
   C. Microscopic intralesional infarcts are not a feature.
   D. Cases of malignant transformation to glioblastoma have been reported.
   E. Recurrence at the resection site is rare.

✅ **Answer C**
- Focal infarcts, microcalcifications, and vascular sclerosis may be seen histologically.
- Due to their midline location and associated proximity to the brainstem and spinal cord, some recommend against aggressive surgical resection to reduce morbidity. However, these are WHO grade I lesions and maximal cytoreduction is significantly conducive to prognosis.

20. **Diffuse leptomeningeal glioneuronal tumor. The FALSE answer is:**
   A. Frequently exhibits *KIAA1549-BRAF* gene fusions.
   B. May demonstrate 1p/19q codeletion.
   C. Frequently shows positive OLIG2 and S100 expression.
   D. Is WHO grade II.
   E. Typically present with signs of increased intracranial pressure.

✅ **Answer D**
- No clear WHO grading has been assigned to these lesions as of yet—this is due to the low number of patients and brief follow-up periods.

21. **Diffuse leptomeningeal glioneuronal tumor. The FALSE answer is:**
   A. Diffuse nodular leptomeningeal enhancement is characteristically seen.
   B. An intraparenchymal component may be present.
   C. There is a male predilection with a median age at presentation of 4 years.
   D. Combined chemoradiotherapy has proven to be effective.
   E. 1p/19q codeletion is associated with reduced chemosensitivity.

✅ **Answer E**
- As in oligodendroglioma, 1p/19q codeletion is associated with improved responsiveness to chemotherapy and chemoradiotherapy.
- In cases where a discrete intraparenchymal lesion exists, the commonest location is within the spinal cord.

❓ 22. **Extraventricular neurocytoma. The FALSE answer is:**
  A. May appear as a cyst with a mural nodule on imaging.
  B. Stippled "salt and pepper" chromatin is seen on microscopy.
  C. Homer Wright rosettes are a histological feature.
  D. Often contains calcified foci.
  E. Negative NeuN expression excludes the diagnosis.

✅ **Answer E**
- NeuN is a marker localized to neuronal nuclei.
- Although it is often positive in extraventricular neurocytoma, it may be negative and such a result does not strictly exclude this diagnosis.

❓ 23. **Extraventricular neurocytoma. The FALSE answer is:**
  A. Atypical histology is associated with significantly poorer outcomes.
  B. Prognosis in typical tumors is akin to typical central neurocytomata.
  C. Prognosis in atypical tumors is akin to atypical central neurocytomata.
  D. Old age is not an independent poor prognostic indicator.
  E. Adjuvant radiotherapy may have a role following subtotal resection.

12

✅ **Answer C**
- Atypical extraventricular neurocytomata have higher rates of recurrence and mortality than those seen in atypical central neurocytoma.
- Central neurocytomata may present sooner than more peripherally located extraventricular tumors—this may, in part, account for the prognostic disparity.
- Patients with histologically atypical tumors may have an up to tenfold increased risk of death in under 10 years.

❓ 24. **Cerebellar liponeurocytoma. The FALSE answer is:**
  A. Is WHO grade III lesions.
  B. Demonstrates low Ki-67 indices.

C. Frequently recurs following surgical resection.

D. May demonstrate necrosis and vascular proliferation.

E. The mean patient age at presentation is 50 years.

✓ **Answer A**

▬ These are considered WHO grade II lesions—they demonstrate recurrence in at least 50% of cases; mitotic figures are scarce or absent.

❓ 25. **Cerebellar liponeurocytoma. The FALSE answer is:**

A. May demonstrate similar features to medulloblastoma or ependymoma.

B. Lipidic cells are positive for neuronal markers.

C. Most commonly present with headache and raised ICP.

D. Typically demonstrates avid contrast enhancement.

E. Surgical resection forms the mainstay of treatment.

✓ **Answer D**

▬ Cerebellar liponeurocytomata are typically hypointense on T1 with patchy or mild contrast uptake.

▬ These lesions may demonstrate small blue cells similar to medulloblastoma, or clear cells reminiscent of ependymoma.

▬ Lipidic cells are typically positive for neuronal cell markers such as synaptophysin, MAP2, and neuron-specific enolase (NSE).

❓ 26. **Paraganglioma. The FALSE answer is:**

A. Typically seen in cauda equina, filum terminale, and jugulotympanic areas.

B. Arises from mesodermal derivatives.

C. Is densely vascular and often bleeds freely.

D. May appear similar to ependymoma or schwannoma.

E. Intimately packed lobules of cells are characteristically seen microscopically.

✓ **Answer B**

▬ Paragangliomata arise from neural crest cells, which are of ectodermal origin.

▬ The appearance of densely arranged lobules of chromaffin cells is known as "zellballen"—this is seen in paraganglioma and pheochromocytoma.

? 27. **Paraganglioma. The FALSE answer is:**
  A. Can be found in the lumbar spine.
  B. Hereditary mutation to the succinate dehydrogenase complex predisposes to these tumors.
  C. May secrete vasoactive substances into the circulation.
  D. Radiotherapy is always ineffective in management.
  E. In the absence of complete resection, recurrence is frequently observed.

✓ Answer D
— Adjuvant radiotherapy may be used in cases in which complete resection could not be achieved.

Bibliography

1. Berger MS, Prados MD. Textbook of neuro-oncology. Philadelphia, PA: Elsevier; 2005.
2. Louis DN, Ohgaki H, Wiestler OD, Cavenee WK. The 2016 World Health organization classification of tumours of the central nervous system. Acta Neuropathol. 2016;131:803–20.
3. Thom M, Blümcke I, Aronica E. Long-term epilepsy-associated tumors. Brain Pathol. 2012;22(3):350–79.
4. Batchelor TT, Nishikawa R, Tarbell NJ, Weller M. Oxford textbook of neuro-oncology. Oxford: Oxford University Press; 2017.
5. Sontowska I, Matyja E, Malejczyk J, Grajkowska W. Dysembryoplastic neuroepithelial tumour: insight into the pathology and pathogenesis. Folia Neuropathol. 2017; 55(1):1–13.
6. Kleinschmidt-DeMasters BK, Rodriguez FJ, Tihan T. Neuropathology. 2nd ed. Philadelphia, PA: Elsevier; 2016.
7. Hoischen A, Ehrler M, Fassunke J, Simon M, Baudis M, Landwehr C, et al. Comprehensive characterization of genomic aberrations in gangliogliomas by CGH, array-based CGH and interphase FISH. Brain Pathol. 2008;18(3):326–37.
8. Ahmed AK, Dawood HY, Gerard J, Smith TR. Surgical resection and cellular proliferation index predict prognosis for patients with papillary glioneuronal tumor: systematic review and pooled analysis. World Neurosurg. 2017;107:534–41.
9. Anyanwu CT, Robinson TM, Huang JH. Rosette forming glioneuronal tumor: an update. Clin Transl Oncol. 2020;22(5):623–30.
10. Lyle MR, Dolia JN, Fratkin J, Nichols TA, Herrington BL. Newly identified characteristics and suggestions for diagnosis and treatment of diffuse leptomeningeal glioneuronal/neuroepithelial tumors: a case report and review of the literature. Child Neurol Open. 2015;2(1):2329048X14567531.
11. Kane AJ, Sughrue ME, Rutkowski MJ, Aranda D, Mills SA, Lehil M, et al. Atypia predicting prognosis for intracranial extraventricular neurocytomas. J Neurosurg. 2012;116(2):349–54.

12

12. Choudhari KA, Kaliaperumal C, Jain A, Sarkar C, Soo MY, Rades D, Singh J. Central neurocytoma: a multi-disciplinary review. Br J Neurosurg. 2009;23(6):585–95.

13. Patel DM, Schmidt RF, Liu JK. Update on the diagnosis, pathogenesis, and treatment strategies for central neurocytoma. J Clin Neurosci. 2013;20(9):1193–9.

14. Reinhardt A, Pfister K, Schrimpf D, Stichel D, Sahm F, Reuss DE, Capper D, Wefers AK, Ebrahimi A, Sill M, Felsberg J. Anaplastic ganglioglioma—a diagnosis comprising several distinct tumour types. Neuropathol Appl Neurobiol. 2022;48(7):e12847.

15. Selvanathan SK, Hammouche S, Salminen HJ, Jenkinson MD. Outcome and prognostic features in anaplastic ganglioglioma: analysis of cases from the SEER database. J Neuro-Oncol. 2011;105:539–45.

16. Zhao RJ, Zhang XL, Chu SG, Zhang M, Kong LF, Wang Y. Clinicopathologic and neuroradiologic studies of papillary glioneuronal tumors. Acta Neurochir. 2016 Apr;158:695–702.

17. Anyanwu CT, Robinson TM, Huang JH. Rosette-forming glioneuronal tumor: an update. Clin Transl Oncol. 2020;22:623–30.

18. Hsu C, Kwan G, Lau Q, Bhuta S. Rosette-forming glioneuronal tumour: imaging features, histopathological correlation and a comprehensive review of literature. Br J Neurosurg. 2012;26(5):668–73.

19. Gardiman MP, Fassan M, Nozza P, Orvieto E, Garre ML, Milanaccio C, Severino M, Perilongo G, Giangaspero F. Diffuse leptomeningeal glioneuronal tumours: clinicopathological follow-up. Pathologica. 2012;104(6):428–31.

20. Gardiman MP, Fassan M, Orvieto E, D'Avella D, Denaro L, Calderone M, Severino M, Scarsello G, Viscardi E, Perilongo G. Diffuse leptomeningeal glioneuronal tumors: a new entity? Brain Pathol. 2010;20(2):361–6.

21. Patil AS, Menon G, Easwer HV, Nair S. Extraventricular neurocytoma, a comprehensive review. Acta Neurochir. 2014;156:349–54.

22. Xu L, Ouyang Z, Wang J, Liu Z, Fang J, Du J, He Y, Li G. A clinicopathologic study of extraventricular neurocytoma. J Neuro-Oncol. 2017;132:75–82.

23. Deora H, Prabhuraj AR, Saini J, Yasha TC, Arimappamagan A. Cerebellar liponeurocytoma: a rare fatty tumor and its literature review. J Neurosci Rural Pract. 2019;10(02):360–3.

24. Patel N, Fallah A, Provias J, Jha NK. Cerebellar liponeurocytoma. Can J Surg. 2009;52(4):E117.

25. Young WF Jr. Paragangliomas: clinical overview. Ann N Y Acad Sci. 2006;1073(1): 21–9.

26. Lee JA, Duh QY. Sporadic paraganglioma. World J Surg. 2008;32:683.

Pituitary Tumors and Tumors of the Sellar Region

Baha'eddin A. Muhsen, Sama Albairmani, and Samer S. Hoz

❓ 1. **Familial mutations associated with pituitary adenoma. The FALSE answer is:**
   A. Multiple endocrine neoplasia type 1.
   B. Multiple endocrine neoplasia type 4.
   C. Familial isolated pituitary adenomas.
   D. Kallman syndrome.
   E. McCune-Albright.

✅ **Answer D**

Familial syndrome	Gene affected (Germline)
Multiple endocrine neoplasia type 1	MEN1, CDKN1B, CDKN2C
Multiple endocrine neoplasia type 4	CDKN1B
Familial isolated pituitary adenomas	AIP
Carney complex	PRKAR1A
McCune-Albright	GNAS

Tumor subtype	Gene affected
Prolactinoma	HMGA2 (a)
Corticotroph	USP8, USP48, BRAF
GH-secreting	GNAS

▬ Familial syndromes are listed in the top part of the table, and subtype-specific somatic alterations and their mechanisms are listed in the bottom portion A the table. A, amplification; all other genes are mutated.

13

❓ 2. **Regarding invasive pituitary adenoma. The FALSE answer is:**
   A. Invasive pituitary adenomas express significantly higher levels of RIZI.
   B. Invasive pituitary adenomas express higher levels of C-myc.
   C. Increased RIZI expression also correlates with significant differences in methylation at four CpG sites.
   D. Correlations between epigenetic modifications and gene expression further affirm the possibility that histone modifications may alter gene expression in pituitary tumors.
   E. P53 missed expression correlates with H3K9 methylation.

✅ **Answer A**

- Invasive pituitary adenomas express lower levels of RIZI than noninvasive ones.

❓ 3. **Regarding the completeness of resection of pituitary adenoma, using transsphenoidal approach, the FALSE answer is:**

A. A large tumor diameter has been shown to be an independent predictor of subtotal resection and higher postoperative complication rates.

B. Tumors that demonstrate marked fibrosis represent dissection challenges.

C. Treatment with radiation therapy adds more obstacles to resection.

D. Laterally extending tumors can be managed safely by this approach.

E. Incomplete resection rarely leads to catastrophic events such as hemorrhage and edema.

✅ **Answer D**

- Lateral extension decreases the likelihood of gross total resection, especially when there is the involvement of the cranial nerves and major blood vessels.

❓ 4. **Factors affecting headaches associated with pituitary adenomas. The FALSE answer is:**

A. Tumor size.

B. Opticochiasm compression.

C. Sellar destruction.

D. Cavernous sinus invasion.

E. The character of the headache is not influenced by biochemical-neuroendocrine factors.

✅ **Answer E**

- Participation of biochemical-neuroendocrine factors, mainly in prolactinomas, seems to be an important associated factor in the origin and determination of the severity of pituitary tumor-related headaches.

❓ 5. **Characteristics of adamantinomatous craniopharyngioma (ACP). The FALSE answer is:**

    A. It exhibits two age peaks in presentation, occurring between 5–15 years and 45–60 years.

    B. It originates from embryonic remnants of Rathke's pouch epithelium.

    C. Has no calcifications.

    D. Causes visual impairment, headache, and endocrine deficiencies.

    E. Has distinctive epithelium that forms satellite reticulum, wet keratin, and basal palisades.

✅ **Answer C**

▬ **ACPs:**

Age of presentation:

Bimodal peaks at 5–15 and 45–60 years.

– Cell of origin: embryonic remnants of the Rathke's pouch epithelium.

– Appearance on MRI: cauliflower-like shape with calcifications (40%), enhancement (90%), and cyst containing cholesterol-rich oily fluid (90%).

– Pathological I features: distinctive epithelium that forms stellate reticulum, wet keratin, and basal palisades • Key symptomology: visual impairment, headache, and endocrine deficiencies.

▬ **PCPs:**

Age of presentation: 40–55 years.

Cell of origin: embryonic remnants of the Rathke's pouch epithelium.

– Appearance on MRI: mostly solid. Rarely cystic and without calcification.

– Pathological feature: fibrovascular cores lined by nonkeratinizing squamous epithelium.

– Key symptomology: headache, hypothalamic symptoms, and psychiatric alterations.

❓ 6. **The Knosp–Steiner classification scheme. The FALSE answer is:**

    A. Grade 1 tumors do not exhibit invasion.

    B. Grade 2 is characterized by invasion extending to but not past the lateral aspect of the common carotid artery (CCA).

    C. Grade 3 is characterized by invasion past the lateral aspect of the CCA but not completely filling the cavernous sinus.

    D. Grade 4 is when the tumor completely fills the CS both medial and lateral to the CCA.

    E. Each cavernous sinus side is graded separately by this classification.

✅ **Answer A**

▬ The Knosp-Steiner classification scheme:
- (0) No invasion and the lesion does not reach the medial aspect of the CCA.
- (1) Invasion extending to but not past, the intercarotid line.
- (2) Invasion extending to but not past, the lateral aspect of the CCA.
- (3) Invasion past the lateral aspect of the CCA but not completely filling the CS.
- (4) Completely filling the CS both medial and lateral to the CCA.

❓ 7. **Pituicytoma. The FALSE answer is:**
- A. Originates from specialized glial cells in the neurohypophysis and infundibulum.
- B. The tumor is slow-growing and benign.
- C. WHO grade II.
- D. It is typically challenging to distinguish from other sellar and suprasellar lesions.
- E. Surgical treatment may be challenging, owing to the hypervascularity of the tumor.

✅ **Answer C**

▬ Pituicytoma is a rare tumor of the sellar and suprasellar regions, originating from specialized glial cells in the neurohypophysis and infundibulum. The tumor is slow-growing and benign and histologically corresponds to World Health Organization (WHO) grade I.

❓ 8. **Spindle cell oncocytoma. The FALSE answer is:**
- A. A spindled-to-epithelioid, oncocytic, nonendocrine neoplasm of the neurohypophysis.
- B. Manifests in adults.
- C. Benign clinical course.
- D. Do not show immunoreactivity for chromogranin, synaptophysin, and pituitary hormones.
- E. Expresses vimentin and S-100 protein.

✅ **Answer A**

▬ SCO is defined as a spindled-to-epithelioid, oncocytic, nonendocrine neoplasm of the anterior hypophysis that manifests in adults and follows a benign clinical course.

? 9. **Pituitary carcinoma. The FALSE answer is:**
A. Defined by a disseminated disease that is noncontiguous with the sellar region and/or extraneural metastases.
B. Histomorphologically distinguishable from pituitary adenomas.
C. The pathogenesis is not entirely clear.
D. In the sequential tumorigenesis model, it follows a step-by-step transformation from nonadenomatous pituitary cells to adenoma cells, then aggressive pituitary adenoma and/or pituitary carcinoma.
E. In the *de novo* transformation model, pituitary carcinoma cells metastasize from an aggressive pituitary adenoma that originates in a normal pituitary gland.

✓ Answer B
− Histomorphologically, pituitary carcinomas are intrinsically indistinguishable from pituitary adenomas. Consequently, appropriate classification of a lesion as "pituitary carcinoma" can sometimes be challenging.

? 10. **Variants considered disadvantageous to the transfrontal approach to the sellar region. The FALSE answer is:**
A. Prefixed chiasm.
B. Normal chiasm with 2 mm or less between the chiasm and tuberculum sellae.
C. An obtuse angle between the optic nerves as they enter the chiasm.
D. Prominent tuberculum sella protruding above a line connecting the optic nerves as they enter the optic canals.
E. Carotid arteries approaching within 4 mm of midline within or above the sella turcica.

✓ Answer C
− An acute angle that is not obtuse between the optic nerves as they enter the chiasm is regarded as disadvantageous to the transfrontal approach to the sellar region.

? 11. **Factors disadvantageous to the transsphenoidal approach. The FALSE answer is:**
A. Large anterior intercavernous sinuses extending anterior to the gland just posterior to the anterior sellar wall (10%).
B. A thin diaphragm (62%), or a diaphragm with a large opening (56%).
C. Carotid arteries exposed in the sphenoid sinus with no bone over them (4%).

13

D. Carotid arteries lying more than 4 mm from midline within the sella (10%).

E. Sphenoid sinuses with no major septum (28%) or a sinus with the major septum well off the midline (47%).

✅ **Answer D**

— Carotid arteries that approach within 4 mm of midline within the sella are considered disadvantageous for the transsphenoidal approach.

❓ 12. **Papillary cranipharyngioma. The FALSE answer is:**

A. Most commonly presents between 5 and 10 years.

B. Cell of origin: embryonic remnants of the Rathke's pouch epithelium.

C. Appearance on MRI: mostly solid, rarely cystic, and without calcifications.

D. Pathological features: fibrovascular cores lined by nonkeratinizing squamous epithelium.

E. Key symptomology includes psychiatric alterations, headache, and hypothalamic symptoms.

✅ **Answer A**

— Papillary craniopharyngioma most commonly presents between 40 and 55 years.

❓ 13. **The side effects of cabergoline (dopamine agonist). The FALSE answer is:**

A. Low blood pressure.

B. Nausea.

C. Cardiac valvular fibrosis.

D. Addictive/compulsive behaviors.

E. Lower GI bleeding.

✅ **Answer E**

❓ 14. **Risks for dopamine agonist-resistant prolactinoma. The FALSE answer is:**

A. Male gender.

B. Large tumor volume.

C. Presence of a hemorrhagic, necrotic, and blood component.

D. Presence of comorbidities.

E. Time for prolactin to normalize after treatment.

✅ **Answer D**

? 15. **Cushing disease (CD). The FALSE answer is:**
   A. CD accounts for approximately 10% of all pituitary adenomas.
   B. CD is eight times more common in women.
   C. The gold-standard treatment for CD is transsphenoidal adeno-mectomy.
   D. Early postoperative remission rates range from 45% to 60%.
   E. It is most commonly found in the third or fourth decade of life.

✓ Answer D
— The early postoperative remission rates range from 67% to 95%.

? 16. **Signs and symptoms of excess growth hormone secretion. The FALSE answer is:**
   A. Hypertension and cardiomegaly.
   B. Sweating and body odor.
   C. Type 2 diabetes mellitus.
   D. It is not associated with an increased risk of cancers.
   E. Sleep apnea.

✓ Answer D
— GH and IGF-1 excess are associated with cancer development in multiple locations.

? 17. **Tumors of sellar origin according to the WHO 2016 classification. The FALSE answer is:**
   A. Craniopharyngioma.
   B. Granular cell tumor of the sellar region.
   C. Spindle cell oncocytoma.
   D. Pituicytoma.
   E. Medulloepithelioma.

13

✓ Answer E

? 18. **Spindle cell oncocytoma. The FALSE answer is:**
   A. Nonfunctioning.
   B. Rare neoplasm of the adenohypophysis.
   C. Radiologically and clinically distinguishable from nonfunction-ing pituitary adenomas.
   D. WHO Grade 1 tumor.
   E. Accounts for 0.1–0.4% of all sellar region tumors.

✅ **Answer C**
- It is very difficult to distinguish these tumors from nonfunctioning adenomas.

❓ 19. **Sellar and parasellar metastatic tumors. The FALSE answer is:**
   A. Breast and lung metastases are the two most common types.
   B. Account for approximately 1% of tumors in the sellar/parasellar region.
   C. Prostate and renal cell metastases have been reported.
   D. Multidisciplinary management includes radiation therapy, chemotherapy, and/or surgery.
   E. Leukemia and lymphoma metastases have not been reported.

✅ **Answer E**

Bibliography

1. Hauser BM, Lau A, Gupta S, Bi WL, Dunn IF. The epigenomics of pituitary adenoma. Front Endocrinol. 2019;10
2. Theodros D, Patel M, Ruzevick J, Lim M, Bettegowda C. Pituitary adenomas: historical perspective, surgical management and future directions. CNS Oncol. 2015;4(6):411–29.
3. Gondim JA, Almeida JPCD, Albuquerque LAFD, Schops M, Gomes É, Ferraz T. Headache associated with pituitary tumors. J Headache Pain. 2008;10(1):15–20.
4. Müller HL, Merchant TE, Warmuth-Metz M, Martinez-Barbera J-P, Puget S. Craniopharyngioma. Nat Rev Dis Primers. 2019;5:1.
5. Woodworth GF, Patel KS, Shin B, Burkhardt J-K, Tsiouris AJ, Mccoul ED, et al. Surgical outcomes using a medial-to-lateral endonasal endoscopic approach to pituitary adenomas invading the cavernous sinus. J Neurosurg. 2014;120(5):1086–94.
6. Yang X, Liu X, Li W, Chen D. Pituicytoma: a report of three cases and literature review. Oncol Lett. 2016;12(5):3417–22.
7. Chandler J, Ogiwara H, Shafizadeh S, Dubner S, Raizer J. Spindle cell oncocytoma of the pituitary and pituicytoma: two tumors mimicking pituitary adenoma. Surg Neurol Int. 2011;2(1):116.
8. Xu L, Khaddour K, Chen J, Rich KM, Perrin RJ, Campian JL. Pituitary carcinoma: two case reports and review of literature. World J Clin Oncol. 2020;11(2):91–102.
9. Renn WH, Rhoton AL. Microsurgical anatomy of the sellar region. J Neurosurg. 1975;43(3):288–98.
10. Borghei-Razavi H, Muhsen BA, Joshi K, Woodard T, Kshettry VR. Endoscopic extracapsular resection of an adrenocorticotropic hormone–secreting macroadenoma with selective resection of the medial cavernous sinus wall. World Neurosurg. 2020;144:199.
11. Castinetti F, Albarel F, Amodru V, Cuny T, Dufour H, Graillon T, Morange I, Brue T. The risks of medical treatment of prolactinoma. Ann Endocrinol (Paris). 2021;82(1):15–9. https://doi.org/10.1016/j.ando.2020.12.008.

12. Vermeulen E, D'Haens J, Stadnik T, et al. Predictors of dopamine agonist resistance in prolactinoma patients. BMC Endocr Disord. 2020;20(1):68. https://doi.org/10.1186/s12902-020-0543-4.
13. Pendharkar AV, Sussman ES, Ho AL, Hayden Gephart MG, Katznelson L. Cushing's disease: predicting long-term remission after surgical treatment. Neurosurg Focus. 2015;38(2):E13. https://doi.org/10.3171/2014.10.FOCUS14682.
14. Asa SL, Ezzat S. An update on pituitary neuroendocrine tumors leading to acromegaly and gigantism. J Clin Med. 2021;10(11):2254. https://doi.org/10.3390/jcm10112254.
15. Louis DN, Perry A, Reifenberger G, von Deimling A, Figarella-Branger D, Cavenee WK, Ohgaki H, Wiestler OD, Kleihues P, Ellison DW. The 2016 World Health Organization Classification of tumors of the central nervous system: a summary. Acta Neuropathol. 2016;131(6):803–20. https://doi.org/10.1007/s00401-016-1545-1.
16. Yip CM, Lee HP, Hsieh PP. Pituitary spindle cell oncocytoma presented as pituitary apoplexy. J Surg Case Rep. 2019;2019(6):rjz179 https://doi.org/10.1093/jscr/rjz179.

13

Tumors of the Pineal Region

Ameya S. Kamat, Zaid Aljuboori, Ignatius N. Esene, and Maliya Delawan

© The Author(s), under exclusive license to Springer Nature Switzerland AG 2024
S. S. Hoz et al. (eds.), *Surgical Neuro-Oncology*,
https://doi.org/10.1007/978-3-031-53642-7_14

1. **Epidemiology of pineal tumors. The FALSE answer is:**
   A. Accounts for less than 1% of CNS tumors in adults.
   B. Accounts for more than 3% of CNS tumors in children.
   C. Male to female ratio is 1:1.
   D. The prevalence is higher in Asian countries.
   E. The prevalence is higher in males.

✅ **Answer C**
— Male to female ratio is 3:1.

2. **Venous flow through the pineal region. The FALSE answer is:**
   A. The precentral cerebellar vein courses through the pineal region.
   B. The thalamostriate vein courses through the pineal region.
   C. The vein of Galen courses through the pineal region.
   D. The internal cerebral vein courses through the pineal region.
   E. The internal occipital veins course through the pineal region.

✅ **Answer B**
— The thalamostriate vein commences in the groove between the corpus striatum and thalamus and unites behind the crus of the fornix with the superior choroid vein to form each of the internal cerebral veins. It does not course through the pineal region.

3. **Classification of pineal region tumors. The FALSE answer is:**
   A. Choriocarcinoma is the most common histological subtype.
   B. Germinomas and nongerminomatous tumors make up 60% of pineal region tumors.
   C. Pineocytomas are WHO I grade tumors.
   D. Pineal parenchymal tumors of intermediate differentiation are WHO II or III tumors.
   E. Pineoblastomas are WHO IV grade tumors.

14

✅ **Answer A**
— Germinomas are overwhelmingly the commonest pineal region tumor subtype.

4. **The following are differential diagnoses for pineal region masses. The FALSE answer is:**
   A. Germ cell tumor.
   B. Meningioma.

C. Macroadenoma.
D. Pineocytoma.
E. Pineoblastoma.

✅ **Answer C**

— Macroadenomas occur in the sellar region.

❓ 5. **Common clinical features associated with pineal region tumors. The FALSE answer is:**
A. Parinaud's syndrome due to quadrigeminal plate compression.
B. Cerebellar dysfunction due to cerebellar compression.
C. Noncommunicating hydrocephalus due to cerebral aqueduct compression.
D. Hearing loss and tinnitus due to inferior colliculus compression.
E. Seizures due to temporal lobe compression.

✅ **Answer E**

— Seizures are a very rare finding in patients with a tumor in the pineal region.

❓ 6. **CSF markers for pineal region tumors. The FALSE answer is:**
A. Alpha-fetoprotein (AFP) predominance suggests endodermal sinus tumor.
B. Beta-HCG predominance suggests choriocarcinoma.
C. Carcinoembryonic antigen (CEA) predominance suggests yolk sac tumor.
D. Negative markers may suggest teratoma or pineal parenchymal tumor.
E. Placental alkaline phosphatase predominance suggests germinoma.

✅ **Answer C**

— CEA is a marker for cancers of the colon, rectum, prostate, ovary, lung, thyroid, or liver and not the pineal region.

❓ 7. **Remote effects of pineal region tumors. The FALSE answer is:**
A. Radiculopathy/myelopathy due to CSF seeding and drop metastases.
B. Diabetes insipidus.
C. Precocious puberty due to beta-HCG secretion.

D. Retinoblastomas may occur in combination with pineocytomas and are referred to as "trilateral" tumors.

E. Tandem suprasellar lesion.

✔ **Answer D**

— Trilateral tumors are retinoblastomas that occur in combination with pineoblastomas.

❓ 8. **Histology of pineal region tumors. The FALSE answer is:**

A. Teratomas and yolk sac tumors are germ cell tumors.

B. Pineocytoma is a pineal parenchyma tumor.

C. Embryonal carcinoma is a germ-cell tumor.

D. Pineoblastomas are sympathetic nerve tumors.

E. Epidermoid and dermoid cysts are remnants of the ectoderm.

✔ **Answer D**

— Chemodectomas are sympathetic nerve tumors.

❓ 9. **Five-year overall survival (OS) rates in pineal region tumors. The FALSE answer is:**

A. Germinoma—80–95%.

B. Mature teratoma—80–95%.

C. Immature teratoma—60–75%.

D. Pineocytoma—80–90%.

E. Pineoblastoma—70–80%.

✔ **Answer E**

— Pineoblastomas have a poor prognosis with five-year OS rates of 10–20%.

❓ 10. **Complete surgical resection may be curative in the following pineal region tumors. The FALSE answer is:**

A. Pineocytoma.

B. Epidermoid.

C. Mature teratoma.

D. Immature teratoma.

E. Intermediately differentiated pineal parenchymal tumor with low-grade features.

✔ **Answer D**

— Immature teratomas require adjuvant therapy.

14

? 11. Infratentorial supracerebellar approach to pineal region tumors. The FALSE answer is:

A. Useful for small- to medium-sized lesions.

B. Useful for lesions that are confined to the pineal region and below the Vein of Galen.

C. Useful for lesions that are confined to the pineal region and above the Vein of Galen.

D. Follows the natural plane between the cerebellum and tentorium which minimizes.

E. brain retraction,

F. If performed using the sitting position, cerebellar retraction and venous pressure can be minimized.

✔ **Answer C**

— Useful for lesions that are confined to the pineal region and below the Vein of Galen.

? 12. Occipital transtentorial approach to pineal region tumors. The FALSE answer is:

A. Contraindicated in lesions extending to the cerebellomesence-phalic cistern.

B. Useful for lesions that are confined to the pineal region and above the Vein of Galen.

C. The prone position with neutral neck flexion allows a surgical trajectory perpendicular to the floor.

D. Allows access to relatively large lesions that extend beyond the pineal region and into the third ventricle.

E. Further contralateral exposure can be achieved by dividing the inferior sagittal sinus and incising the falx.

✔ **Answer A**

— The occipital transtentorial approach may be more appropriate for large lesions extending beyond the pineal region and into the third ventricle, or into cerebellomesencephalic cistern.

? 13. Parinaud's syndrome consists of the following. The FALSE answer is:

A. Convergence-retraction nystagmus.

B. Eyelid retraction.

C. Light-near dissociation.

D. Argyll-Robertson pupil.

E. Supranuclear paralysis of conjugate upward gaze.

✅ **Answer D**
- Parinauds presents with a pseudo-Argyll-Robertson pupil where accommodative paresis ensues, and pupils become mid-dilated and show light-near dissociation.

❓ 14. **Pineal region tumors. The FALSE answer is:**
   A. In the pineal region, the most common glial cell tumor is diffuse glioma.
   B. In the pineal region, the least common glial cell tumor is pilocytic astrocytoma.
   C. Glial cell tumor in the pineal area tends to occur in younger patients with slight male predominance.
   D. Recurrent hemorrhage may occur in pineal region meningiomas.
   E. Pineal region meningioma accounts for 30% of pineal tumors.

✅ **Answer E**
- Pineal-region meningiomas are uncommon, accounting for 2–8% of all tumors in this area. These tumors are characterized by meningioma occupying the quadrigeminal cistern and showing little or no dural attachment.

❓ 15. **Pineal regional metastases. The FALSE answer is:**
   A. The most frequently reported histological type of lung cancer metastasizing to the pineal region is adenocarcinoma.
   B. Gastrointestinal malignancy can metastasize to the pineal region.
   C. Colorectal carcinoma may present as Parinaud's syndrome without GIT symptoms.
   D. Pineal metastases are usually asymptomatic and diagnosed on autopsy.
   E. Metastases to the pineal region comprise only 0.4% of intracranial metastatic tumors.

14

✅ **Answer A**
- The most frequently reported histological type of lung cancer metastasizing to the pineal region is small cell carcinoma, although other histological types, including squamous cell carcinoma and adenocarcinoma have also been reported.

? 16. **In pineal cysts (PCs), The FALSE answer is:**
   A. Most are asymptomatic.
   B. PC wall consists of three layers: glial, pineal, and collagenous.
   C. In cases of atypical MRI appearance, surgery might be justified to obtain tissue samples.
   D. Are histologically similar to pineoblastomas.
   E. A stereotactic approach enables puncture and aspiration of the PC.

✔️ **Answer D**
▬ Pineocytomas and pineal cysts appear similar histologically.

? 17. **Pineal region tumors. The FALSE answer is:**
   A. Pure germinomas have a good prognosis.
   B. Mature teratoma has a five-year survival rate of over 90%.
   C. GCTs in the pineal region have a better prognosis.
   D. Endodermal sinus tumor is the most likely pineal region tumor to metastasize.
   E. Bone and lung are the commonest metastasis sites for GCT.

✔️ **Answer D**
▬ Choriocarcinoma is the most likely pineal region tumor to metastasize.

? 18. **Pineal parenchymal tumor of intermediate differentiation (PPTID). The FALSE answer is:**
   A. It comprises 10–45% of tumors in the pineal region.
   B. PPTID has a female predominance.
   C. The rate of local recurrence is around 40%.
   D. PPTIDs have craniospinal dissemination in approximately 10% of cases.
   E. PPTIDs are classified as grade II or grade III.

✔️ **Answer C**
▬ The rate of local recurrence is around 80%.

? 19. **Dermoid and epidermoid cysts. The FALSE answer is:**
   A. There is no gender predilection.
   B. They are remnants of the ectoderm.
   C. The imaging modality of choice is a DWI MRI at b1000.
   D. Epidermoids lack dermal appendages.
   E. Dermoids are usually nonmidline lesions.

✅ **Answer E**
— Dermoids are midline lesions. Epidermoids are midline and nonmidline.

❓ 20. **Papillary tumor of the pineal region. The FALSE answer is:**
   A. Usually occurs between the third and fifth decades of life.
   B. Biological behavior ranges from WHO grade II to III.
   C. Microscopically, it shows an epithelial-looking tumor with papillary features and dense cellular areas, often exhibiting ependymal-like differentiation (true rosettes).
   D. Microvascular proliferation is common.
   E. Higher global methylation is associated with shorter progression-free survival.

✅ **Answer D**
— Microvascular proliferation is usually absent.

❓ 21. **Pineal apoplexy. The FALSE answer is:**
   A. The blood supply of pineal and pituitary glands is different.
   B. Apoplexy may occur in the presence of tumor, PC, or adjacent cavernoma.
   C. There is an increased risk of apoplexy in patients on anticoagulation therapy.
   D. Typical clinical presentation includes headache, gaze paresis, nausea/vomiting, syncope, and ataxia.
   E. Treatment of mild cases of pineal apoplexy is primarily symptomatic.

✅ **Answer A**
— Pineal apoplexy shares some similarities with pituitary apoplexy due to the similar anatomy and blood supply of both glands.

14

❓ 22. **Calcification of the pineal gland. The FALSE answer is:**
   A. Calcification rates vary widely by country and correlate with an increase in age.
   B. Calcification occurs in an estimated 90% of patients by the age of 17 years.
   C. Pineal calcifications are often seen on plain skull radiographs and are considered normal.

D. In children under the age of 10 years, pineal calcification is unusual and might be suggestive of the presence of a neoplasm, such as germinoma or teratoma.
E. Has been observed in children as young as two years of age.

✔️ **Answer B**
— 40% of patients have calcified glands by age 17, and 90% by age 40.

❓ 23. **Transcortical transventricular approach to the pineal region. The FALSE answer is:**
A. Can only be used in patients with acute hydrocephalus.
B. This approach adds morbidity from cortical incision with a limited view.
C. It could be useful with ventricular extension and with dilated ventricles.
D. The cortical incision is placed in the posterior part of the superior temporal gyrus or parietal cortex.
E. Favored over the infratentorial supracerebellar approach in cases where the tumor is below the Vein of Galen (VoG).

✔️ **Answer E**
— The infratentorial supracerebellar approach is favored for tumors below the VoG and the occipital transtentorial approach is favored for tumors above the VoG.

❓ 24. **Endoscopic transventricular approach. The FALSE answer is:**
A. Very useful technique in the presence of hydrocephalus.
B. ETV can also be done to treat hydrocephalus.
C. Contraindicated in patients without hydrocephalus.
D. Endoscopy adds the benefit of tissue sampling, increasing the accuracy of biopsy in addition to CSF sampling.
E. Around 90% of patients with pineal tumors have hydrocephalus at the time of presentation.

✔️ **Answer C**
— The technical limitation of this technique is the presence or absence of hydrocephalus although Yamamoto et al. reported their experience with a flexible endoscope and Souweidane and Luther reported a series of patients with biopsy without hydrocephalus.

? 25. Transcallosal approach to pineal region tumors. The FALSE answer is:

  A. It is associated with higher rates of mortality and morbidity.

  B. Useful in large pineal region tumors or posterior third ventricular tumors when most of tumor is above the tent or vein of Galen.

  C. Approach modifications were made from the original Dandy approach including the retrocallosal approach, falcine incision, and tentorial incision which makes this approach safer and more versatile.

  D. Corpus callosotomy greater than 2.5 cm is associated with increased morbidity.

  E. Contraindicated in patients with hydrocephalus.

✓ Answer E

– Hydrocephalus is neither an indication nor a contraindication for this approach.

Bibliography

1. Bailey S, Skinner R, Lucraft HH, Perry RH, Todd N, Pearson AD. Pineal tumours in the north of England 1968–93. Arch Dis Child. 1996;75(3):181–5.

2. Perry A, Brat DJ. Practical surgical neuropathology: a diagnostic approach. Philadelphia, PA: Churchill Livingstone/Elsevier; 2010.

3. Louis DN. WHO Classification of tumours of the central nervous system. 4th ed. Lyon: International Agency for Research on Cancer; 2007.

4. Tamrazi B, Nelson M, Bluml S. Pineal region masses in pediatric patients. Neuroimaging Clin N Am. 2017;27(1):85–97.

5. Erlich SS, Apuzzo ML. The pineal gland: anatomy, physiology, and clinical significance. J Neurosurg. 1985;63:321–41.

6. Perkins GL, Slater ED, Sanders GK, Prichard JG. Serum tumor markers. Am Fam Physician. 2003;68:1075–82.

7. Louis DN, Perry A, Reifenberger G, Von Deimling A, Figarella-Branger D, Cavenee WK, Ohgaki H, Wiestler OD, Kleihues P, Ellison DW. The 2016 World Health Organization Classification of Tumors of the central nervous system: a summary. Acta Neuropathol. 2016;131(6):803–20.

8. Bruce JN. Pineal tumors. In: Winn HR, editor. Youmans neurological surgery, vol. 2. 6th ed. Philadelphia, PA: Elsevier Saunders; 2011. p. 1359–72.

9. Bernstein M, Berger MS. Neuro-oncology: the essentials. 2nd ed. New York, NY: Thieme; 2008.

10. Bruce JN, Stein BM. The infratentorial supracerebellar approach. In: Apuzzo MLJ, editor. Surgery of the third ventricle. 2nd ed. Baltimore, MD: Williams & Wilkins; 1998. p. 697–719.

14

11. Hankinson EV, Lyons CJ, Hukin J, Cochrane DD. Ophthalmological outcomes of patients treated for pineal region tumors. J Neurosurg Pediatr. 2016;17(5):558–63.

12. Lozier AP, Bruce JN. Meningiomas of the velum interpositum: surgical considerations. Neurosurg Focus. 2003;15:1–9. https://doi.org/10.3171/foc.2003.15.1.11.

13. Fain JS, Tomlinson FH, Scheithauer BW, Parisi JE, Fletcher GP, Kelly PJ, Miller GM. Symptomatic glial cysts of the pineal gland. J Neurosurg. 1994;80(3):454–60.

14. Mottolese C, Szathmari A, Beuriat PA. Incidence of pineal tumors. A review of the literature. Neurochirurgie. 2015;61(2–3):65–9.

15. Wang CC, Turner J, Steel T. Spontaneous pineal apoplexy in a pineal parenchymal tumor of intermediate differentiation. Cancer Biol Med. 2013;10(1):43.

16. Gelabert-González M. Quistes dermoides y epidermoides intracraneales [Intracranial epidermoid and dermoid cysts]. Rev Neurol. 1998;27(159):777–82. (Spanish)

17. Mattogno PP, Frassanito P, Massimi L, Tamburrini G, Novello M, Lauriola L, Caldarelli M. Spontaneous regression of pineal lesions: ghost tumor or pineal apoplexy? World Neurosurg. 2016;88:64–9.

18. Zimmerman RA. Age-related incidence of pineal calcification detected by computed tomography (PDF). Radiology. 1982;142(3):659–62. https://doi.org/10.1148/radiology.142.3.7063680.

19. Choudhry O, Gupta G, Prestigiacomo CJ. On the surgery of the seat of the soul: the pineal gland and the history of its surgical approaches. Neurosurg Clin. 2011;22(3): 321–33.

20. Yamamoto M, Oka K, Takasugi S, Hachisuka S, Miyake E, Tomonaga M. Flexible neuroendoscopyfor percutaneous treatment of intraventricular lesions in the absence of hydrocephalus. Minim Invasive Neurosurg. 1997;40(04):139–43.

21. Soweidane M, Luther N. Endoscopic resection of solid intraventricular tumors. J Neurosurg. 2006;105:271–8.

22. Little KM, Friedman AH, Fukushima T. Surgical approaches to pineal region tumors. J Neuro-Oncol. 2001;54(3):287–99.

23. McComb JG, Levy ML, Apuzzo ML. The posterior intrahemispheric retrocallosal and transcallosal approaches to the third ventricle region. In: Apuzzo MLJ, editor. Surgery of the third ventricle. Baltimore, MD: Williams & Wilkins; 1998. p. 743.

24. Azab WA, Nasim K, Salaheddin W. An overview of the current surgical options for pineal region tumors. Surg Neurol Int. 2014:5.

25. Hu X, Ren YM, Yang X, Liu XD, Huang BW, Chen TY, Jv Y, Lan ZG, Liu WK, Liu XS, Hui XH. Surgical treatment of pineal region tumors: an 18 year-experience at a single institution. World Neurosurg. 2023;172:e1-1.

Germ Cell Tumors

*Oday Atallah, Osama M. Al-Awadi,
Almutasimbellah K. Etaiwi, Younus M. Al-Khazaali,
Khalid M. Alshuqayfi, Ahmed Muthana,
and Maliya Delawan*

? 1. **Germ cell tumors: classification. The FALSE answer is:**
   A. Germinoma.
   B. Embryonal cell carcinoma.
   C. Atypical teratoid/rhabdoid tumor.
   D. Teratoma.
   E. Yolk sac tumor.

Answer C
— Atypical teratoid/rhabdoid tumor is not a germ cell tumor.

? 2. **Germ cell tumors: epidemiology. The FALSE answer is:**
   A. They constitute approximately 1% of all primary intracranial neoplasms.
   B. The highest occurrence is observed between the ages of 10 and 14 years.
   C. The incidence is more prevalent in Far East Asia in comparison to the West.
   D. Exhibit a preference toward females.
   E. The majority of teratomas (90%) occur in males.

Answer D
— They have a preference toward males.

? 3. **Germ cell tumors: percentage. The FALSE answer is:**
   A. Choriocarcinoma: 25%.
   B. Teratoma: 18%.
   C. Yolk sac tumor: 7%.
   D. Embryonal cell carcinoma: 5%.
   E. Germinoma: 60–70%.

Answer A
— Choriocarcinoma constitutes around 5% of all germ-cell cancers.

? 4. **Germ cell tumors: clinical presentation. The FALSE answer is:**
   A. Hydrocephalus.
   B. Pseudoprecocious puberty.
   C. Headaches.
   D. Nausea and vomiting.
   E. Gerstmann syndrome.

15

✅ **Answer E**
━ Gerstmann syndrome is typically attributed to the presence of a lesion in close proximity to the angular gyrus.

❓ 5. **Germ cell tumors: imaging. The FALSE answer is:**
A. Teratoma: prominent homogenous contrast enhancement.
B. Choriocarcinoma: intratumoral hemorrhage.
C. Yolk sac tumor: iso- or hyperdense lesion.
D. Germinoma: vivid contrast enhancement.
E. Embryonal cell carcinoma: isointense in T1 and T2.

✅ **Answer A**
━ Because it has all three germinal layers, it is more heterogeneous.

❓ 6. **Germ cell tumors: tumor marker. The FALSE answer is:**
A. Choriocarcinoma: ß-hCG.
B. Mature teratoma: AFP.
C. Yolk sac tumor: ß-hCG.
D. Embryonal cell carcinoma: AFP.
E. Germinoma: PLAP.

✅ **Answer B**
━ AFP is secreted by immature teratoma but not by mature teratoma.

❓ 7. **Germ cell tumors: Location. The FALSE answer is:**
A. There is a midline predilection.
B. Pineal region.
C. Suprasellar region.
D. Fourth ventricle.
E. Foramen of Monro.

✅ **Answer E**
━ The foramen of Monro has a propensity for other tumors, such as colloid cysts.

❓ 8. **Germ cell tumors: radiotherapy. The FALSE answer is:**
A. Teratomas are among the most radiosensitive germ cell tumors.
B. Prophylactic spinal irradiation is controversial.
C. Germinomas exhibit radiosensitivity.

D. Radiosurgery is not advised.

E. The cure rate for germinoma patients with radiation therapy is around 80%.

✅ **Answer A**

➖ Germinomas are the most radiosensitive germ cell tumors.

❓ 9. **Germ cell tumors: chemotherapy. The FALSE answer is:**

A. Chemotherapy can be effective in treating germ cell tumors.

B. The effectiveness of chemotherapy is higher for nongerminomas.

C. In the majority of germinoma cases, chemotherapy is not necessary.

D. In cases of nongerminomas, chemotherapy must be given following radiation.

E. Chemotherapy for germinomas is particularly recommended for young children.

✅ **Answer D**

➖ Chemotherapy is required before radiation treatment for nongerminomas.

❓ 10. **Germ cell tumors: surgery. The FALSE answer is:**

A. Initial surgical treatment for germinomas could be unnecessary.

B. Biopsy is frequently required in order to establish the diagnosis.

C. Aggressive surgical debulking has been demonstrated to be beneficial in most cases.

D. Surgery is recommended for residual tumors with normal tumor markers following radiation and chemotherapy.

E. Surgery can also help to relieve symptoms by reducing intracranial pressure.

✅ **Answer C**

➖ Severe surgical debulking has a high morbidity rate and little proof of benefit.

15

❓ 11. **Germ cell tumors: approaches for the pineal region. The FALSE answer is:**

A. Occipital transtentorial.

B. Infratentorial supracerebellar.

C. Parietal-interhemispheric-transcallosal.

D. Combined supratentorial-infratentorial.

E. Telovelar.

✅ **Answer E**
— The telovelar approach is more appropriate for tumors in the fourth ventricle.

❓ 12. **Germinoma: general information. The FALSE answer is:**
   A. It is the most prevalent pineal tumor.
   B. Calcification exhibits a lateral distribution.
   C. It is also referred to as intracranial seminoma.
   D. The incidence peaks between the ages of 10 and 30 years.
   E. The cells are derived from the endoderm of the yolk sac.

✅ **Answer B**
— As opposed to pineocytoma and pineoblastoma, calcification is central.

❓ 13. **Teratoma: general information. The FALSE answer is:**
   A. It is derived from all three germinal layers.
   B. The third most common germ cell tumor.
   C. It can contain bone, muscle, nerve, and skin tissue.
   D. Categorized into mature and immature types.
   E. It can be found in intra- and extra-axial locations.

✅ **Answer B**
— Teratomas are the second most common germ cell tumor behind germinomas.

❓ 14. **Choriocarcinoma: general information. The FALSE answer is:**
   A. It is derived from trophoblastic tissue.
   B. It comprises 5% of total pineal masses.
   C. It can be located in the pineal and suprasellar areas.
   D. The tumor is highly vascular.
   E. It cannot expand to other regions of the body.

✅ **Answer E**
— It has the potential to metastasize hematogenously.

❓ 15. **Yolk sac tumor: general information. The FALSE answer is:**
   A. Due to the location of the tumor, hydrocephalus is a common symptom.
   B. An elevated AFP level is mandatory for diagnosis.
   C. Can be associated with Down syndrome.

D. It contributes to a small fraction of all germ cell tumors.

E. It can lead to Parinaud's syndrome.

✅ **Answer B**

— Although AFP is usually increased, it can also be normal.

❓ 16. **Embryonal cell carcinoma: general information. The FALSE answer is:**

A. It features zones of necrosis and a high rate of mitosis.

B. The tumor is characterized by a high degree of malignancy.

C. Both AFP and ß-hCG levels have the potential to be increased.

D. Surgery is considered to be the preferred therapeutic option.

E. It is able to metastasize systemically.

✅ **Answer D**

— First-choice treatments include radiation therapy and chemotherapy.

Bibliography

1. Jennings MT, Gelman R, Hochberg F. Intracranial germ cell tumors: natural history and pathogenesis. J Neurosurg. 1985;63(2):155–67.
2. Sato K, Takeuchi H, Kubota T. Pathology of intracranial germ cell tumors. Prog Neurol Surg. 2009;23:59–75.
3. Brandes AA, Pasetto LM, Monfardini S. The treatment of cranial germ cell tumours. Cancer Treat Rev. 2000;26(4):233–42.
4. Lo AC, Hodgson D, Dang J, Tyldesley S, Bouffet E, Bartels U, Cheng S, Hukin J, Bedard PL, Goddard K, Laperriere N. Intracranial germ cell tumors in adolescents and young adults: a 40-year multi-institutional review of outcomes. Int J Radiat Oncol Biol Phys. 2020;106(2):269–78.
5. Kyritsis AP. Management of primary intracranial germ cell tumors. J Neuro-Oncol. 2010;96(2):143–9.
6. Kurucu N, Akyüz C, Varan A, Zorlu F, Aydin B, Söylemezoglu F, Yalcin B, Kutluk T, Büyükpamukcus M. Primary intracranial germ cell tumors in children 36-year experience of a single center. J Cancer Res Ther. 2020;16(6):1459–65.
7. Sahay A, Epari S, Chinnaswamy G, Chatterjee A, Goda JS, Patil V, Moyiadi A, Shetty P, Singh V, Sahu A, Choudhary A, Janu A, Gupta T. Primary intracranial germ cell tumors: a study with an integrated clinicopathological approach. Neurol India. 2023;71(3):500–8.
8. Aoyama H. Radiation therapy for intracranial germ cell tumors. Prog Neurol Surg. 2009;23:96–105.
9. Khafaga Y, El Weshi A, Nazmy M, Hassounah M, Alshail E, Moussa E, Allam A, Alkofide A, Jamshed A, Elhusseiny G, Ezzat I, Jenkin D. Intracranial germ cell tumors: a single-institution experience. Ann Saudi Med. 2012;32(4):359–65.
10. Matsutani M. Pineal germ cell tumors. Prog Neurol Surg. 2009;23:76–85.

15

11. Bowzyk Al-Naeeb A, Murray M, Horan G, Harris F, Kortmann RD, Nicholson J, Ajithkumar T. Current management of intracranial germ cell tumours. Clin Oncol (R Coll Radiol). 2018;30(4):204–14.

12. Balmaceda C, Finlay J. Current advances in the diagnosis and management of intracranial germ cell tumors. Curr Neurol Neurosci Rep. 2004;4(3):253–62.

13. Kakkar A, Biswas A, Kalyani N, Chatterjee U, Suri V, Sharma MC, Goyal N, Sharma BS, Mallick S, Julka PK, Chinnaswamy G, Arora B, Sridhar E, Chatterjee S, Jalali R, Sarkar C. Intracranial germ cell tumors: a multi-institutional experience from three tertiary care centers in India. Childs Nerv Syst. 2016;32(11):2173–80.

14. Plant AS, Chi SN, Frazier L. Pediatric malignant germ cell tumors: a comparison of the neuro-oncology and solid tumor experience. Pediatr Blood Cancer. 2016;63(12):2086–95.

15. Osorio DS, Allen JC. Management of CNS germinoma. CNS Oncol. 2015;4(4):273–9.

Cysts and Tumor-Like Lesions

Wardan A. Tamer and Samer S. Hoz

© The Author(s), under exclusive license to Springer Nature Switzerland AG 2024
S. S. Hoz et al. (eds.), *Surgical Neuro-Oncology*,
https://doi.org/10.1007/978-3-031-53642-7_16

❓ 1. Epidermoid cysts (EC).
   Definition. The FALSE answer is:
   A. Primary epidermoid cysts are also called cholesteatomas.
   B. Primary epidermoid cysts are neoplastic cystic lesions.
   C. Epidermoid cysts are lined with a simple stratified squamous epithelium.
   D. Epidermoid cysts are congenital.
   E. Epidermoid cysts arise from misplaced epidural cells.

✅ Answer B
— Primary epidermoid cysts are nonneoplastic cystic lesions.

❓ 2. Epidermoid cysts (EC).
   Definition. The FALSE answer is:
   A. EC reflects an abnormality at the blastulation stage of development.
   B. There is a primary disruption of tissues derived from one or more of the three germ cell layers.
   C. EC reflects an abnormality of the surface ectoderm.
   D. Spinal epidermoid cysts are frequently associated with one or more mesodermal malformations.
   E. The mesodermal malformations particularly involve the vertebrae.

✅ Answer A
— EC reflects a problem at the gastrulation stage of development.

❓ 3. Epidermoid cysts (EC).
   Definition. The FALSE answer is:
   A. ECs are benign lesions that may arise in the spine or intracranially.
   B. EC may be intradural (usually extra-axial) or extradural (in the diploic space).
   C. Intracranial ECs account for 0.2–1.8% of all intracranial tumors.
   D. EC usually occurs in the pineal region or in the floor of the anterior cranial fossa.
   E. Most intraspinal ECs are subdural and extramedullary.

16

✅ Answer D
— EC usually occurs in the cerebellopontine angle or in the parasellar cisterns.

? 4. **Epidermoid cysts (EC).**
   Definition. The FALSE answer is:
   A. ECs are derived from ectopic inclusions of epithelial cells during neural tube closure.
   B. It is due to gastrulation dysembryogenesis.
   C. It occurs during the sixth to eighth weeks of gestation.
   D. EC represents malformations of surface ectoderm.
   E. EC has been reported in patients from infancy to adulthood.

✓ **Answer C**
– EC occurs due to the secondary disruption of neural tube closure during the third to fifth weeks of gestation.

? 5. **Epidermoid cysts (EC).**
   Pathology. The FALSE answer is:
   A. EC is positive for CA19–9.
   B. CA19–9 staining occurs in the epithelial cells of the cyst wall.
   C. CA19–9 staining occurs in subepithelial collagenous and keratinous tissues.
   D. CA19–9 can present as a tumor marker in colon cancer.
   E. CA19–9 serum values cannot be used for EC recurrence or progression after surgery.

✓ **Answer E**
– CA19–9 serum values can be used to evaluate patients for tumor recurrence or progression.

? 6. **Epidermoid cysts (EC).**
   Pathology: macroscopic appearance. The FALSE answer is:
   A. ECs are well-demarcated, encapsulated lesions.
   B. ECs often have a striking white capsule with a mother-of-pearl sheen.
   C. The outer surface of EC is usually flat.
   D. ECs may be easily shelled out from adjacent structures.
   E. ECs may sometimes be firmly anchored as a result of local inflammation.

✓ **Answer C**
– The outer surface of EC may be smooth, nodular, or lobulated.

? 7. **Epidermoid cysts (EC).**
   Pathology: macroscopic appearance. The FALSE answer is:
   A. EC in the ventricles or subarachnoid space is liable to rupture and cause hemorrhage.
   B. The interior is filled with soft, flaky material.
   C. The content may be brownish-gray.
   D. Calcification is rare.
   E. The capsule of EC may enclose nerves and blood vessels.

✅ **Answer A**
— EC in the ventricles or in the subarachnoid space is liable to rupture and can cause meningitis. Hemorrhage is not a common characteristic of epidermoid cysts.

? 8. **Epidermoid cysts (EC).**
   Clinical presentation. The FALSE answer is:
   A. Pediatric patients with EC are usually symptomatic in the early phase of life.
   B. EC has an insidious onset.
   C. EC grows linearly.
   D. Patients may present with features of aseptic meningitis.
   E. Aseptic meningitis may be caused by leakage of the debris into the subarachnoid spaces.

✅ **Answer A**
— Although ECs are congenital lesions, patients are usually not symptomatic until they are aged 30–40 years.

? 9. **Epidermoid cysts (EC).**
   Radiology. The FALSE answer is:
   A. On FLAIR, EC is hyperintense to CSF.
   B. Calcification is common.
   C. On DW1, there is restricted diffusion.
   D. They are mostly isointense to CSF on T1.
   E. Most are hyperintense to gray matter on T2.

16

✅ **Answer B**
— EC rarely shows calcification on CT.

? 10. **Epidermoid cysts (EC).**
Surgery. The FALSE answer is:
A. Both symptomatic and asymptomatic ECs should be removed surgically.
B. There is no role for radiotherapy or chemotherapy.
C. Total excision is not always possible.
D. Spillage of the contents may cause severe chemical meningitis.
E. Rinsing with hydrocortisone in ringer solution helps remove residual cyst contents.

✅ **Answer A**
– Incidentally discovered asymptomatic cysts do not need to be removed but must be followed up regularly.

? 11. **Epidermoid cysts (EC).**
Complications: chemical meningitis. The FALSE answer is:
A. Spilling the contents of the cyst may cause chemical meningitis.
B. Preoperative administration of antibiotics and irrigation of the surgical field with antibiotics help in alleviating meningitis.
C. Postop administration of steroids helps in reducing the risk of chemical meningitis.
D. Lumbar puncture helps in alleviating the headache and pyrexia due to chemical meningitis.
E. Chemical meningitis may lead to basal arachnoiditis and communicating hydrocephalus.

✅ **Answer B**
– Preoperative administration of steroids and irrigation of the surgical field with steroids help in alleviating meningitis.

? 12. **Cysts and tumor-like lesions, dermoid cysts (DCs).**
Definition. The FALSE answer is:
A. DCs account for 0.04–0.6% of all intracranial tumors.
B. DCs tend to occur at the midline.
C. DCs occur at the blastulation stage of development.
D. DCs are benign lesions.
E. DCs are associated with a dermal sinus in the midline.

✅ **Answer C**
– DC occurs at the gastrulation phase, with secondary dysraphism.

? 13. **Cysts and tumor-like lesions, dermoid cysts (DCs).**
   Definition. The FALSE answer is:
   A. DC involves the scalp.
   B. Scalp dermoids typically present as subcutaneous nodules that are elastic and tender.
   C. DC lesions often erode into the skull.
   D. DC may be present in the intracranial space.
   E. DC may be intradural or extradural.

✓ Answer B
   — Scalp dermoids typically present as subcutaneous nodules that are firm and nontender.

? 14. **Cysts and tumor-like lesions, dermoid cysts (DCs).**
   Presentation. The FALSE answer is:
   A. The average age of presentation for DC is about 15 years of age.
   B. Patients may present with local neural deficits.
   C. DCs are usually found at midline.
   D. There is a male predominance.
   E. DC is associated with Klippel-Feil syndrome.

✓ Answer D
   — As with epidermoid cysts, there is a female predominance.

? 15. **Cysts and tumor-like lesions, dermoid cysts (DCs).**
   Clinical Features. The FALSE answer is:
   A. DC may rupture with head trauma.
   B. Spontaneous rupture may occur due to a progressive increase in ICP.
   C. Rupture of the cyst may result in chemical meningitis.
   D. Rupture of the cyst may result in hydrocephalus.
   E. Spinal dermal cysts with dermal sinus tracts may lead to secondary spinal subdural hematoma.

✓ Answer E
   — Spinal dermal cysts with dermal sinus tracts can lead to secondary spinal subdural abscesses resulting from infection spreading from the dermal cyst.

16

❓ 16. **Cysts and tumor-like lesions, dermoid cysts (DCs).**
Pathology: macroscopic appearance. The FALSE answer is:
A. Are well-demarcated, smooth, round, or oval masses.
B. The walls may have papillary projections.
C. Contain thick yellowish material.
D. Hair is often found, but teeth are rare.
E. The connection of dermoid cysts with dermal sinuses occurs in spinal but not intracranial DCs.

✅ **Answer E**
— The connection of dermoid cysts with dermal sinuses is known to occur in both intracranial and spinal cases.

❓ 17. **Cysts and tumor-like lesions, dermoid cysts (DCs).**
Pathology: microscopy. The FALSE answer is:
A. DC lining is composed of stratified squamous epithelium mounted on collagenous connective tissue.
B. Thicker parts of the wall contain hair follicles and sebaceous and sweat glands.
C. Bone and cartilage are common findings.
D. The epithelial cell lining may be less differentiated in DC than in epidermoids.
E. CA19–9 may be elevated in DC.

✅ **Answer C**
— Bone and cartilage are rare, their presence being more typical of classic teratomas.

❓ 18. **Cysts and tumor-like lesions, dermoid cysts (DCs).**
Pathology: biological behavior. The FALSE answer is:
A. DCs are typically slow-growing and benign.
B. Dermal sinuses penetrating the dura may be the route of pyogenic infection.
C. Cyst rupture may lead to the dissemination of fat into CSF.
D. Malignant transformation is common.
E. The rupture of DC into the CSF may lead to granulomatous meningitis with foreign body-type giant cells.

✅ **Answer D**
— These lesions are slow-growing and benign but are likely to recur when incompletely removed. Malignant transformation is extremely rare.

? 19. **Cysts and tumor-like lesions, dermoid cysts (DCs).**
Spinal dermal sinus (SDS): general information. The FALSE answer is:
A. SDS may appear with or without hair.
B. Is usually very close to the midline.
C. The skin surrounding the opening of SDS may be normal or pigmented.
D. There is no connection between SDS and the dura of the thecal sac.
E. May lead to meningitis or intrathecal abscess.

✅ **Answer D**
− The sinus may terminate superficially, may connect with the coccyx, or may traverse between normal vertebrae or through bifid spines to the dural tube.

? 20. **Cysts and tumor-like lesions, dermoid cysts (DCs).**
Spinal dermal sinus (SDS): radiological evaluation. The FALSE answer is:
A. The tract may be probed or injected with contrast to evaluate it.
B. Clinical examination is directed toward detecting abnormalities in sphincter function, reflexes, and lower extremities sensation.
C. When SDS is seen at birth, ultrasound is the best means to evaluate for spina bifida.
D. When SDS is seen at birth, an MRI should be obtained.
E. Plain X-rays and CT are unable to demonstrate the fine tract that may exist between the skin and the dura.

✅ **Answer A**
− These tracts should NOT be probed or injected with contrast as this can precipitate infection or sterile meningitis.

? 21. **Cysts and tumor-like lesions, dermoid cysts (DCs).**
Spinal dermal sinus (SDS): surgical technique. The FALSE answer is:
A. The sinus must be followed deep until the termination of the tract is encountered.
B. The use of a lacrimal duct probe under direct vision may facilitate excision without violating the tract.

16

C. If the tract penetrates the spine, laminectomy must be performed.
D. If the tract enters the dura, it usually does so on the lateral side of the thecal sac.
E. There is a risk of cyst content spilling into the subdural space.

Answer D
- If the tract enters the dura, it usually does so in the midline, and in these cases the dura should be opened and inspected.

22. **Cysts and tumor-like lesions, dermoid cysts (DCs).**
Cranial dermal sinus (CDS): general information. The FALSE answer is:
A. Stalk begins with a dimple in the occipital or nasal region.
B. Cutaneous stigmata of hemangioma, subcutaneous DC, or abnormal hair formation may occur.
C. Occipital sinuses extend caudally.
D. Presentation may include recurrent bacterial (usually S. aureus) or aseptic meningitis.
E. Occipital sinuses enter the skull superior to the torcular herophili.

Answer E
- Occipital sinuses extend cranially, and if they enter the skull, they do so caudal to the torcular herophili.

23. **Cysts and tumor-like lesions, dermoid cysts (DCs).**
Radiological features. The FALSE answer is:
A. On CT, the DC appearance is hyperdense to CSF.
B. On MRI T1W, they are typically hyperintense.
C. They do not show enhancement.
D. MRI DW1 shows restricted diffusion.
E. There is high signal loss on MRI with fat saturation sequence.

Answer A
- On CT, DCs appear hypodense, similar to CSF. They exhibit lobulated margins with no enhancement.

? 24. **Cysts and tumor-like lesions, dermoid cysts (DCs).**
Management: surgical technique. The FALSE answer is:
   A. A plane between the capsule and overlying arachnoid tissue can be easily established.
   B. CUSA can be used in the removal of DC.
   C. DC is avascular.
   D. There is a risk of cranial nerve injury.
   E. The presence of a granulomatous reaction can cause dense adherence between the capsule and adjacent structures.

✓ Answer B
— The CUSA is not used with DC for fear of causing inadvert injury to cranial nerves that have become involved in the tumor mass.

? 25. **Cysts and tumor-like lesions, neurenteric cysts (NCs).**
Definition. The FALSE answer is:
   A. Are also known as enterogenous, neuroepithelial, and foregut cysts, as well as gastrocytoma.
   B. May occur intracranially or in the spinal canal.
   C. Represent approximately 0.7% to 1.3% of all spinal cord tumors.
   D. Are most commonly intramedullary.
   E. Arise in the pontomedullary and parasellar regions, CPA, craniocervical junction and spinal axis.

✓ Answer D
— Although intramedullary lesions have been reported, they are more commonly extramedullary. They arise in the pontomedullary and parasellar regions, CPA, craniocervical junction, and spinal axis.

? 26. **Cysts and tumor-like lesions, neurenteric cysts (NCs).**
Definition. The FALSE answer is:
   A. Develop as early as embryonic days 12–14.
   B. Are considered a form of split notochord syndrome.
   C. Most are ventral and extra-axial.
   D. Spinal NCs are associated with vertebral anomalies.
   E. Up to 5% of patients with Klippel–Feil syndrome and vertebral fusion abnormalities have NCs and fistulas.

16

✓ Answer A
— These cysts develop as early as embryonic days 16–17.

? 27. **Cysts and tumor-like lesions, neurenteric cysts (NCs).**
   Embryology. The FALSE answer is:
   A. Can be seen anywhere along the gastrointestinal tract.
   B. Extend into the intradural compartment.
   C. Occur due to disturbance in the interrelations between the meso-
   derm and endoderm.
   D. Associated with midline fusion abnormalities of the vertebral
   column.
   E. May develop at the end of the third embryonic week.

✓ **Answer C**
   ▬ NCs occur due to a disturbance in the interrelations between the ectoderm, notochord, and endoderm.

? 28. **Cysts and tumor-like lesions, neurenteric cysts (NCs).**
   Presentation. The FALSE answer is:
   A. May manifest as early as prenatally and as late as adulthood.
   B. Spinal NCs are seen more often in females.
   C. Intracranial NCs are more common in females.
   D. The disease course in adults is slow and insidious, and is more
   rapid in children.
   E. When a fistula persists, patients may present with recurrent men-
   ingitis.

✓ **Answer B**
   ▬ Spinal NCs are seen more often in males, whereas 60% of the intracranial
   cysts have been reported in females.

? 29. **Cysts and tumor-like lesions, neurenteric cysts (NCs).**
   Imaging. The FALSE answer is:
   A. Display high density on CT due to high mucin content.
   B. Are nonenhancing on CT.
   C. On T1 MRI, the appearance is isointense or slightly hyperintense
   to CSF.
   D. On T2 MRI, the appearance is isointense to CSF.
   E. Are nonenhancing on MRI.

✓ **Answer A**
   ▬ NCs display low density on CT due to high mucin content.

? 30. **Cysts and tumor-like lesions, neurenteric cysts (NCs).**
   Pathology: macroscopic appearance. The FALSE answer is:
   A. Most cases of spinal NC are encountered in the extradural extra-medullary spinal compartment.
   B. Solitary NCs occur most frequently in the cervical region.
   C. Lumbosacral cases of NC are often associated with dysraphic defects.
   D. Ventral location of NC is more common than dorsal lesions.
   E. NCs can occur in the cranial cavity.

✓ **Answer A**
— Most cases are encountered in the intradural extramedullary spinal compartment.

? 31. **Cysts and tumor-like lesions, neurenteric cysts (NCs).**
   Histopathology. The FALSE answer is:
   A. Lined by a single-layered or pseudostratified cuboidal or columnar epithelium.
   B. The epithelium may be ciliated or nonciliated.
   C. Lined by transitional epithelium.
   D. The epithelium is mounted on a basement membrane.
   E. Some NCs contain mucous or serous glands and smooth muscle.

✓ **Answer C**
— NC is typically lined by a single-layered or pseudostratified cuboidal or columnar epithelium.

? 32. **Cysts and tumor-like lesions, neurenteric cysts (NCs).**
   Treatment. The FALSE answer is:
   A. Treatment is primarily surgical excision.
   B. They can be strongly adherent to adjacent structures.
   C. Aspiration or a cyst-subarachnoid shunt may be used.
   D. Conventional radiotherapy for residual tumor can be effective.
   E. Chemotherapy has not been shown to be effective.

✓ **Answer D**
— Conventional radiotherapy for residual tumor is not likely to be effective.

16

33. Cysts and tumor-like lesions, colloid cysts (CCs).
Definition. The FALSE answer is:
A. Are benign.
B. Are mostly intraventricular.
C. Account for 0.5–2% of all intracranial mass lesions.
D. Are most commonly found in the posterior portion of the lateral ventricles.
E. Are usually associated with obstructive hydrocephalous of the lateral ventricles.

✅ **Answer D**
– CCs are most commonly found in the anterior portion of the third ventricle.

34. Cysts and tumor-like lesions, colloid cysts (CCs).
Definition. The FALSE answer is:
A. Are also known as neuroepithelial cysts.
B. Are slow-growing benign tumors.
C. Comprise 2% of gliomas.
D. Usually diagnosed between 20 and 50 years of age.
E. Are most commonly found in the fourth ventricle.

✅ **Answer E**
– CCs are most commonly found in the third ventricle in the region of the foramina of Monro, but may be seen elsewhere, e.g., in the septum pellucidum.

35. Cysts and tumor-like lesions, colloid cysts (CCs).
Pathogenesis. The FALSE answer is:
A. Are normally located anteriorly in the third ventricle at the level of the foramen of Monro.
B. There is no gender predilection.
C. Familial cases have been also reported.
D. Most are found as multiple lesions.
E. Can range from a few millimeters to up to 9 cm in diameter.

✅ **Answer D**
– Most cases of CC are found as an isolated lesion, although multiple cysts have been also described.

? 36. **Cysts and tumor-like lesions, colloid cysts (CCs).**
Pathology: microscopic appearance. The FALSE answer is:
A. Electron microscopy reveals ciliated and nonciliated epithelial cells.
B. The cyst content is Periodic acid–Schiff positive.
C. The epithelium contains goblet cells.
D. Originate from the endoderm.
E. The cyst content is composed of amorphous debris with necrotic leukocytes and lipid droplets.

✓ Answer D
— CCs originate from the ectoderm.

? 37. **Cysts and tumor-like lesions, colloid cysts (CCs).**
Presentation. The FALSE answer is:
A. Hydrocephalus can be chronic.
B. Obstruction to CSF flow can be intermittent.
C. Patients commonly present with headache and vomiting.
D. Sudden death is most commonly due to spontaneous cyst rupture.
E. Other symptoms include gait disturbance and short memory loss.

✓ Answer D
— Sudden death is most commonly due to acute CSF outflow obstruction associated with interventions such as lumbar punctures and ventriculography. However, decompensation and death can also occur in patients with chronic hydrocephalus.

? 38. **Cysts and tumor-like lesions, colloid cysts (CCs).**
Diagnostic imaging. The FALSE answer is:
A. Most are hyperdense on CT.
B. Around half of them enhance slightly on CT.
C. On T1W1, the appearance is hypointense.
D. On T2W1, the appearance is hypointense.
E. The signal on T2 may be hyperintense as a result of increased water content of the expanding cyst.

16

✓ Answer C
— CCs are usually hyperintense on T1W1.

? 39. **Cysts and tumor-like lesions, colloid cysts (CCs).**
   Surgical treatment options. The FALSE answer is:
   A. Transcallosal approach.
   B. Transcortical approach.
   C. Stereotactic drainage.
   D. Ventriculoscopic removal.
   E. LP shunt if associated with hydrocephalus.

✔ **Answer E**
− LP shunt is a contraindication in the case of CCs associated with hydrocephalus.

? 40. **Cysts and tumor-like lesions, colloid cysts (CCs).**
   Microneurosurgery: transcortical approach. The FALSE answer is:
   A. Is indicated if the cyst is located in the posterior part of the third ventricle.
   B. Has a higher rate of postoperative epilepsy.
   C. A transient attention deficit may result from anterior frontal incision.
   D. Short-term memory loss may occur.
   E. Transient hemiparesis may occur in the case of more posterior frontal cortical incision.

✔ **Answer A**
− This approach is suitable for lesions of the anterosuperior part of the third ventricle.

? 41. **Cysts and tumor-like lesions, colloid cysts (CCs).**
   Microneurosurgery: transcortical approach. The FALSE answer is:
   A. The transcortical approach was first used by Dandy on a CC in the third ventricle.
   B. Is useful in the case of normal-sized ventricles.
   C. The CC in the third ventricle could be dissected through the dilated foramen of Monro.
   D. Avoids injury to the frontal draining veins of the sagittal sinus.
   E. Decreases the chance of injury to the pericallosal arteries.

✔ **Answer B**
− The transcortical approach is useful if the ventricles are enlarged and access to the foramen of Monro and third ventricle can be readily obtained.

? 42. **Cysts and tumor-like lesions, colloid cysts (CCs).**
Microneurosurgery: transcallosal transventricular approach. The FALSE answer is:
A. Is indicated in the case of normal-sized lateral ventricles.
B. A direct approach may be made between the fornices.
C. The septum pellucidum is incised.
D. The interforniceal approach is only used when the fornices are spread apart by CC.
E. A transforaminal approach is employed when the foramen of Monro is enlarged.

✓ **Answer C**
– In transcallosal approach, to enter the third ventricle, the tela choroidea has to be incised to enter the third ventricle.

? 43. **Cysts and tumor-like lesions, colloid cysts (CCs).**
Stereotactic aspiration. The FALSE answer is:
A. May be used urgently in the setting of acute raised intracranial pressure.
B. The aspirability of the cyst may be predicted by the density appearance on CT.
C. Successful aspiration is more likely for hypodense or isodense lesions.
D. Associated with low mortality and morbidity.
E. CC may recur even after successful aspiration.

✓ **Answer A**
– Stereotactic aspiration is contraindicated in cases of acute raised intracranial pressure.

? 44. **Cysts and tumor-like lesions, colloid cysts (CCs).**
Endoscopic management. The FALSE answer is:
A. The skin incision is made 4 cm lateral to the midline.
B. The skin incision is made 4 cm anterior to the coronal suture.
C. A left-sided approach is the most common.
D. It is important that after identification of the foramen, the endoscopic sheath remains in the lateral ventricle.
E. When a large part of the cyst content is aspirated, the capsule is caught by forceps and slowly pulled out.

✅ **Answer C**
- A right-sided approach is chosen unless the cyst is far more prominent through the left foramen of Monro or the right ventricle is too small.

❓ 45. **Cysts and tumor-like lesions, colloid cysts (CCs).**
Endoscopic management complications. The FALSE answer is:
A. Septic or aseptic meningitis.
B. Transient memory deficit.
C. Transient hemiparesis.
D. Postop slit ventricular syndrome.
E. Transient postoperative seizures.

✅ **Answer D**
- No cases of slit ventricular syndrome have been reported as a complication of endoscopic treatment of CCs.

Bibliography

1. Richard Winn H. Youmans neurological surgery, vol. 2., Chapter 152. 7th ed. Elsevier; 2017.
2. Love S, Louis DN, Ellison DW. Greenfield's neuropathology, vol. 2., Chapter 42. 8th ed. CRC Press; 2015.
3. Thamburaj VA. Textbook of contemporary neurosurgery, vol. 2. Chapter 81. Jaypee Brothers Medical Publishers; 2012.
4. Narain TP. Ramamurthi and Tandon's, textbook of neurosurgery. 3rd ed. Jaypee Brothers Medical Publisher Pvt. Limited; 2012. Chapter 159
5. Richard G. Ellenbogen, principles of neurological surgery. 4th ed. Elsevier; 2018. p. 227. (Chapter 13)
6. Kirollos RW. Oxford textbook of neurological surgery., Chapter 16. Oxford University Press; 2019.
7. Yasargil MG. Microneurosurgery IVB., Chapter 11A. Thieme; 1996.
8. ten Donkelaar HJ, Lammens M, Hori A. Clinical neuroembryology. Berlin, Heidelberg: Springer-Verlag; 2006. p. 253.
9. Sekhar LN, Fessler RG. Atlas of neurosurgical techniques: brain, vol. 2. 2nd ed. Thieme; 2016.
10. Sindou M. Practical handbook of neurosurgery, from leading neurosurgeons, vol. 2. New York: Springer; 2009.
11. Ganko R, Rodriguez M, Magnussen J, Simons M, Myint E, Assaad N. Do prophylactic steroids prevent chemical meningitis in surgery for epidermoid cysts? case report and literature review. Surg Neurol Int. 2020:11.
12. Prior A, Anania P, Pacetti M, Secci F, Ravegnani M, Pavanello M, Piatelli G, Cama A, Consales A. Dermoid and epidermoid cysts of scalp: case series of 234 consecutive patients. World Neurosurg. 2018;120:119–24.

13. Velho V, Khan S, Agarwal V, Sharma M. Intra-axial CNS dermoid cyst. Asian J Neurosurg. 2012;7(01):42–4.

14. Tan LA, Kasliwal MK, Harbhajanka A, Kellogg RG, Arvanitis LD, Munoz LF. Hyperdense suprasellar mass: an unusual radiological presentation of intracranial dermoid cyst. J Clin Neurosci. 2015;22(7):1208–10.

15. Orakcioglu B, Halatsch ME, Fortunati M, Unterberg A, Yonekawa Y. Intracranial dermoid cysts: variations of radiological and clinical features. Acta Neurochir. 2008;150:1227–34.

16. Ray MJ, Barnett DW, Snipes GJ, Layton KF, Opatowsky MJ. Ruptured intracranial dermoid cyst. In: Baylor University medical center proceedings 2012 Jan 1, vol. 25, No. 1. Taylor & Francis. p. 23–5.

17. Ren X, Lin S, Wang Z, Luo L, Jiang Z, Sui D, Bi Z, Cui Y, Jia W, Zhang Y, Yu L. Clinical, radiological, and pathological features of 24 atypical intracranial epidermoid cysts. J Neurosurg. 2012;116(3):611–21.

18. Jacków J, Tse G, Martin A, Sąsiadek M, Romanowski C. Ruptured intracranial dermoid cysts: a pictorial review. Pol J Radiol. 2018;83:e465.

19. Mishra SS, Panigrahi S. Thoracic congenital dermal sinus associated with intramedullary spinal dermoid cyst. J Pediatr Neurosci. 2014;9(1):30.

20. Vadivelu S, Desai SK, Illner A, Luerssen TG, Jea A. Infected lumbar dermoid cyst mimicking intramedullary spinal cord tumor: observations and outcomes. J Pediatr Neurosci. 2014;9(1):21.

21. Venkatesh R, Rajasekar G, Jeevarajan S. Spectrum of spinal dermal sinus: analysis and outcome evaluation. J Spinal Surg. 2018;5(1):4–9.

22. Choi JS, Bae YC, Lee JW, Kang GB. Dermoid cysts: epidemiology and diagnostic approach based on clinical experiences. Arch Plast Surg. 2018;45(06):512–6.

23. Balasundaram P, Garg A, Prabhakar A, Joseph Devarajan LS, Gaikwad SB, Khanna G. Evolution of epidermoid cyst into dermoid cyst: embryological explanation and radiological-pathological correlation. Neuroradiol J. 2019;32(2):92–7.

24. Liu JK, Gottfried ON, Salzman KL, Schmidt RH, Couldwell WT. Ruptured intracranial dermoid cysts: clinical, radiographic, and surgical features. Neurosurgery. 2008;62(2):377–84.

25. de Oliveira RS, Cinalli G, Roujeau T, Sainte-Rose C, Pierre-Kahn A, Zerah M. Neurenteric cysts in children: 16 consecutive cases and review of the literature. J Neurosurg Pediatr. 2005;103(6):512–23.

26. Chen CT, Lee CY, Lee ST, Chang CN, Wei KC, Wu CT. Neurenteric cysts: risk factors and management of recurrence. Acta Neurochir. 2016;158:1325–31.

27. Tubbs RS, Salter EG, Oakes WJ. Neurenteric cyst: case report and a review of the potential dysembryology. Clin Anat. 2006;19(7):669–72.

28. Yang T, Wu L, Fang J, Yang C, Deng X, Xu Y. Clinical presentation and surgical outcomes of intramedullary neurenteric cysts. J Neurosurg Spine. 2015;23(1):99–110.

29. Preece MT, Osborn AG, Chin SS, Smirniotopoulos JG. Intracranial neurenteric cysts: imaging and pathology spectrum. Am J Neuroradiol. 2006;27(6):1211–6.

30. Chakraborty S, Priamo F, Loven T, Li J, Insinga S, Schulder M. Supratentorial neurenteric cysts: case series and review of pathology, imaging, and clinical management. World Neurosurg. 2016;85:143–52.

31. Savage JJ, Casey JN, McNeill IT, Sherman JH. Neurenteric cysts of the spine. J Craniovertebr Junction Spine. 2010;1(1):58–63.

16

32. Wang L, Zhang J, Wu Z, Jia G, Zhang L, Hao S, Geng S. Diagnosis and management of adult intracranial neurenteric cysts. Neurosurgery. 2011;68(1):44–52.
33. Lagman C, Rai K, Chung LK, Nagasawa DT, Beckett JS, Tucker AM, Yang I. Fatal colloid cysts: a systematic review. World Neurosurg. 2017;107:409–15.
34. Beaumont TL, Limbrick DD, Rich KM, Wippold FJ, Dacey RG. Natural history of colloid cysts of the third ventricle. J Neurosurg. 2016;125(6):1420–30.
35. Turillazzi E, Bello S, Neri M, Riezzo I, Fineschi V. Colloid cyst of the third ventricle, hypothalamus, and heart: a dangerous link for sudden death. Diagn Pathol. 2012; 7(1):1–5.
36. Sayehmiri F, Starke RM, Eichberg DG, Ghanikolahloo M, Rahmatian A, Fathi M, Vakili K, Ebrahimzadeh K, Rezaei O, Samadian M, Mousavinejad SA. Comparison of microscopic and endoscopic resection of third-ventricular colloid cysts: a systematic review and meta-analysis. Clin Neurol Neurosurg. 2022;215:107179.
37. Ravnik J, Bunc G, Grcar A, Zunic M, Velnar T. Colloid cysts of the third ventricle exhibit various clinical presentation: a review of three cases. Bosn J Basic Med Sci. 2014;14(3):132.
38. Algin O, Ozmen E, Arslan H. Radiologic manifestations of colloid cysts: a pictorial essay. Can Assoc Radiol J. 2013;64(1):56–60.
39. Sheikh AB, Mendelson ZS, Liu JK. Endoscopic versus microsurgical resection of colloid cysts: a systematic review and meta-analysis of 1278 patients. World Neurosurg. 2014;82(6):1187–97.
40. Elshamy W, Burkard J, Gerges M, Erginoglu U, Aycan A, Ozaydin B, Dempsey RJ, Baskaya MK. Surgical approaches for resection of third ventricle colloid cysts: meta-analysis. Neurosurg Rev. 2021:1–10.
41. Heller RS, Heilman CB. Colloid cysts: evolution of surgical approach preference and management of recurrent cysts. Oper Neurosurg. 2020;18(1):19–25.
42. Vazhayil V, Sadashiva N, Nayak N, Prabhuraj AR, Shukla D, Somanna S. Surgical management of colloid cysts in children: experience at a tertiary care center. Childs Nerv Syst. 2018;34:1215–20.
43. Rajshekhar V. Rate of recurrence following stereotactic aspiration of colloid cysts of the third ventricle. Stereotact Funct Neurosurg. 2012;90(1):37–44.
44. Greenlee JD, Teo C, Ghahreman A, Kwok B. Purely endoscopic resection of colloid cysts. Oper Neurosurg. 2008;62(3):51–6.
45. Zohdi A, El Kheshin S. Endoscopic approach to colloid cysts. Minim Invasive Neurosurg. 2006;49(05):263–8.

Tumors of the Cranial Nerves

Viraat Harsh, Manoj Kumar, Anil Kumar, Sadeem A. Albulaihed, and Samer S. Hoz

❓ 1. **Cerebellopontine (CP) angle surgical anatomy. The FALSE answer is:**
   A. It is laterally bound by the petrous bone.
   B. The floor is formed by the middle cerebellar peduncle.
   C. The pons forms the medial boundary.
   D. It has two neurovascular complexes.
   E. The superior border is formed by the tentorium.

✅ **Answer D**
— CP angle has three neurovascular complexes: upper, middle, and lower.

❓ 2. **CP angle surgical anatomy. The FALSE answer is:**
   A. There are three neurovascular complexes.
   B. The upper complex is formed by the trigeminal nerve, SCA, and superior petrosal vein.
   C. The middle complex is formed by the facial nerve, vestibulocochlear nerve, and anterior inferior cerebellar artery.
   D. The lower complex is formed by the glossopharyngeal, vagus, and spinal accessory nerves, as well as the posterior inferior cerebellar artery.
   E. From the foramen of Luschka, a tuft of choroid plexus protrudes and lies above the flocculus.

✅ **Answer E**
— The tuft of choroid plexus lies below the flocculus and is just inferior to the junction of the facial and vestibulocochlear nerves with the brainstem.

❓ 3. **CP angle surgical anatomy. The FALSE answer is:**
   A. CN 7 and CN 8 arise from the pontomedullary junction and course toward the internal acoustic meatus.
   B. CN 7 is inferomedial to CN 8 at the brainstem.
   C. At the lamina cribrosa, CN 7 lies anterosuperior separated from the cochlear nerve by the falciform crest (transverse crest).
   D. The CN 7 is separated from the superior vestibular never by a vertical crest known as Bill's bar.
   E. The inferior vestibular nerve lies anteroinferiorly to CN 7.

✅ **Answer E**
— The inferior vestibular nerve lies posteroinferiorly to CN 7.

17

❓ 4. **Vestibular schwannoma (VS) pathology. The FALSE answer is:**
   A. Most commonly arises from the inferior vestibular nerve.
   B. Originates from the Obersteiner-Redlich zone where central and peripheral myelin meet.
   C. CN 7 runs posterior to the tumor in most instances.
   D. The neurovascular structures lie between a double arachnoid layer.
   E. A loculation of the CSF may present as an arachnoid cyst dorso-lateral to the tumor.

✔️ **Answer C**
━ CN 7 runs anterior to the tumor in most instances.

❓ 5. **VS pathology. The FALSE answer is:**
   A. The relative amounts of Antoni A and B types of tissue determine the tumor consistency.
   B. Grows at a rate of less than 2 mm per year.
   C. Antoni A tissue is compact with elongated bipolar cells and a classical palisading pattern.
   D. Tumors with softer consistency are easier to excise.
   E. Antoni B type of tissue is seen mostly in large tumors and is believed to be the result of ischemia.

✔️ **Answer D**
━ Firm tumors push the surrounding vascular and neural structures that lie stretched over it and thus are easier to excise than softer varieties, which have a tendency to grow all around the neurovascular structures and creep into the crevices.
━ Antoni B tissue has random cells clustered around cystic areas, necrotic tissue, and hemorrhagic tissue.

❓ 6. **VS clinical features. The FALSE answer is:**
   A. Sudden severe hearing loss is due to compression on the cochlear nerve or labyrinthine artery.
   B. Tinnitus is the earliest and most frequent symptom.
   C. Acute presentation may be seen in cases of rapid expansion of the cystic lesion or intratumoral hemorrhage.
   D. The most common vestibular symptom is imbalance with movement of the head.
   E. Unilateral lid lag is an early indication of CN 7 involvement.

✅ **Answer B**

- Hearing loss is the earliest and most frequent symptom, seen in more than 90% of patients. Tinnitus alone is seen in about 30% of patients.

❓ 7. **Hearing loss in VS. The FALSE answer is:**
   A. Higher frequency hearing loss.
   B. Speech discrimination is affected more than pure tone.
   C. It is often preceded by tinnitus.
   D. The recruitment phenomenon is present.
   E. Roll-over phenomenon is often seen.

✅ **Answer D**

- Vestibular schwannoma presents with high-frequency retrocochlear sensorineural hearing loss.
- The recruitment phenomenon is seen in the cochlear type of sensorineural hearing loss.

❓ 8. **Nystagmus seen in VS. The FALSE answer is:**
   A. Nystagmus is usually due to vestibular involvement in the early stages and brainstem involvement in later stages.
   B. The most common nystagmus seen is horizontal jerk nystagmus.
   C. Large tumors may present with Brun's nystagmus.
   D. Brun's nystagmus is a bidirectional nystagmus.
   E. Downbeat nystagmus may be seen.

✅ **Answer E**

- Downbeat nystagmus is seen in patients with Chiari or craniovertebral junction anomalies.
- Brun's nystagmus is a bidirectional nystagmus with high amplitude low-frequency coarse nystagmus ipsilateral to the lesion and low amplitude high-frequency fine nystagmus contralateral to the lesion.
- The most common nystagmus seen is fine horizontal jerk nystagmus directed away from the side of the lesion due to unilateral labyrinthine dysfunction.

❓ 9. **Clinical features of VS. The FALSE answer is:**
   A. Female preponderance with equal male-female predilection in children.
   B. Bimodal age distribution.

17

C. The sensory features of CN 5 and CN 7 appear before the motor features of CN 5 and CN 7.
D. The trigeminal nerve is involved when the tumor reaches extra-canalicular size of 3 cm.
E. The most common abnormality due to involvement of CN 5 is impaired corneal reflex.

✓ **Answer B**

— Most vestibular schwannomas are present between the fourth and sixth decades and do not have a bimodal age distribution.

❓ 10. **Extent of the tumor in VS. The FALSE answer is:**
A. Trigeminal involvement indicates superior extension up to the tentorium and petrous apex.
B. Intracranial hypertension indicates medial extension up to the brainstem.
C. Lower cranial nerve involvement indicates inferior extension down to the cerebellomedullary cistern.
D. Trigeminal involvement indicates tumor >2 cm in size.
E. Hydrocephalus with intracranial hypertension occurs when tumor size is >4 cm.

✓ **Answer D**

— Trigeminal involvement indicates tumor > 3 cm in size.

❓ 11. **Neuro-otological workup in VS. The FALSE answer is:**
A. Level of hearing impairment helps in deciding the course of management.
B. Modified Gardner and Robertson classification for hearing loss is the most common grading system used.
C. Bekesy audiometry and speech discrimination scores are used to classify hearing loss by modified Gardner and Robertson Grading.
D. Serviceable hearing is defined as pure tone loss of less than 50 dB and speech discrimination score greater than 50 % (50-50 rule).
E. Aidable ear is defined as pure tone loss of less than 70 dB and speech discrimination score greater than 70%.

✅ **Answer C**
- Pure tone, and not Bekesy audiometry, is used to classify hearing loss.
- Electronystagmography assesses the superior vestibular nerve.
- Vestibular-evoked myogenic potential assesses the inferior vestibular nerve.

❓ 12. **Imaging in VS. The FALSE answer is:**
  A. In the pre-CT era, the Stenvers view on X-ray was most commonly used as it showed the canal and meatus in actual form and size in one film.
  B. The trumpeted internal acoustic meatus sign implies a widening of the porus acusticus from an intracanalicular tumor.
  C. The ice cream cone appearance is seen when tumor grows in the extra-meatal space.
  D. Solid portions of the tumor are usually isodense, while cystic portions are hypodense on plain imaging.
  E. About 30% of tumors show ring enhancement.

✅ **Answer A**
- The transorbital Caldwell view on X-ray showed the canal and meatus in actual form and size in one film.
- In the Stenvers view, the internal acoustic canal is visualized in a shortened form.
- Other views used are Schuller and Towne.

❓ 13. **Imaging in VS. The FALSE answer is:**
  A. Contrast-enhanced CT along with BAER has a sensitivity of 99% in the diagnosis.
  B. A prominent jugular tubercle may be mistaken for a tumor on contrast-enhanced CT.
  C. Internal acoustic canal widening is the earliest sign of tumor growth on MRI.
  D. Tractography and diffusion tensor imaging help to identify the location and course of facial nerve preoperatively.
  E. On enhanced MRI, Antoni type A tissue enhances homogeneously, while type B tissue shows irregular enhancement.

✅ **Answer C**
- Focal swelling and CN 8 obscuration are the earliest signs of tumor growth on MRI.
- IAC widening is the earliest sign of tumor growth on CT.

17

❓ 14. **Differential diagnosis of VS. The FALSE answer:**
   A. In meningiomas, CN 7 is involved earlier in the course of the disease.
   B. Epidermoid generally presents with early features of intracranial hypertension.
   C. Irritative features of trigeminal neuralgia are seen in the CP angle epidermoid.
   D. Tumor passing from the posterior fossa to the middle fossa through the tentorial incisura is highly suggestive of epidermoid.
   E. In trigeminal schwannoma, the involvement of motor features of CN 5 is present early in the course of the disease.

✅ **Answer B**
▬ Epidermoid generally presents with multiple nerve involvement and very late features of intracranial hypertension.

❓ 15. **Indications for conservative management in VS. The FALSE answer is:**
   A. Elderly with comorbidities and with minimal/no life-threatening symptoms.
   B. Small tumor with only hearing and minimal neurological symptoms.
   C. In patients with NF2 without mass effect and intracranial hypertension and with preserved hearing.
   D. Patient choice.
   E. Non-growing tumors.

✅ **Answer E**
▬ Conservative management carries a significant risk of hearing loss even in non-growing tumors; hence, when hearing preservation is considered, earlier intervention is indicated.

❓ 16. **Poor prognosticators of hearing preservation in VS. The FALSE answer is:**
   A. Abnormal auditory brainstem response latency.
   B. Inferior vestibular nerve origin and fundus opacification.
   C. Hypotension caused by trigeminocardiac reflex (TCR).
   D. Intraoperative wave V latency of 1 ms.
   E. Intraoperative wave II latency of 2 ms.

✅ **Answer E**

- Changes in waves I, III, and V are most significant. Decreased amplitudes and/or increased inter-peak latencies should warn the surgeon of impending hearing loss.
- TCR is defined as a decrease in mean arterial blood pressure of $\geq 20\%$ associated with bradycardia of < 60 bpm after handling CN 5 during surgery.

❓ 17. **Indications for surgery in VS. The FALSE answer is:**
   A. Large tumor with brainstem compression or hydrocephalus.
   B. Cystic tumor.
   C. Age < 50 years.
   D. Complete unilateral hearing loss.
   E. With NF2 and mass effect.

✅ **Answer D**

- Hearing loss does not guide the surgery for VS although it may direct the surgeon to prefer one approach over the other especially when the involved side is the only hearing ear.
- Patients with vestibular symptoms due to the tumor have a progressively declining quality of life and warrant surgical intervention.

❓ 18. **Retromastoid suboccipital approach for VS. The FALSE answer is:**
   A. Good exposure with direct visualization of major CP angle vessels.
   B. Option to preserve CN 7 and 8 function.
   C. Familiarity and preference among neurosurgeons.
   D. Complete exposure of IAC contents.
   E. Risk of cerebellar retraction injury, especially in large tumors.

✅ **Answer D**

- The retromastoid approach allows for incomplete exposure of IAC contents in comparison with a middle cranial fossa approach, which provides better IAC decompression.

❓ 19. **Middle cranial fossa approach for VS. The FALSE answer is:**
   A. Indicated in large tumors.
   B. Low morbidity due to extradural subtemporal dissection.
   C. Early exposure of CN 7.
   D. Limited access to the posterior fossa.
   E. Risk of seizures from temporal lobe injury.

17

✅ **Answer A**
- Indicated in small laterally placed tumors.

❓ 20. **Translabyrinthine approach for VS. The FALSE answer is:**
   A. Indicated when hearing preservation (HP) is not possible.
   B. Extracranial approach, hence low morbidity.
   C. Early identification of CN 7 allows for nerve repair in the primary procedure itself.
   D. Lesser chances of postoperative CSF leak and meningitis as compared to other approaches.
   E. Contraindicated in middle ear infection, perforated tympanic membrane, and in patients with externalized mastoid cavity.

✅ **Answer D**
- With this approach, there is less cerebellar/brainstem retraction but higher chances of postoperative CSF leak and meningitis as compared to other approaches.

❓ 21. **Surgical management for VS. The FALSE answer is:**
   A. The transcanal approach exposes IAC through EAC and is therefore preferred by ENT surgeons.
   B. The suboccipital translabyrinthine approach allows for very limited exposure of the tumor.
   C. The retrolabyrinthine approach exposes the cerebellopontine angle space anterior to the sigmoid sinus hence limiting exposure to the tumor.
   D. The subtemporal transtentorial approach is an intradural procedure and requires tentorial incision behind the petrosal sinus for tumor exposure.
   E. With the subtemporal transtentorial approach, small intracanalicular tumors cannot be reached and are not suitable for inferiorly extending tumors.

✅ **Answer B**
- The suboccipital translabyrinthine approach overcomes the disadvantages of both the retromastoid suboccipital and translabyrinthine approaches by allowing to work on both sides of the sigmoid sinus and thus allows for a wide exposure to the tumor.

? 22. Postoperative complications in VS. The FALSE answer is:
   A. Mortality of 1% in small tumors and 5% in large tumors.
   B. CSF leak occurs in about 10% of patients.
   C. Facial nerve preservation in <40%.
   D. HP in about 40%.
   E. GTR is possible in more than 90%.

✓ Answer C
— Anatomical preservation of facial nerve is reported in >90% with >50% functional preservation. The middle cranial fossa approach allows for better preservation of CN 7 than the retromastoid suboccipital approach (2).

? 23. Facial nerve preservation in VS. The FALSE answer is:
   A. In cystic lesions, CN 7 is better preserved.
   B. Dissection should always proceed from known to unknown structures.
   C. Excessive cerebellar retraction leads to increased tension on CN 7.
   D. In the event of nerve transection, primary end-to-end anastomosis, with or without glue or the use of cable graft, may be attempted.
   E. Injury to CN 7 results from trauma, stretching, thermal/cautery injury, or vascular injury.

✓ Answer A
— In cystic lesions, nerve preservation is worse due to adhesions.

? 24. Postoperative facial nerve weakness in VS. The FALSE answer is:
   A. Nimodipine and hydroxyethyl starch may be used.
   B. Lateral tarsorrhaphy for orbicularis oculi and temporal fascia sling may be done.
   C. The incidence of facial nerve weakness is more than 30% of patients.
   D. Re-animation technique can be utilized if there is no sign of improvement in 12-18 months.
   E. As a secondary procedure, reconstruction with hypoglossal, spinal accessory, or phrenic nerves has been described.

✓ Answer C
— In the hands of an experienced surgeon and with the use of intraoperative monitoring facial nerve weakness has been reported in less than 10% of patients (2).

❓ 25. **Hearing preservation (HP) in VS surgery. The FALSE answer is:**
   A. BAER prognosticates the chance of HP.
   B. There is approximately a 30% chance of HP in tumors with extracanalicular extension of <5 mm.
   C. HP is better in cystic lesions than in solid lesions.
   D. HP is better via the middle cranial fossa approach than with the retromastoid suboccipital approach in small tumors (<15 mm).
   E. Delayed postoperative hearing loss may also be seen.

✅ **Answer B**
- There is approximately 60% chance of HP in tumors with extracanalicular extension of <5 mm; 35% HP in tumors with extracanalicular extension of 5–15 mm and very poor HP when extension is >20 mm.
- Delayed postoperative hearing loss is hypothesized to be due to a combination of the effect of edema from cerebellar retraction, disturbance in the microcirculation in the vasa nervosum, or increased permeability of endo-neuronal vessels after mechanical compression and exhaustion of residual neurotransmitters over time.

❓ 26. **Gamma knife surgery (GKS) for VS. The FALSE answer is:**
   A. Indicated only in young patients with tumor size < 3 cm.
   B. HP is possible in up to 90% of intracanalicular tumors.
   C. Limited to tumor volume of < 19 cc.
   D. The marginal dose is 12.6 Gy and the mean maximal dose to the tumor center is 25.4 Gy.
   E. The biggest disadvantage is that it may take up to 18 to 24 months for radiological improvement.

✅ **Answer A**
- Indicated in tumors < 3 cm regardless of age or comorbidities.
- Post-GKS facial palsy incidence is < 2%.

❓ 27. **Cystic VS. The FALSE answer is:**
   A. Acute expansion of cystic component may cause sudden severe hearing loss.
   B. Patients have a shorter duration of symptoms.
   C. Postoperative hearing preservation is better than in solid tumors.
   D. Rarely shows IAC enlargement on imaging.
   E. Radiosurgery shows better results than microsurgery.

✅ **Answer E**

— Surgery shows better results than radiosurgery. Also, cyst formation is still predictive of worse surgical outcomes compared with solid tumors.

❓ 28. **Nonsurgical management of VS. The FALSE answer is:**
   A. In VS with NF2, bevacizumab and anti-VEGF monoclonal antibodies have shown promising results.
   B. Cyberknife may be used (18-21 Gy in three fractions).
   C. Fractionated multidose radiotherapy is preferred over single-shot radiosurgery.
   D. Fractionated radiotherapy is used in a dose of 1.8 Gy for 5/7 days per week for 6 weeks.
   E. LINAC uses a dose of 12.5 Gy.

✅ **Answer C**

— The most commonly used radiosurgery is single-shot stereotactic radiosurgery, especially in smaller tumors or for residual tumors.

❓ 29. **Trigeminal schwannomas. The FALSE answer is:**
   A. More commonly presents with facial hypoesthesia than pain.
   B. Since it often extends above and below the tentorium it is also known as an "hourglass tumor."
   C. Facial hypoesthesia associated with dissociated sensory loss is commonly seen.
   D. The middle cranial fossa approach with the Kawase approach is the most commonly used.
   E. Other surgical approaches are retrosigmoid and pre-sigmoid.

✅ **Answer C**

— Facial hypoesthesia associated with dissociated sensory loss is seen in intramedullary cervical spinal tumors, which forms an important differential diagnosis.

❓ 30. **Nonvestibular schwannomas. The FALSE answer is:**
   A. Incidence: CN 5 (40%) > CN 7 (23%) > lower cranial nerves (20%).
   B. Lower cranial nerve (LCN) schwannomas usually present as a jugular foramen mass.
   C. Among LCN schwannomas, those from CN 9 are most common, followed by CN 10 and CN 11.

17

    D. Trochlear nerve schwannoma arises most commonly from the pre-cavernous segment of the nerve.

    E. Surgery is the mainstay of all jugular foramen schwannomas irrespective of age.

✅ **Answer E**

▬ Most jugular foramen schwannomas are managed conservatively or with stereotactic radiosurgery, especially in older patients who cannot tolerate rapid change in cranial nerve function.

▬ Oculomotor and abducens nerve schwannomas arise from both cisternal and cavernous segments.

❓ 31. **Facial nerve schwannoma. The FALSE answer is:**

    A. The most common site of origin is the geniculate ganglion and the adjoining labyrinthine segment.

    B. Gradually progressive facial paresis and hearing deficit are the most common symptoms.

    C. Hearing loss is exclusively sensorineural.

    D. It may be differentiated from VS by the eccentricity of the tumor mass to the axis of the IAC.

    E. Microsurgical excision with end-to-end anastomosis with or without interposition cable graft is the surgery of choice.

✅ **Answer C**

▬ Both conductive and sensorineural hearing loss may be seen depending on the site of the tumor.

▬ With end-to-end anastomosis, improvement beyond House-Brackmann grade III is rarely seen postoperatively.

❓ 32. **Optic nerve glioma. The FALSE answer is:**

    A. Common in children below 10 years of age.

    B. Gliomas account for two-thirds of optic nerve tumors.

    C. Chiasmal tumors are more common than optic nerve tumors.

    D. Malignant transformation is more common in children than in adults.

    E. More commonly occurs in association with NF1 than with NF2.

✅ **Answer D**

▬ Malignant transformation is more common in adults than in children.

❓ 33. Optic nerve glioma. The FALSE answer is:
   A. Spontaneous regression has been reported and manifests either as shrinkage of the tumor size or a change in signal intensity on imaging.
   B. The wait-and-watch approach is applied to patients with preserved vision, minimal proptosis, and those with NF1.
   C. Should be treated only if the tumor or symptoms are progressive as surgery may lead to further visual diminution.
   D. Chemotherapy for younger children and radiotherapy for older patients are effective in achieving long-term tumor control.
   E. Post-therapy, diabetes insipidus is the most common endocrine abnormality.

✅ Answer E
— Post-therapy, growth hormone deficiency is the most common endocrine abnormality.

❓ 34. Optic nerve glioma. The FALSE answer is:
   A. Pilocytic astrocytoma is the most common histopathological variety.
   B. Fat-suppressed T1W images with contrast help in better delineation of the tumor tissue.
   C. The "Tram-track" sign on MRI refers to a hyperintense core in T1W images surrounded by a lower signal intensity with exact opposite features on T2W MRI.
   D. Cisplatin-based regimens are mostly used for chemotherapy.
   E. Radiotherapy is given as 45-50 Gy in 2 Gy daily fractions to the tumor and the surrounding 10 mm margin.

✅ Answer D
— Carboplatin-based regimens are mostly used for chemotherapy.

❓ 35. Optic nerve glioma. The FALSE answer is:
   A. Children may present with diencephalic syndrome of infancy due to dysregulation in the leptin-ghrelin system.
   B. Spasmus nutans may be seen in a few patients.
   C. Primary optic atrophy is seen in 60% of patients.

    D. Hypothalamic symptoms are mostly seen in NF1 optic pathway gliomas.

    E. Chiasmal gliomas are often unable to be differentiated from hypothalamic gliomas and are therefore clubbed as hypothalamic-chiasmal gliomas.

✅ **Answer D**

— Hypothalamic symptoms are more common in non-NF1 optic pathway gliomas.

❓ 36. **Optic nerve glioma: indications for surgery. The FALSE answer is:**
    A. Biopsy has no role.
    B. Disfiguring or painful proptosis.
    C. Total vision loss.
    D. Excision of chiasmal exophytic mass.
    E. To decrease mass effect.

✅ **Answer A**

— Biopsy may be done for atypical imaging findings.

❓ 37. **Surgical approaches for chiasmal hypothalamic gliomas. The FALSE answer is:**
    A. Pterional.
    B. Anterior subfrontal.
    C. Trans-nasal trans-sphenoidal endoscopic surgery.
    D. Anterior interhemispheric trans-lamina terminalis.
    E. Endoscopic transventricular.

✅ **Answer C**

— Interhemispheric transcallosal transventricular approach is used. Trans-nasal trans-sphenoidal endoscopic surgery would not be useful in the complete excision of large tumors.

Bibliography

1. Samii M, Gerganov V, Samii M, Gerganov V. History of cerebellopontine angle surgery. In: Surgery of cerebellopontine lesions. Berlin, Heidelberg: Springer; 2013. p. 1–8.

2. Rahimpour S, Zomorodi AR, Codd PJ, Krucoff MO, Friedman AH, Gonzalez LF. Approaches to the Cerebellopontine Angle. In: Surgery of the cerebellopontine angle. Cham: Springer International Publishing; 2023. p. 61–70.

3. Yuguang L, Chengyuan W, Meng L, Shugan Z, Wandong S, Gang L, Xingang L. Neuroendoscopic anatomy and surgery of the cerebellopontine angle. J Clin Neurosci. 2005;12(3):256–60.
4. Akamatsu Y, Murakami K, Watanabe M, Jokura H, Tominaga T. Malignant peripheral nerve sheath tumor arising from benign vestibular schwannoma treated by gamma knife radiosurgery after two previous surgeries: a case report with surgical and pathological observations. World Neurosurg. 2010;73(6):751–4.
5. Brodhun M, Stahn V, Harder A. Pathogenesis and molecular pathology of vestibular schwannoma. HNO. 2017;65:362–72.
6. Huang X, Xu J, Xu M, Zhou LF, Zhang R, Lang L, Xu Q, Zhong P, Chen M, Wang Y, Zhang Z. Clinical features of intracranial vestibular schwannomas. Oncol Lett. 2013;5(1):57–62.
7. Lassaletta L, Calvino M, Morales-Puebla JM, Lapunzina P, Rodriguez-De La Rosa L, Varela-Nieto I, Martinez-Glez V. Biomarkers in vestibular schwannoma–associated hearing loss. Front Neurol. 2019;10:978.
8. Lloyd SK, Baguley DM, Butler K, Donnelly N, Moffat DA. Bruns' nystagmus in patients with vestibular schwannoma. Otol Neurotol. 2009;30(5):625–8.
9. Harati A, Scheufler KM, Schultheiss R, Tonkal A, Harati K, Oni P, Deitmer T. Clinical features, microsurgical treatment, and outcome of vestibular schwannoma with brainstem compression. Surg Neurol Int. 2017;8.
10. Li D, Tsimpas A, Germanwala AV. Analysis of vestibular schwannoma size: a literature review on consistency with measurement techniques. Clin Neurol Neurosurg. 2015;138:72–7.
11. Gimsing S. Vestibular schwannoma: when to look for it? J Laryngol Otol. 2010;124(3):258–64.
12. Dang L, Tu NC, Chan EY. Current imaging tools for vestibular schwannoma. Curr Opin Otolaryngol Head Neck Surg. 2020;28(5):302–7.
13. Connor SE. Imaging of the vestibular schwannoma: diagnosis, monitoring, and treatment planning. Neuroimaging Clin. 2021;31(4):451–71.
14. Goldbrunner R, Weller M, Regis J, Lund-Johansen M, Stavrinou P, Reuss D, Evans DG, Lefranc F, Sallabanda K, Falini A, Axon P. EANO guideline on the diagnosis and treatment of vestibular schwannoma. Neuro Oncol. 2020;22(1):31–45.
15. Ferri GG, Modugno GC, Pirodda A, Fioravanti A, Calbucci F, Ceroni AR. Conservative management of vestibular schwannomas: an effective strategy. Laryngoscope. 2008;118(6):951–7.
16. Malhotra PS, Sharma P, Fishman MA, Grumbine FL, Tholey R, Dam VQ, Dasgupta A, Pequignot E, Willcox TO. Clinical, radiographic, and audiometric predictors in conservative management of vestibular schwannoma. Otol Neurotol. 2009;30(4):507–14.
17. Ansari SF, Terry C, Cohen-Gadol AA. Surgery for vestibular schwannomas: a systematic review of complications by approach. Neurosurg Focus. 2012;33(3):E14.
18. Sahu RN, Mehrotra N, Tyagi I, Banerji D, Jain VK, Behari S. Management strategies for bilateral vestibular schwannomas. J Clin Neurosci. 2007;14(8):715–22.
19. Arts HA, Telian SA, El-Kashlan H, Thompson BG. Hearing preservation and facial nerve outcomes in vestibular schwannoma surgery: results using the middle cranial fossa approach. Otol Neurotol. 2006;27(2):234–41.
20. Nickele CM, Akture E, Gubbels SP, Başkaya MK. A stepwise illustration of the translabyrinthine approach to a large cystic vestibular schwannoma. Neurosurg Focus. 2012;33(3):E11.

21. Nicoucar K, Momjian S, Vader JP, De Tribolet N. Surgery for large vestibular schwannomas: how patients and surgeons perceive quality of life. J Neurosurg. 2006;105(2):205–12.

22. Mahboubi H, Ahmed OH, Yau AY, Ahmed YC, Djalilian HR. Complications of surgery for sporadic vestibular schwannoma. Otolaryngol—Head Neck Surg. 2014;150(2):275–81.

23. Yang I, Sughrue ME, Han SJ, Fang S, Aranda D, Cheung SW, Pitts LH, Parsa AT. Facial nerve preservation after vestibular schwannoma Gamma Knife radiosurgery. J Neurooncol. 2009;93:41–8.

24. Samii M, Gerganov V, Samii A. Improved preservation of hearing and facial nerve function in vestibular schwannoma surgery via the retrosigmoid approach in a series of 200 patients. J Neurosurg. 2006;105(4):527–35.

25. Yang I, Aranda D, Han SJ, Chennupati S, Sughrue ME, Cheung SW, Pitts LH, Parsa AT. Hearing preservation after stereotactic radiosurgery for vestibular schwannoma: a systematic review. J Clin Neurosci. 2009;16(6):742–7.

26. Hasegawa T, Kida Y, Kobayashi T, Yoshimoto M, Mori Y, Yoshida J. Long-term outcomes in patients with vestibular schwannomas treated using gamma knife surgery: 10-year follow up. J Neurosurg. 2005;102(1):10–6.

27. Piccirillo E, Wiet MR, Flanagan S, Dispenza F, Giannuzzi A, Mancini F, Sanna M. Cystic vestibular schwannoma: classification, management, and facial nerve outcomes. Otol Neurotol. 2009;30(6):826–34.

28. Arribas L, Chust ML, Menéndez A, Arana E, Vendrell JB, Crispín V, Pesudo C, Mengual JL, Mut A, Arribas M, Guinot JL. Non surgical treatment of vestibular schwannoma. Acta Otorrinolaringol (English Ed). 2015;66(4):185–91.

29. Neff BA, Carlson ML, O'Byrne MM, Van Gompel JJ, Driscoll CL, Link MJ. Trigeminal neuralgia and neuropathy in large sporadic vestibular schwannomas. J Neurosurg. 2017;127(5):992–9.

30. Malone JP, Lee WJ, Levin RJ. Clinical characteristics and treatment outcome for nonvestibular schwannomas of the head and neck. Am J Otolaryngol. 2005;26(2):108–12.

31. Quesnel AM, Santos F. Evaluation and management of facial nerve schwannoma. Otolaryngol Clin North Am. 2018;51(6):1179–92.

32. Shapey J, Danesh-Meyer HV, Kaye AH. Diagnosis and management of optic nerve glioma. J Clin Neurosci. 2011;18(12):1585–91.

33. Mishra MV, Andrews DW, Glass J, Evans JJ, Dicker AP, Shen X, Lawrence YR. Characterization and outcomes of optic nerve gliomas: a population-based analysis. J Neurooncol. 2012;107:591–7.

34. Farazdaghi MK, Katowitz WR, Avery RA. Current treatment of optic nerve gliomas. Curr Opin Ophthalmol. 2019;30(5):356.

35. Nair AG, Pathak RS, Iyer VR, Gandhi RA. Optic nerve glioma: an update. Int Ophthalmol. 2014;34:999–1005.

36. Yilmaz E, Emengen A, Ceylan EC, Cabuk B, Anik I, Ceylan S. Endoscopic transnasal surgery in optic pathway gliomas located in the chiasma-hypothalamic region: case series of ten patients in a single-center experience and endoscopic literature review. Childs Nerv Syst. 2022;38(11):2071–82.

Tumors of Spinal and Peripheral Nerves

Ahmed A. Farag, Mohammed A. Al-Dhahir, Maliya Delawan, and Samer S. Hoz

© The Author(s), under exclusive license to Springer Nature Switzerland AG 2024
S. S. Hoz et al. (eds.), *Surgical Neuro-Oncology*,
https://doi.org/10.1007/978-3-031-53642-7_18

18

? 1. **Tumors involving the peripheral nerve. The FALSE answer is:**
   A. Schwannomas.
   B. Neurofibromas.
   C. Perineurioma.
   D. Malignant teratoma.
   E. Peripheral non-neural sheath tumors.

✓ **Answer E**
— Malignant peripheral nerve sheath tumors (MPNSTs).

? 2. **Peripheral non-neural sheath tumors. The FALSE answer is:**
   A. Lipomas.
   B. Ganglion cysts.
   C. Desmoid tumors.
   D. Ganglioneuromas.
   E. Cavernoma.

✓ **Answer E**
— Cavernomas are not peripheral non-neural sheath tumors.

? 3. **Peripheral nerve sheath tumors (PNSTs). Benign types, 2016 WHO classification. The FALSE answer is:**
   A. Schwannoma (cellular and plexiform).
   B. Melanotic schwannoma.
   C. Neurofibroma (atypical and plexiform).
   D. Neuroma.
   E. Hybrid nerve sheath tumors.

✓ **Answer D**
— Perineurioma.

? 4. **Inherited conditions associated with PNSTs. The FALSE answer is:**
   A. Costello syndrome.
   B. NF1 mostly develops neurofibroma.
   C. NF2 dominantly affects the spine and the cranial nerves.
   D. Schwannomatosis.
   E. Carney complex.

✓ **Answer A**

5. PNSTs: schwannoma incidence. The FALSE answer is:
A. The most common tumors of peripheral nerves.
B. 5% of all soft-tissue tumors.
C. 95% occur sporadically.
D. More common in schwannomatosis than NF2.
E. Can occur in NF1.

Answer D
— More common in NF2 (3%) than schwannomatosis.

6. PNSTs: schwannoma pathology. The FALSE answer is:
A. Benign neoplasms of Schwann cell origin.
B. Displace the nerve fascicle.
C. Large tumors have an eccentric position in relation to the nerve.
D. Well-encapsulated.
E. Rapidly growing.

Answer E
— Slow growing.

7. PNSTs: schwannoma histologic features. The FALSE answer is:
A. Uniphasic architecture.
B. Spindle cells.
C. Hyaline vessel walls.
D. Nuclear palisading (Verocay bodies).
E. Fibrous capsule with displaced parent nerve fascicles.

Answer A
— Biphasic architecture (Antoni A and Antoni B areas).

8. Schwannoma tumor cells are immunopositive for the following. The FALSE answer is:
A. Desmin.
B. Podoplanin.
C. Calretinin.
D. SOX10.
E. Leu-7.

Answer A
— Tumor cells are strongly immunopositive for S-100.

18

❓ 9. **Schwannoma: clinical variants. The FALSE answer is:**
   A. Conventional.
   B. Cellular.
   C. Plexiform.
   D. Melanotic schwannomas.
   E. Hypomelanotic.

✅ **Answer E**

❓ 10. **Cellular schwannoma: clues to diagnosis. Includes all. The FALSE answer is:**
   A. A well-formed capsule containing lymphoid aggregates.
   B. Foamy histiocyte aggregate.
   C. Diffuse strong S-100 protein.
   D. Pericellular collagen III expression.
   E. Increased mitotic activity.

✅ **Answer D**
— Pericellular collagen IV expression.

❓ 11. **Cellular schwannoma behavior. The FALSE answer is:**
   A. Local recurrence seldom occurs.
   B. Lacks malignant potential.
   C. Never metastasizes.
   D. Occasionally, locally destructive.
   E. Better prognosis than plexiform.

✅ **Answer A**
— May have a high local recurrence rate (5–40%).

❓ 12. **Plexiform schwannoma: features. The FALSE answer is:**
   A. Usually occurs in superficial locations.
   B. Defined by an intraneural nodular pattern of growth.
   C. Deeply localized lesions are better than superficial ones.
   D. May show widespread S-100 protein.
   E. Collagen IV immunoreactivity is a reassuring sign.

✅ **Answer C**
— Lesions that arise in deep anatomic locations are more problematic as they demonstrate increased cellularity and mitotic activity.

❓ 13. **Melanotic schwannoma: features. The FALSE answer is:**
   A. <1% of all nerve sheath tumors.
   B. A predilection for spinal nerves.
   C. Potentially benign.
   D. Epithelioid cells with marked accumulation of melanin.
   E. Psammoma bodies are present in 50% of cases with Carney complex.

✅ **Answer C**
— Melanotic schwannomas are malignant neoplasms and can metastasize.

❓ 14. **PNSTs: schwannoma clinical picture. The FALSE answer is:**
   A. Painless, firm, round masses.
   B. Tinel's sign on percussion.
   C. The mass can be moved laterally but not longitudinally.
   D. Neurological function mostly remains intact.
   E. Loss of function from smaller schwannomas is common.

✅ **Answer E**
— Loss of function from smaller benign schwannomas is rare unless a prior biopsy had injured the involved nerve or an unsuccessful attempt at tumor removal had been performed.

❓ 15. **Schwannomas. Syndromic cases: features. The FALSE answer is:**
   A. NF1 schwannomas involve large peripheral nerve trunks.
   B. Schwannomatosis has multiple nonvestibular, non-cutaneous schwannomas.
   C. The hallmark of NF2 is the presence of bilateral vestibular schwannomas.
   D. The most common symptom of schwannomatosis is pain (68%).
   E. Nonvestibular intracranial schwannoma is the most common lesion in schwannomatosis.

✅ **Answer E**
— Peripheral schwannomas are the most common lesion in schwannomatosis (89%).

❓ 16. **Schwannoma features on MR neurography (MRN). The FALSE answer is:**
   A. The tail sign can be eccentrically located.
   B. Hyperintense to skeletal muscle on T1WI.

18

    C. Heterogeneously hyperintense on T2WI.
    D. Variable contrast enhancement.
    E. Can show target sign.

✅ **Answer B**
— Isointense to skeletal muscle on T1WI.

❓ 17. **Schwannoma features on MRN. The FALSE answer is:**
    A. Cystic changes.
    B. Hemorrhage.
    C. Calcification.
    D. Fascicular sign.
    E. Split muscle sign.

✅ **Answer E**
— Split fat sign.

❓ 18. **Neurofibromas: incidence. The FALSE answer is:**
    A. Account for 5% of all benign soft-tissue tumors.
    B. Occurring sporadically in 95% of cases.
    C. Young to middle age.
    D. Occur at older age with NF1.
    E. There is no sex predilection.

✅ **Answer D**
— Occur at younger age with NF1.

❓ 19. **Neurofibromas: general features. The FALSE answer is:**
    A. Slow-growing lesion.
    B. The growth pattern is either intraneural or diffuse infiltrative.
    C. Clinically can be localized, diffuse, or plexiform.
    D. Localized type is common at superficial cutaneous sites.
    E. Diffuse neurofibromas usually occur in major nerve trunks.

✅ **Answer E**
— Diffuse neurofibromas usually occur in the head and neck region.

❓ 20. **Neurofibromas: pathology. The FALSE answer is:**
    A. Are encapsulated tumors.
    B. Result in a fusiform expansion of the nerve trunk.

C. Involve the cross-section of a nerve fascicle.

D. Cut surface is tan-white and glistening.

E. No surgical cleavage plane between the normal nerve fibers.

✅ **Answer A**

— Are unencapsulated tumors.

❓ 21. **Neurofibromas: histologic features. The FALSE answer is:**

A. Proliferation of all elements of peripheral nerves.

B. Spindle cells dispersed in fibromyxoid stroma.

C. Schwann cells with wire-like collagen fibrils.

D. Verocay bodies.

E. Intense staining with reticulin.

✅ **Answer D**

— No Verocay bodies, nuclear palisading, or hyalinized thickening of vessel walls.

❓ 22. **Neurofibroma cells can be immunopositive for the following. The FALSE answer is:**

A. Factor XIII.

B. CD34.

C. SOX10.

D. Desmin.

E. Collagen type IV.

✅ **Answer D**

— Neurofibroma cells are negative for desmin. They are also immunopositive for S-100; however, they stain poorly compared with schwannomas.

❓ 23. **Neurofibromas: MRN features. The FALSE answer is:**

A. Tail sign can be centrally located.

B. Target sign.

C. Split fat sign.

D. Fascicular sign.

E. Can differentiate between neurofibroma and schwannoma.

✅ **Answer E**

— MRN does not reliably differentiate between neurofibroma and schwannoma.

18

? 24. Plexiform neurofibroma: general features. The FALSE answer is:
    A. The rarest form of neurofibroma.
    B. Almost always associated with NF1.
    C. Usually affects major nerve trunks.
    D. Grossly described as a bag of worms.
    E. Malignant degeneration never occurs.

✓ Answer E
— The plexiform neurofibroma is a recognized precursor for malignant peripheral nerve sheath tumor (MPNST) in NF1 patients.

? 25. Neurofibroma: clinical picture. The FALSE answer is:
    A. Tend to present with pain.
    B. Loss of function is rare compared with schwannomas.
    C. Tinel's sign is usually present.
    D. Can be moved laterally but not longitudinally.
    E. Neurological deficit may result from prior biopsy or attempted removal.

✓ Answer B
— Loss of function is common compared with schwannomas.

? 26. Peripheral nerve sheath tumors (PNSTs): rapid progression of size. The FALSE answer is:
    A. Can be due to cyst formation.
    B. Can be due to hemorrhage.
    C. May lead to malignant transformation.
    D. Occur infrequently.
    E. More in sporadic cases.

✓ Answer E
— More common in syndromic (NF1) cases than sporadic cases due to the increased incidence of the plexiform type in NF1.

? 27. Perineuriomas: general features. The FALSE answer is:
    A. Two distinct types: intraneural and soft tissue.
    B. Soft-tissue perineuriomas almost always lack an associated nerve.
    C. The intraneural type is characterized by the solitary expansion of peripheral nerves.

D. Histologically, the intraneural type shows "pseudo-onion bulbs."
E. Histologically, soft-tissue perineuriomas show ovoid cells with thick processes.

✅ **Answer E**
— Histologically, soft-tissue perineuriomas show slender cells with very delicate, overlapping elongated cellular processes, arranged in loose fascicles.

❓ 28. **Perineuriomas are immunonegative for the following. The FALSE answer is:**
A. S-100 protein.
B. Desmin.
C. Vimentin.
D. Muscle-specific actin.
E. CD34.

✅ **Answer C**
— **Perineurioma** cells express **vimentin** and epithelial membrane antigen (**EMA**).

❓ 29. **Hybrid nerve sheath tumors (HNSTs): general features. The FALSE answer is:**
A. Neurofibroma/perineurioma.
B. Schwannoma/perineurioma.
C. Neurofibroma/schwannoma.
D. Are almost exclusively in the digits and extremities.
E. Tend to be solitary in nature.

✅ **Answer E**
— HNSTs are typically multifocal.

❓ 30. **MPNST: incidence. The FALSE answer is:**
A. Sporadic cases: 40–50 years of age.
B. In NF1: 60 years of age.
C. 5–10% of all soft-tissue sarcomas.
D. 50% are associated with NF1.
E. Up to 11% arise in the post-irradiation setting.

✅ **Answer B**
— In NF1, MPNST is usually diagnosed 10 years earlier than in sporadic cases.

❓ 31. **MPNST: general pathology. The FALSE answer is:**
   A. Can arise from extraneural soft tissue.
   B. Epithelioid MPNST.
   C. MPNST with perineurial differentiation.
   D. A gain in distal 17q and a loss of 13q14-q21 are common.
   E. The most common mesenchymal element identified in MPNSTs is osteosarcoma.

✅ **Answer E**
— The most common heterogeneous mesenchymal element identified in MPNSTs is rhabdomyosarcoma (so-called malignant triton tumor).

❓ 32. **MPNST: histology. The FALSE answer is:**
   A. Absence of necrosis.
   B. Fascicles of alternating cellularity.
   C. Palisades.
   D. Rosette-like arrangements.
   E. Subendothelial accentuation of tumor cells.

✅ **Answer A**
— Large areas of geographic-like necrosis.

❓ 33. **MPNST: gross pathology. The FALSE answer is:**
   A. MPNSTs typically have a true capsule.
   B. Cut surface can be tan, fleshy, necrotic, or hemorrhagic.
   C. Cut surface can be firm and fibrous.
   D. Depends on the histologic grade.
   E. Is usually >5 cm at presentation.

✅ **Answer A**
— MPNSTs typically have a pseudocapsule.

❓ 34. **MPNST immunohistochemistry may include the following. The FALSE answer is:**
   A. S-100 protein is expressed in almost all cases.
   B. Most are immunopositive for TP53.
   C. EGFR amplification.
   D. Deletions of NF1.
   E. Deletions of CDKN2A.

✅ **Answer A**
- S-100 protein is expressed in 50–70% of cases.
- **MPNST** lacks a diagnostic cytogenic signature.

❓ 35. **Epithelioid MPNST: features. The FALSE answer is:**
   A. Rare subtype of MPNST.
   B. Common in deep sites.
   C. Are typically diffuse.
   D. Express S-100 protein strongly.
   E. Most arise in preexisting benign schwannomas.

✅ **Answer B**
- Common in superficial sites.

❓ 36. **MPNST: clinical picture. The FALSE answer is:**
   A. A rapid increase in size.
   B. Painless lesions.
   C. Rapid symptom progression.
   D. New-onset neurological deficit.
   E. Autonomic dysfunction.

✅ **Answer B**
- New or intensified pain.

❓ 37. **MPNST: MRN features. The FALSE answer is:**
   A. Early arterial enhancement on dynamic MRI.
   B. Irregular or round in shape.
   C. Enhance homogeneously.
   D. Areas of hemorrhage or necrosis.
   E. Perilesional edema.

✅ **Answer C**
- MRI features include T1 and T2 heterogeneity, heterogeneous enhancement, and lack of a targetoid appearance.

❓ 38. **MPNSTs may arise in the following. The FALSE answer is:**
   A. Plexiform neurofibromas.
   B. Ganglioneuromas.
   C. Ganglioglioma.
   D. Phaeochromocytomas.
   E. Schwannomas.

18

✅ **Answer C**
— Ganglioneuroblastomas.

❓ 39. **EMG and NCS roles. The FALSE answer is:**
    A. Localization of the lesion.
    B. Detect subclinical deficits.
    C. Document baseline function.
    D. No role in plexus lesions.
    E. Repeated postoperatively to assess outcome.

✅ **Answer D**
— EMG and NCS are especially useful in plexus-level tumors involving multiple nerves to the extremities to localize involved nerves.

❓ 40. **Nerve tumor surgery: general principles. The FALSE answer is:**
    A. Wide exposure.
    B. Muscle relaxants should be used.
    C. An operating microscope is often required.
    D. Loupe magnification may be used.
    E. Neurophysiological monitoring is mandatory.

✅ **Answer B**
— The use of muscle relaxants must be avoided.

❓ 41. **Nerve tumor surgery: exposure. The FALSE answer is:**
    A. The skin incision is 2–4 cm both proximal and distal to the tumor.
    B. Dissection is performed through the subcutaneous tissues.
    C. Exposure of the nerve begins within the tumor.
    D. Identify the normal proximal and distal limits of the tumor.
    E. The tumor is isolated from the surrounding neurovascular structures.

✅ **Answer C**
— Exposure of the nerve begins within an area of normal anatomy.

❓ 42. **Nerve tumor surgery: tumor dissection. The FALSE answer is:**
    A. A nerve stimulator helps identify a fascicular entry points.
    B. An afascicular dissection plane is established by gently elevating and separating the fascicles from the tumor capsule.

C. Internal neurolysis is not required.

D. Internal debulking of the tumor with an ultrasonic aspirator may facilitate dissection in very large tumors.

E. Meticulous hemostasis is of paramount importance.

✅ **Answer C**

— Internal neurolysis may be required to identify the fascicles coursing over the tumor.

❓ 43. **Schwannoma surgery: general considerations. The FALSE answer is:**

A. Nonfunctioning single fascicles entering and exiting a schwannoma may need to be divided to remove the tumor.

B. Most schwannomas are removed piecemeal.

C. It is not necessary to remove the tumor capsule of schwannomas as it is not associated with tumor recurrence.

D. Involved and uninvolved fascicles at both the proximal and distal poles are identified by interfascicular dissection, intraoperative stimulation, and recording.

E. Wound closure is performed in layers with care taken not to entrap nerves in a tight compartment.

✅ **Answer B**

— Most schwannomas can be rolled out of their capsule and removed en bloc.

❓ 44. **Neurofibroma surgery: general considerations. The FALSE answer is:**

A. Fascicles enlarged by neurofibromas are often still functioning, and removal of the tumor inevitably requires the sacrifice of one or more fascicles.

B. Nerve grafting should be considered on occasions when a significant fascicle is sacrificed.

C. The sural nerve commonly serves as the donor nerve.

D. The surgical goal in the plexiform type is total excision.

E. In the plexiform type, frozen sections should be obtained to determine whether a malignancy is present.

✅ **Answer D**

— The surgical goal in the plexiform type is often debulking to alleviate symptoms caused by neural compression.

18

❓ 45. **MPNST management: general considerations. The FALSE answer is:**
   A. In localized disease, complete surgical excision with clear margins is the treatment of choice.
   B. Resectability rates depend on the age of the patient.
   C. Wide resection often requires complete en bloc resection of major nerves and acceptance of potentially significant functional loss.
   D. Postop radiotherapy can reduce local recurrence.
   E. Multidisciplinary team management is mandatory.

✅ **Answer B**
   — Resectability rates depend on location.
   — Resectability ranges from 20% (paraspinal) to 95% (extremity).

❓ 46. **Surgery for MPNSTs of the brachial plexus. The FALSE answer is:**
   A. Excision of tumors may result in unpredictable neurological deficits.
   B. Good three-dimensional clearance is mandatory for a successful outcome.
   C. May result in no change or improvement in pain or weakness.
   D. Routine nodal dissection is not indicated.
   E. Resection of the sciatic, peroneal, or tibial nerves should not be done.

✅ **Answer E**
   — Resection of the sciatic, peroneal, or tibial nerves may be carried out as necessary with acceptable functional deficits that may be managed with appropriate rehabilitation.

❓ 47. **Surgery for extremity MPNSTs: amputation. The FALSE answer is:**
   A. In most cases, **amputation** is required for complete resection.
   B. Indicated when a wide excision is not feasible with a compromised limb function.
   C. Indicated for recurrence after apparently adequate excision.
   D. Both amputation and a less radical tumor excision may lead to comparable survival rates.
   E. A multimodality approach favoring limb salvage is advisable.

✅ **Answer A**
   — In most cases, a complete resection may be accomplished with limb preservation.

❓ 48. Brachial plexus tumor: location and approach. The FALSE answer is:

A. An anterior subclavicular approach for tumors on most roots and trunks.

B. An infraclavicular approach for tumors on cords and distal elements.

C. A posterior approach for tumors within spinal foramina.

D. The posterior approach for a residual or recurrent tumor or after radiotherapy.

E. A posterior approach for C8-T1 roots and the lower trunk.

✅ Answer A

━ An anterior supraclavicular approach for tumors on most roots and trunks.

❓ 49. Radiotherapy for MPNSTs. The FALSE answer is:

A. May be administered intraoperatively.

B. A cumulative dose of >60 Gy is required to achieve local control.

C. Has not been demonstrated to improve survival.

D. Brachytherapy may be an effective treatment in combination with external beam radiotherapy for local control.

E. Used for high-grade MPNSTs only.

✅ Answer E

━ The Oncology Consensus Group, as part of a uniform treatment policy for MPNSTs, recommends adjuvant radiotherapy for "intermediate- to high-grade lesions and for low-grade tumors after a marginal excision."

❓ 50. Chemotherapy for MPNSTs. The FALSE answer is:

A. MPNSTs remain largely insensitive to chemotherapy.

B. Its role is mainly confined to the treatment of systemic disease.

C. Can be administered in both the preoperative and postoperative settings.

D. Preoperative neoadjuvant chemotherapy may reduce tumor size.

E. Monotherapy is favored to avoid myelotoxicity.

18

✅ Answer E

— The recently reported SARC006 phase II trial conducted by the Sarcoma Alliance for Research Through Collaboration (SARC) evaluated the role of chemotherapy with doxorubicin, ifosfamide, and etoposide in 48 locally advanced metastatic MPNST patients. It revealed encouraging disease stabilization rates with responses accruing from neoadjuvant chemotherapy that rendered subsequent local therapy feasible, in most patients with localized disease (Widemann et al. 2013).

❓ 51. MPNSTs: prognostic factors. The FALSE answer is:
   A. Tumor size is the least consistent prognostic factor.
   B. Tumor grade.
   C. Surgical margin status.
   D. Local recurrence.
   E. Truncal location.

✅ Answer A

— Tumor size (>5 cm) has been the most consistent adverse prognostic factor.

❓ 52. MPNSTs: molecular factors with poor outcomes. The FALSE answer is:
   A. Nuclear p53 expression.
   B. AKT pathway suppression.
   C. TOR pathway activation.
   D. MET activation.
   E. 17 q 11.2 co-deletion.

✅ Answer B

— AKT pathway activation; however, there are no well-defined or widely reproducible molecular prognostication factors [10].

❓ 53. MPNSTs in NF1. The FALSE answer is:
   A. One of the most frequent causes of death.
   B. Lifetime risk is 10%.
   C. Worse outcomes compared to sporadic.
   D. Postop radiotherapy should be used cautiously.
   E. MRI is the modality of choice.

✅ **Answer E**
- 18FDG PET/CT is currently the most efficient imaging modality in the detection of MPNST and staging in NF1 patients.
- SUV_{MAX} values have also been correlated with histologic grade.

❓ 54. **Local recurrence for MPNSTs: rate and risk factors. The FALSE answer is:**
   A. Up to 65% recur after a median interval of 5 to 32.2 months.
   B. 75% of recurrences occur within the first 5 years of surgery.
   C. Positive resection margins increase the risk of recurrence.
   D. MPNSTs in NF1 patients have a higher risk of recurrence.
   E. Location in the head and neck increases the risk of recurrence.

✅ **Answer B**
- 75% of recurrences occur within the first 2 years of surgery.

❓ 55. **PNST surgery outcome. The FALSE answer is:**
   A. Complete excision of benign lesions can be done safely.
   B. MPNSTs have high metastatic potential.
   C. Recurrence is rare in benign lesions.
   D. The 5-year survival of MPNST is <50%.
   E. > 50% RECIST response rate.

✅ **Answer E**
- The response evaluation criteria in solid tumors (RECIST) response rate was reported to be 21% in a multi-institution retrospective study pooling MPNST patients from across multiple soft-tissue sarcoma trials [3].

Bibliography

1. Das S, Ganju A, Tiel RL, Kline DG. Tumors of the brachial plexus. Neurosurg Focus. 2007;22(6):E26.
2. Kolberg M, Høland M, Agesen TH, et al. Survival meta-analyses for >1800 malignant peripheral nerve sheath tumor patients with and without neurofibromatosis type 1. Neuro-Oncology. 2013;15(2):135–47.
3. Kroep JR, Ouali M, Gelderblom H, et al. First-line chemotherapy for malignant peripheral nerve sheath tumor (MPNST) versus other histological soft tissue sarcoma subtypes and as a prognostic factor for MPNST: an EORTC soft tissue and bone sarcoma group study. Ann Oncol. 2011;22(1):207–14.

4. Louis DN, Perry A, Reifenberger G, et al. The 2016 World Health Organization Classification of Tumors of the Central Nervous System: a summary. Acta Neuropathol. 2016;131(6):803–20.

5. Rodriguez FJ, Folpe AL, Giannini C, Perry A. Pathology of peripheral nerve sheath tumors: diagnostic overview and update on selected diagnostic problems. Acta Neuropathol. 2012;123(3):295–319.

6. Brahmi M, Thiesse P, Ranchere D, et al. Diagnostic accuracy of PET/CT-guided percutaneous biopsies for malignant peripheral nerve sheath tumors in neurofibromatosis type 1 patients. PLoS One. 2015;10(10):e0138386.

7. Carney JA. Psammomatous melanotic schwannoma. A distinctive, heritable tumor with special associations, including cardiac myxoma and the Cushing syndrome. Am J Surg Pathol. 1990;14(3):206–22.

8. Combemale P, Valeyrie-Allanore L, Giammarile F, et al. Utility of 18F-FDG PET with a semi-quantitative index in the detection of sarcomatous transformation in patients with neurofibromatosis type 1. PLoS One. 2014;9(2):e85954.

9. Dunn GP, Spiliopoulos K, Plotkin SR, et al. Role of resection of malignant peripheral nerve sheath tumors in patients with neurofibromatosis type 1. J Neurosurg. 2013;118(1):142–8.

10. Farid M, Demicco EG, Garcia R, et al. Malignant peripheral nerve sheath tumors. Oncologist. 2014;19(2):193–201. https://doi.org/10.1634/theoncologist.2013-0328.

11. Fine SW, McClain SA, Li M. Immunohistochemical staining for calretinin is useful for differentiating schwannomas from neurofibromas. Am J Clin Pathol. 2004;122(4):552–9.

12. Goldblum J, Folpe A, Weiss S, Enzinger F. Enzinger and Weiss's soft tissue tumors. 7th ed. Philadelphia: Elsevier; 2019. p. 892–994.

13. Winn H. Youmans & Winn neurological surgery. 7th ed. Philadelphia: Elsevier; 2017. p. 2103–16.

14. Batchelor T, Nishikawa R, Tarbell N, Weller M. Oxford textbook of neuro-oncology. 1st ed. Oxford: Oxford University Press; 2017. p. 169–85.

15. Batchelor T, Nishikawa R, Tarbell N, Weller M. Oxford textbook of neuro-oncology. 1st ed. Oxford: Oxford University Press; 2017. p. 1–13.

16. Yuk Kwan Tang C, Fung B, Fok M, Zhu J. Schwannoma in the Upper Limbs. Biomed Res Int. 2013;2013:1–4.

17. Kransdorf M. Benign soft-tissue tumors in a large referral population: distribution of specific diagnoses by age, sex, and location. Am J Roentgenol. 1995;164(2):395–402.

18. Wippold FJ 2nd, Lubner M, Perrin RJ, et al. Neuropathology for the neuroradiologist: Antoni A and Antoni B tissue patterns. AJNR Am J Neuroradiol. 2007;28:1633–8.

19. Jokinen C, Dadras S, Goldblum J, van de Rijn M, West R, Rubin B. Diagnostic implications of Podoplanin expression in peripheral nerve sheath neoplasms. Am J Clin Pathol. 2008;129(6):886–93.

20. Nonaka D, Chiriboga L, Rubin B. Sox10: a Pan-Schwannian and melanocytic marker. Am J Surg Pathol. 2008;32(9):1291–8.

21. Perentes E, Rubenstein LJ. Immunohistochemical recognition of human nerve sheath tumors by anti-leu 7 (HNK-1) monoclonal antibody. Acta Neuropathol (Berl). 1985;68:319–24.

22. Kirollos R, Helmy A, Thomson S, Hutchinson P. Oxford textbook of neurological surgery. 1st ed. Oxford: Oxford University Press; 2019. p. 555–61.

23. Batchelor T, Nishikawa R, Tarbell N, Weller M. Oxford textbook of neuro-oncology. 1st ed. Oxford: Oxford University Press; 2017. p. 108–13.

24. Vindhyal M, Elshimy G. Carney complex. Statpearls.com; 2020 (cited 21 November 2020). https://www.statpearls.com/kb/viewarticle/18953/

25. Adani R, Tarallo L, Mugnai R, Colopi S. Schwannomas of the upper extremity: analysis of 34 cases. Acta Neurochir. 2014;156(12):2325–30.

26. Merker VL, Esparza S, Smith MJ, Stemmer-Rachamimov A, Plotkin SR. Clinical features of schwannomatosis: a retrospective analysis of 87 patients. Oncologist. 2012;17(10):1317–22.

27. Ahlawat S, Chhabra A, Blakely J. Magnetic resonance neurography of peripheral nerve tumors and tumorlike conditions. Neuroimaging Clin N Am. 2014;24(1):171–92.

28. Murphey MD, Smith WS, Smith SE, Kransdorf MJ, Temple HT. From the archives of the AFIP. Imaging of musculoskeletal neurogenic tumors: radiologic-pathologic correlation. Radiographics. 1999;19(5):1253–80.

29. Ferner R, O'Doherty M. Neurofibroma and schwannoma. Curr Opin Neurol. 2002;15(6):679–84.

30. Tagliafico AS, Isaac A, Bignotti B, Rossi F, Zaottini F, Martinoli C. Nerve tumors: what the MSK radiologist should know. Semin Musculoskelet Radiol. 2019;23(1):76–84.

31. Lang S, Zager E, Coyne T, Nangunoori R, Kneeland J, Nathanson K. Hybrid peripheral nerve sheath tumor. J Neurosurg. 2012;117(5):897–901.

32. Demehri S, Belzberg A, Blakeley J, et al. Conventional and functional MR imaging of peripheral nerve sheath tumors: initial experience. AJNR Am J Neuroradiol. 2014;35:1615–20.

33. Warbey VS, Ferner RE, Dunn JT, et al. [18F] FDG PET/CT in the diagnosis of malignant peripheral nerve sheath tumours in neurofibromatosis type-1. Eur J Nucl Med Mol Imaging. 2009;3(60):751–7.

34. Ferner RE, Lucas JD, O'Doherty MJ, et al. Evaluation of 18fluorodeoxyglucose positron emission tomography (18FDGPET) in the detection of malignant peripheral nerve sheath tumours arising from within plexiform neurofibromas in neurofibromatosis 1. J Neurol Neurosurg Psychiatry. 2000;68:353–7.

35. Bredella MA, Torriani M, Hornicek F, et al. Value of PET in the assessment of patients with neurofibromatosis type 1. AJR Am J Roentgenol. 2007;189:928–35.

36. Ferner RE, Golding JF, Smith M, et al. [18F]2-fluoro-2-deoxy-Dglucose positron emission tomography (FDG PET) as a diagnostic tool for neurofibromatosis 1 (NF1) associated malignant peripheral nerve sheath tumours (MPNSTs): a long-term clinical study. Ann Oncol. 2008;919:390–4.

37. Bastiaannet E, Groen H, Jager PL, et al. The value of FDG-PET in the detection, grading and response to therapy of soft tissue and bone sarcomas: a systematic review and meta-analysis. Cancer Treat Rev. 2004;30:83–101.

38. Kumar V, Nath K, Berman CG, et al. Variance of SUVs for FDG-PET/CT is greater in clinical practice than under ideal study settings. Clin Nucl Med. 2013;38:175–82.

39. De Langen AJ, Vincent A, Velasquez LM, et al. Repeatability of 18 F-FDG uptake measurements in tumors: a metaanalysis. J Nucl Med. 2012;53:701–8.

40. Khiewvan B, Macapinlac HA, Lev D, et al. The value of 18F-FDG PET/CT in the management of malignant peripheral nerve sheath tumors. Eur J Nucl Med Mol Imaging. 2014;41:1756–66.

41. Grobmyer SR, Reith JD, Shahlaee A, et al. Malignant peripheral nerve sheath tumor: molecular pathogenesis and current management considerations. J Surg Oncol. 2008;97:340–9.

42. Kacerovska D, Michal M, Kuroda N, et al. Hybrid peripheral nerve sheath tumors, including a malignant variant in type 1 neurofibromatosis. Am J Dermatopathol. 2013;35(6):641–9.

43. Sato K, Ueda Y, Miwa S, et al. Low-grade malignant soft-tissue perineurioma: interphase fluorescence in situ hybridization. Pathol Int. 2008;58(11):718–22.

44. Agaimy A. Microscopic intraneural perineurial cell proliferations in patients with neurofibromatosis type 1. Ann Diagn Pathol. 2014;18(2):95–8.

45. Miettinen MM, Antonescu CR, Fletcher CDM, et al. Histopathologic evaluation of atypical neurofibromatous tumors and their transformation into malignant peripheral nerve sheath tumor in patients with neurofibromatosis 1: a consensus overview. Hum Pathol. 2017;67:1–10.

46. Yu J, Deshmukh H, Payton JE, et al. Array-based comparative genomic hybridization identifies CDK4 and FOXM1 alterations as independent predictors of survival in malignant peripheral nerve sheath tumor. Clin Cancer Res. 2011;17(7):1924–34.

18

Lymphomas, Hematopoietic Tumors, and Histiocytic Tumors

Husain A. Abdali, Alkawthar M. Abdulsada, Rania H. Al-Taie, and Samer S. Hoz

S. S. Hoz et al. (eds.), *Surgical Neuro-Oncology*,
https://doi.org/10.1007/978-3-031-53642-7_19

19

? 1. **Primary central nervous system lymphoma (PCNSL): definition. The FALSE answer is:**
   A. It is an uncommon lymphoma.
   B. It is an extranodal non-Hodgkin lymphoma.
   C. It is a diffuse large B-cell lymphoma in 90% of cases.
   D. May have systemic involvement.
   E. May be seen in the spinal cord.

✅ **Answer D**
— PCNSL is confined to the craniospinal axis, and before diagnosis of PCNS, the patient should be investigated for systemic sources to rule out secondary CNS lymphoma.

? 2. **Secondary CNS lymphoma (SCNSL). The FALSE answer is:**
   A. More common than PCNSL.
   B. It is a systemic non-Hodgkin lymphoma.
   C. Mostly disseminated to basal ganglia and periventricular areas.
   D. Associated with multiple cranial nerve deficits more frequently than PCNSL.
   E. More commonly results in hydrocephalus compared to PCNSL.

✅ **Answer C**
— SCNSL is usually in the form of leptomeningeal dissemination. Therefore, CN deficits and hydrocephalus are more frequent than in PCNSL.

? 3. **Epidemiology of PCNSL. The FALSE answer is:**
   A. It is a rare brain tumor.
   B. The overall median age at diagnosis is 60 years.
   C. The HIV pandemic led to an increase in PCNSL incidence.
   D. Affects males more than females.
   E. It accounts for <1% of non-Hodgkin lymphoma.

✅ **Answer B**
— The median age at diagnosis for immunocompromised patients is 34 years.

? 4. **Clinical presentation of PCNSL. The FALSE answer is:**
   A. The average duration of symptoms is 2.7–7 months.
   B. Headache is the most common presentation.
   C. Can present with seizures.
   D. Neuropsychiatric signs are common.
   E. Multiple cranial nerve deficits are not uncommon.

✅ **Answer B**

- Changes in mental status and cognition with neuropsychiatric signs and focal deficit are the most common presentation. In such patients, PCNSL should be ruled out.
- Increased ICP symptoms, e.g., headache, are less common.

❓ 5. **Clinical presentation of PCNSL. The FALSE answer is:**
   A. Seizure is as common as in other types of brain tumors.
   B. No typical B symptoms of lymphoma such as weight loss, fever, and night sweating.
   C. Presents with subacute encephalitis if there is subependymal infiltration.
   D. Multiple sclerosis-like histological findings with steroid-induced remission.
   E. May present with uveocyclitis.

✅ **Answer A**

- PCNSL usually affects deep brain structures and spares the cortex, making seizures less common at presentation.

❓ 6. **Clinical presentation of PCNSL. The FALSE answer is:**
   A. Symptoms are nonspecific and rapidly progressive.
   B. Ocular symptoms are common.
   C. Symptoms of raised ICP are not common.
   D. 50% of patients have focal neurological deficits.
   E. Personal changes and cognition impairment are among the most common presentations.

✅ **Answer B**

- Ocular symptoms are seen in only 4% of patients with PCNSL. Ocular symptoms, resulting from involvement of the retina, choroid, or vitreous, manifest as floaters and/or blurred vision. These symptoms can occur either in isolation (10%) or concurrently with cerebral symptoms (10–20%).

❓ 7. **International PCNSL Collaboration Group (IPCG) guidelines for diagnostic evaluation of PCNSL. The FALSE answer is:**
   A. All patients should be evaluated for HIV serology and serum LDH levels.
   B. Bone marrow biopsy is part of the baseline evaluation.

19

    C. A slit-lamp eye examination should be done.
    D. Renal ultrasound should be done early.
    E. CSF cytology, flow cytometry, and IgH PCR should be done.

✅ **Answer D**
- Testicular ultrasound should be considered early because testicular lymphoma has a predilection to spread to the CNS.
- CT abdomen will assess the kidneys better than ultrasound.

❓ 8. **Neuroimaging of PCNSL. The FALSE answer is:**
    A. Usually enhances homogeneously in all patients.
    B. Contrast-enhanced cranial MRI is the modality of choice.
    C. Cerebral hemispheres are the most commonly affected sites.
    D. Isolated spinal involvement is rare.
    E. Brainstem involvement is rare.

✅ **Answer A**
- Homogenous enhancement is usually seen in immunocompetent patients, while ring enhancement is seen in immunocompromised patients.

❓ 9. **Neuroimaging of PCNSL. The FALSE answer is:**
    A. The frontal lobe is the most commonly involved lobe.
    B. Multifocal involvement is seen only in immunocompromised patients.
    C. Most patients have more than one affected lobe.
    D. Periventricular involvement is less common than cortical involvement in both immunocompromised and immunocompetent patients.
    E. Occipital lobe involvement is rare.

✅ **Answer B**
- Multifocal involvement is seen in both immunocompromised and immunocompetent patients.
- 35% of PCNSL in immunocompetent patients is multifocal, and 51% of PCNSL in immunocompromised patients is multifocal.
- Periventricular involvement is seen in 12% of PCNSL in immunocompetent patients and 56% in immunocompromised patients, while cortical involvement is 65% in both patients.

10. Neuroimaging of PCNSL. The FALSE answer is:
A. MRI brain shows restricted diffusion.
B. Cerebral angiography shows an avascular mass in 60%.
C. The vanishing phenomenon is pathognomonic for PCNSL.
D. MRI spectrograph typically demonstrates extremely high lipids.
E. MRI spectrograph shows high choline and lactate and low N-acetyl aspartate and creatine.

Answer C

− Vanishing of the tumor in the images after steroids is not only seen with PCNSL. It is also seen in demyelinating diseases, infarcts, sarcoidosis, and renal cell carcinoma.

11. Investigation for PCNSL. The FALSE answer is:
A. 13% of patients have concomitant disease in the eye.
B. 16% of patients have CSF involvement.
C. In infratentorial involvement, the brainstem is the most common site.
D. 35–50% of PCNSL are multifocal.
E. Deep brain involvement is seen in 40% of patients.

Answer C

− The cerebellum is the most common infratentorial site affected.

12. Lumbar puncture (LP) for PCNSL investigation. The FALSE answer is:
A. Obtained if there is no mass effect.
B. CSF usually shows nonspecific abnormalities.
C. CSF may show elevated protein and cell counts.
D. CSF flow cytometry is mainly for staging and long-term follow-up rather than for primary diagnosis.
E. Finding of lymphoma cells in the CSF does not omit the need for tissue biopsy.

Answer E

− Genetic analysis of the identified lymphoma cells in the CSF, in association with typical neuroimaging, allows a faster and less invasive method to confirm the diagnosis, potentially obviating the need for a stereotactic brain biopsy.

19

? 13. Lumbar puncture (LP) in PCNSL investigation. The FALSE answer is:
   A. Has a low yield in diagnosis.
   B. Cytology is positive for lymphoma cells in only 10% of cases.
   C. Increased sensitivity with periventricular involvement.
   D. Repeating the LP up to three times will increase its yield.
   E. CSF is investigated for cytology, flow cytometry, and IgH PCR.

✓ Answer C
- Leptomeningeal involvement as seen commonly in SCNSL is associated with higher LP sensitivity rather than periventricular involvement.
- In patients with positive LP for lymphoma, SCNSL should be ruled out.

? 14. Ocular involvement in PCNSL. The FALSE answer is:
   A. PCNSL is highly likely if the tumor is seen in association with uveitis.
   B. 15%–25% of PCNSLs also have intraocular lymphoma.
   C. Less responsive to low-dose methotrexate.
   D. Responds to low-dose ocular radiotherapy.
   E. Intrathecal and intraventricular chemotherapy is part of the first-line treatment of PCNSL with ocular involvement.

✓ Answer E
- Intrathecal and intraventricular chemotherapy is for cases that are refractory to treatment with intravenous chemotherapy, as well as for recurrent ocular lymphoma.

? 15. Immunodeficiency-associated PCNSL. The FALSE answer is:
   A. Among patients with immunodeficiency, HIV infection has the highest risk for PCNSL.
   B. Declined dramatically with the introduction of highly active antiretroviral therapy (HAART).
   C. The most common primary brain tumor in AIDS patients.
   D. The most common cerebral mass lesion in HIV-infected patients.
   E. Almost 100% associated with Epstein-Barr virus infection.

✓ Answer D
- It is the second most common cerebral lesion in HIV-infected patients after toxoplasmosis, which could mimic PCNSL and should be ruled out before the diagnosis of PCNSL.

? 16. **Steroids in PCNSL. The FALSE answer is:**
   A. Have lymphotoxic properties.
   B. Avoid prior to tissue diagnosis unless there is raised ICP.
   C. Induce radiographic response in up to 40% of cases.
   D. Mostly results in a complete temporary response.
   E. Response to steroids is a positive prognostic marker.

✓ **Answer D**
– Response of PCNSL to steroids is variable, and complete response is rare.
– Most of the time the response to steroids is temporary.

? 17. **Histopathology of PCNSL in immunocompetent patients. The FALSE answer is:**
   A. Lymphoid clustering around small cerebral vessels (angiocentric pattern of growth).
   B. High proliferation rate (KI-67 > 70%).
   C. The majority are high-grade diffuse large B-cell lymphomas.
   D. PCNSL and SCNSL cannot be differentiated on the basis of immunophenotype.
   E. Associated with Epstein-Barr virus (EBV) infection.

✓ **Answer E**
– PCNSL in immunocompromised patients is associated with EBV, not in those who are immunocompetent.

? 18. **Histopathology of PCNSL when treated with steroids. The FALSE answer is:**
   A. Is mostly low-yield in diagnosis.
   B. High yield if contrast enhancement persists.
   C. Presence of lymphoma cell debris.
   D. Extensive macrophage infiltrate.
   E. May mimic demyelination diseases.

✓ **Answer A**
– The effect of steroids is variable, and in most cases, histopathology will show scattered apoptotic bodies among tumor cells that are still valid for diagnosis.
– Total disappearance of the tumor cells (true vanishing phenomenon) is rare.

? 19. **Lymphomatosis cerebri. The FALSE answer is:**
  A. Widespread and diffuse infiltration of PCNSL in the cerebral white matter.
  B. No formation of a discrete tumor mass.
  C. Commonly presents with personality changes and cognition impairment.
  D. Imaging shows well-enhanced diffuse leukoencephalopathy in both hemispheres.
  E. Gliomatosis cerebri is the main differential diagnosis.

✅ **Answer D**
— Imaging of lymphomatosis cerebri typically reveals diffuse leukoencephalopathy in both hemispheres without enhancement.

? 20. **Surgery for PCNSL. The FALSE answer is:**
  A. Its role is limited to biopsy, shunting, or insertion of an Ommaya Reservoir.
  B. Gross total excision is difficult to achieve.
  C. Gross total excision, if possible, leads to a better prognosis.
  D. Is indicated if PCNSL is causing raised ICP and brain hernia.
  E. Median survival after surgery alone is only 1–4 months.

✅ **Answer C**
— The extent of excision has no prognostic impact, and it may even be detrimental if the PCNSL is deep in the brain.
— Since the tumor is very sensitive to chemotherapy, most of the time the role of surgery is limited to biopsy to establish the diagnosis and to start chemotherapy.

? 21. **Biopsy for PCNSL. The FALSE answer is:**
  A. It is the standard diagnostic method.
  B. Usually obtained using a stereotactic needle.
  C. Recommended to be from the most superficial lesion.
  D. Should be obtained from the center of the lesion in HIV-related PCNSL.
  E. Utilize the least invasive approach from non-eloquent brain areas.

✅ Answer D
- HIV-related PCNSL lesions exhibit ring enhancement on imaging due to the presence of necrosis in the center of the lymphoma, and biopsy from that central necrosis is low yield.
- The recommendation is to take the biopsy from enhancing peripheral areas.

❓ 22. Chemotherapy treatment of PCNSL. The FALSE answer is:
- A. Modern treatment of PCNSL includes induction and consolidation phases.
- B. The recommended frontline therapy consists of high-dose methotrexate-based monochemotherapy.
- C. Alkylating agents and rituximab have a role in the induction phase.
- D. Most elderly patients can tolerate high-dose methotrexate.
- E. High-dose methotrexate is effective in HIV-related PCNSL.

✅ Answer B
- The frontline therapy in the induction phase is high-dose methotrexate combined with an alkylating agent and rituximab (polychemotherapy).

❓ 23. Intrathecal/intraventricular chemotherapy for PCNSL. The FALSE answer is:
- A. Not for patients who are suitable candidates for full-dose induction therapy.
- B. The intraventricular route is preferred over the intrathecal route for chemotherapy.
- C. Is the preferable first choice in patients with meningeal involvement.
- D. A choice for patients with insufficient response to intravenous chemotherapy.
- E. A choice for patients who are unable to receive high-dose methotrexate.

✅ Answer C
- Intravenous chemotherapy is still the first choice of treatment for PCNSL with meningeal involvement.
- Intrathecal and intraventricular chemotherapy is reserved for patients who are not responding to or are not candidates for intravenous chemotherapy.

19

? 24. **Radiotherapy for PCNSL. The FALSE answer is:**
  A. Elderly patients in poor neurological condition with contraindications to chemotherapy should be treated with primary radiotherapy alone.
  B. Plays a central role in the consolidation phase.
  C. Not effective in patients with poor response to induction chemotherapy.
  D. It is not curative when used alone.
  E. Unavoidable option for poor autologous peripheral blood stem cell mobilizers.

✓ Answer C
— Radiotherapy serves as the primary treatment during consolidation, and it also serves as a salvage treatment for patients who do not respond to or are not candidates for induction chemotherapy.

? 25. **Radiotherapy for PCNSL. The FALSE answer is:**
  A. Associated with significantly better progression-free survival where there is no difference in overall survival.
  B. Associated with increased risk of severe neurotoxicity.
  C. It is the only approved effective consolidation treatment.
  D. The dose is less than 50 Gy with a standard fraction.
  E. The whole brain, the first two segments of the spinal and the eye should be irradiated, with or without a tumor bed boost.

✓ Answer C
— High-dose chemotherapy supported by autologous stem cell transplantation (HDC/ASCT) and whole-brain radiotherapy are two effective consolidation treatments.

? 26. **The treatment outcome of PCNSL. The FALSE answer is:**
  A. If left untreated leads to death within weeks to months.
  B. Overall, with treatment, the median survival rate is between 7 and 19 months in young patients.
  C. The prognosis has improved in the last decades.
  D. Poor clinical performance has a strong negative impact on prognosis.
  E. The International Extranodal Lymphoma Study Group (IELSG) score predicts the prognosis.

✅ **Answer B**
- The prognosis of PCNSL has improved significantly over the last decades. In young patients, long-term remission can be achieved with a median survival of ≥26 months. In the elderly, the median survival rate is 14–31 months.

❓ 27. **Prognostic markers for PCNSL. The FALSE answer is:**
   A. Age older than 60 years carries a poor prognosis.
   B. Elevated serum lactate dehydrogenase (LDH) carries a poor prognosis.
   C. High CSF protein is a poor prognostic marker.
   D. Multifocal PCNSL has a poor prognosis.
   E. PCNSL confined to the cerebral lobes has a poor prognosis.

✅ **Answer E**
- PCNSL confined to the cerebral lobes, and cortex has a better prognosis than cases involving deep brain structures.

❓ 28. **Erdheim-Chester disease. The FALSE answer is:**
   A. Is a rare non-Langerhans histiocytosis.
   B. Diagnosed by histopathology demonstrating the infiltration of CD68+ and CD1a foamy histiocytes with fibrosis.
   C. Is a multisystemic disorder commonly involving the CNS, lungs, hearts, long bones, and orbits.
   D. Neuroradiology may show single or multiple enhancing dural masses.
   E. Headache is the most common presentation of intracranial involvement.

✅ **Answer E**
- Diabetes insipidus (DI) due to pituitary involvement is the most common presentation with intracranial involvement.
- Meningioma-like lesions in the presence of DI should raise the possibility for diagnosis of Erdheim-Chester disease.

❓ 29. **Erdheim-Chester disease: clinical presentation. The FALSE answer is:**
   A. Motor weakness is due to cortical involvement.
   B. Exophthalmos and diplopia are due to a retro-orbital mass.
   C. Hypopituitarism and loss of vision are due to sellar and supra-sellar involvement.

D. Cerebellar signs.
E. Brain stem sings.

19 ✅ **Answer A**
   − Motor weakness is usually due to cortical compression by a dural-based mass.

❓ 30. **Rosai-Dorfman disease. The FALSE answer is:**
   A. Uncommon histiocytic disorder.
   B. Most frequently presents as bilateral cervical lymphadenopathy.
   C. CNS involvement is predominantly at the dura.
   D. CNS involvement is usually associated with nodal disease.
   E. Elevated erythrocyte sedimentation rate, leukocytosis, and auto-immune hemolytic anemia are seen in laboratory studies.

✅ **Answer D**
   − CNS involvement in Rosai-Dorfman disease is mainly dural and mimics meningioma clinically and radiologically. It is not usually associated with lymphadenopathy.

❓ 31. **Juvenile xanthogranuloma. The FALSE answer is:**
   A. Rare non-Langerhans cell histiocytosis that mainly involves the skin.
   B. CNS and systemic involvement are common.
   C. The whole neuroaxis can be affected.
   D. May result in seizure, cranial nerve deficit, diabetes insipidus, spinal cord or nerve compression, and leptomeningeal involvement.
   E. For symptomatic lesions, surgery is the choice of treatment.

✅ **Answer B**
   − Extracutaneous involvement of juvenile xanthogranuloma is uncommon and seen in only 10% of the cases.

❓ 32. **Primary histiocytic sarcoma. The FALSE answer is:**
   A. It is a benign neoplasm with rare CNS involvement.
   B. The most common site of involvement is the lymph node, intestine, skin, and soft tissue.
   C. CNS involvement is in the form of localized parenchymal or dural mass.

D. Can mimic lymphoma, meningioma, and demyelination.

E. Treatment modalities include surgery, chemotherapy, and radiotherapy.

✅ **Answer A**

▬ It is a malignant disease with rapidly evolving neurological symptoms and an aggressive clinical course.

▬ The survival rate ranges between 3 and 16 months with the best treatment.

Bibliography

1. Korfel A, Schlegel U. Diagnosis and treatment of primary CNS lymphoma. Nat Rev Neurol. 2013;9(6):317Y327.

2. Nayak L, Pentsova E, Batchelor TT. Primary CNS lymphoma and neurologic complications of hematologic malignancies. Continuum (Minneapolis, Minn). 2015;21:355–72.

3. O'Neill BP, Decker PA, Tieu C, Cerhan JR. The changing incidence of primary central nervous system lymphoma is driven primarily by the changing incidence in young and middle-aged men and differs from time trends in systemic diffuse large B-cell non-Hodgkin's lymphoma. Am J Hematol. 2013;88(12):997–1000.

4. Bataille B, Delwail V, Menet E, Vandermarcq P, Ingrand P, Wager M, et al. Primary intracerebral malignant lymphoma: report of 248 cases. J Neurosurg. 2000;92(2):261–6.

5. Giovanni C, Michele R, Gemma G, Andrés J. Primary central nervous system lymphoma. Crit Rev Oncol Hematol. 2017;113:97–110.

6. Chan CC, Rubenstein JL, Coupland SE, Davis JL, Harbour JW, Johnston PB, et al. Primary vitreoretinal lymphoma: a report from an international primary central nervous system lymphoma collaborative group symposium. Oncologist. 2011;16(11):1589–99.

7. Ferreri AJM, Blay JY, Reni M, Pasini F, Spina M, Ambrosetti A, et al. Prognostic scoring system for primary CNS lymphomas: the international extranodal lymphoma study group experience. J Clin Oncol. 2003;21(2):266–72.

8. Bühring U, Herrlinger U, Krings T, Thiex R, Weller M, Küker W. MRI features of primary central nervous system lymphomas at presentation. Neurology. 2001;57(3):393–6.

9. Yap KK, Sutherland T, Liew E, Tartaglia CJ, Pang M, Trost N. Magnetic resonance features of primary central nervous system lymphoma in the immunocompetent patient: a pictorial essay. J Med Imaging Radiat Oncol. 2012;56(2):179–86.

10. Giannini C, Dogan A, Salomão DR. CNS lymphoma: a practical diagnostic approach. J Neuropathol Exp Neurol. 2014;73(6):478–94.

11. Küker W, et al. Primary central nervous system lymphomas (PCNSL): MRI features at presentation in 100 patients. J Neuro-Oncol. 2005;72(2):169–77.

12. Rimelen V, Ahle G, Pencreach E, Zinniger N, Debliquis A, Zalmaï L, Harzallah I, Hurstel R, Alamome I, Lamy F, Voirin J. Tumor cell-free DNA detection in CSF for primary CNS lymphoma diagnosis. Acta Neuropathol Commun. 2019;7(1):43.

13. Scott BJ, Douglas VC, Tihan T, Rubenstein JL, Josephson SA. A systematic approach to the diagnosis of suspected central nervous system lymphoma. JAMA Neurol. 2013;70(3):311–9.

14. Tang LJ, Gu CL, Zhang P. Intraocular lymphoma. Int J Ophthalmol. 2017;10(8):1301.

15. Acosta MC, Kundro M, Viloria G, Peressín Paz A, Morello F, Latorre F, Seoane E, Toibaro J, Losso M. The role of brain biopsy in the clinical management of HIV-related focal brain lesions. HIV Med. 2018;19(10):673–8.

16. Hoang-Xuan K, et al. Diagnosis and treatment of primary CNS lymphoma in immunocompetent patients: guidelines from the European Association for Neuro-Oncology. Lancet Oncol. 2015;16(7):e322–32.

17. Ferreri AJ. Therapy of primary CNS lymphoma: role of intensity, radiation, and novel agents. Hematol Am Soc Hematol Educ Program Book. 2017;2017(1):565–77.

18. von Baumgarten L, et al. The diagnosis and treatment of primary CNS lymphoma: an interdisciplinary challenge. Deutsches Ärzteblatt Int. 2018;115(25):419.

19. Starkebaum G, Hendrie P. Erdheim–Chester disease. Best Pract Res Clin Rheumatol. 2020;34(4):101510.

20. Bruce-Brand C, Schneider JW, Schubert P. Rosai-Dorfman disease: an overview. J Clin Pathol. 2000;73(11):697–705.

21. Wolfe C, et al. Intradural Juvenile Xanthogranuloma with involvement of multiple nerve roots: a case report and review of the literature. World Neurosurg. 2018;119: 189–96.

22. So H, et al. Primary histiocytic sarcoma of the central nervous system. Cancer Res Treat. 2015;47(2):322.

23. Löw S, Han CH, Batchelor TT. Primary central nervous system lymphoma. Ther Adv Neurol Dis. 2018;11:1756286418793562.

24. Han CH, Batchelor TT. Diagnosis and management of primary central nervous system lymphoma. Cancer. 2017;123(22):4314–24.

25. Correa DD, Maron L, Harder H, Klein M, Armstrong CL, Calabrese P, Bromberg JE, Abrey LE, Batchelor TT, Schiff D. Cognitive functions in primary central nervous system lymphoma: literature review and assessment guidelines. Ann Oncol. 2007;18(7): 1145–51.

26. Campochiaro C, Tomelleri A, Cavalli G, Berti A, Dagna L. Erdheim-chester disease. Eur J Intern Med. 2015;26(4):223–9.

27. Munoz J, Janku F, Cohen PR, Kurzrock R. Erdheim-Chester disease: characteristics and management. In: Mayo clinic proceedings July 1, vol. 89, No. 7. Elsevier; 2014. p. 985–96.

28. Stover DG, Alapati S, Regueira O, Turner C, Whitlock JA. Treatment of juvenile xanthogranuloma. Pediatr Blood Cancer. 2008;51(1):130–3.

29. So H, Kim SA, Yoon DH, Khang SK, Hwang J, Suh CH, Suh C. Primary histiocytic sarcoma of the central nervous system. Cancer Res Treat. 2015;47(2):322–8.

Metastatic and Melanocytic Tumors

Baha'eddin A. Muhsen, Hazem Madi, Maliya Delawan, and Samer S. Hoz

© The Author(s), under exclusive license to Springer Nature Switzerland AG 2024
S. S. Hoz et al. (eds.), *Surgical Neuro-Oncology*,
https://doi.org/10.1007/978-3-031-53642-7_20

? 1. Brain metastases. The FALSE answer is:
  A. Cerebral metastases are the most common brain tumors seen clinically.
  B. 20–40% of patients with cancer develop cerebral metastasis.
  C. At the onset of neurological symptoms, approximately 20% will show multiple lesions on MRI.
  D. The cortex is the only detectable site of spread in 9% of cases.
  E. In the case of a solitary lesion, a biopsy should almost always be performed, as 11% of these lesions may not be metastatic.

✓ Answer C
— At the time of the onset of neurological symptoms, 70% will have multiple lesions on MRI, while 50% will appear solitary on a CT scan.

? 2. Brain metastases originating from the lung. The FALSE answer is:
  A. The lungs are the most common source of cerebral metastases, which are usually multiple.
  B. Small cell lung cancer (SCLC) is considered radiosensitive.
  C. SCLC is known as oat cell cancer.
  D. SCLC is less likely to produce cerebral metastases than other bronchogenic cell types.
  E. SCLC is strongly associated with cigarette smoking.

✓ Answer D
— Although SCLC comprises only about 20% of primary lung cancers, it is more likely to produce cerebral metastasis than other bronchogenic cell types.

? 3. Intracranial metastatic melanoma. The FALSE answer is:
  A. It is often a hemorrhagic lesion surrounded by substantial vasogenic edema.
  B. Melanoma is the third most common cancer in men and the fourth most common in women.
  C. The most common sites of origin include the skin and retina.
  D. The primary site cannot be identified in up to approximately 14% of cases.
  E. Melanomas originating intraocularly and from the GI mucosa are difficult to locate.

✅ **Answer B**

▬ Melanoma is the fifth most common cancer in men and the seventh most common in women.

❓ 4. **The spread of primary CNS tumors (CSF seeding) occurs in the following. The FALSE answer is:**
   A. Medulloblastoma.
   B. Pineal region germ cell tumor.
   C. Ependymoma.
   D. Choroid plexus tumors.
   E. Meningioma.

✅ **Answer E**

▬ Meningioma rarely metastasizes outside the brain. However, a few reports have shown that meningiomas can metastasize to the heart or the lung, but this occurs via the bloodstream.

❓ 5. **Predictors of poor outcome in melanoma. The FALSE answer is:**
   A. More than 3 brain mets.
   B. Development of brain mets before the diagnosis of extracranial disease.
   C. Elevated lactate dehydrogenase >2 times the normal value.
   D. Presence of bone metastases.
   E. Multiple brain mets and extensive visceral disease.

✅ **Answer B**

▬ Development of brain mets after the diagnosis of extracranial disease is a poor prognostic factor in melanoma.

❓ 6. **Survival in metastatic brain tumors. The FALSE answer is:**
   A. Median survival with the best treatment is only approximately 6 months, which is worse than with glioblastoma.
   B. Median survival among untreated patients is approximately 1 month.
   C. The use of steroids alone, to control edema, doubles survival to 2 weeks.
   D. Whole-brain radiation therapy (WBXRT) combined with steroids increases survival to 3–6 months.
   E. The recurrence of the tumor is significantly less frequent and delayed with the use of post-op WBXRT.

✓ Answer C

▬ The use of steroids alone, to control edema, doubles survival to 2 months.

❓ 7. Indications favoring surgical excision of metastatic lesions. The FALSE answer is:
   A. The primary tumor is known to be relatively radioresistant.
   B. The lesion is symptomatic or life-threatening.
   C. Recurrent SCLC following XRT.
   D. Metastases usually have an ill-defined border; thus, a plane of separation from normal brain tissue is difficult.
   E. Total excision of all metastases, if feasible, results in survival similar to those who have a single metastasis removed.

✓ Answer D

▬ Metastases usually have a well-defined border; thus, a plane of separation from normal brain tissue may be exploited, often allowing gross total removal.

❓ 8. Surgical management of metastatic brain tumors. The FALSE answer is:
   A. The mortality associated with removing multiple metastases at a single sitting is significantly higher than that for a single metastasis.
   B. Is indicated in cases involving multiple symptomatic and/or life-threatening lesions, including posterior fossa lesions.
   C. Stereotactic biopsy is indicated for deep lesions.
   D. Most lesions present themselves on the surface of the brain or protrude through the dura.
   E. The median survival is 7.5 months with SRS, compared to 16.4 months with surgery, and there is a higher mortality from cerebral disease in the SRS group.

✓ Answer A

▬ The mortality associated with removing multiple metastases at a single sitting is not statistically significantly higher than removing a single metastasis.

❓ 9. Surgical resection for brain metastases. The FALSE answer is:
   A. The main aim of surgery in patients with brain metastases is to lengthen the survival time.
   B. Surgery can manage medically refractory seizures caused by tumors.

C. Piecemeal resection of tumors is associated with a significant increase in the risk of local recurrence.

D. Surgery combined with WBRT resulted in longer functionally independent survival compared to WBRT alone.

E. Class III evidence supports the combination of surgical resection plus postoperative WBRT, as compared with WBRT alone in patients with good performance status.

✅ **Answer E**

▬ Class I evidence supports the combination of surgical resection plus postoperative WBRT, as compared with WBRT alone in patients with good performance status.

❓ 10. **Radiosensitive brain metastases. The FALSE answer is:**
   A. Small-cell lung cancer.
   B. Germ cell tumors.
   C. Renal cell carcinoma.
   D. Lymphoma.
   E. Multiple myeloma.

✅ **Answer C**

▬ Renal cell carcinoma is highly resistant to WBXRT.

❓ 11. **Radioresistant brain metastases. The FALSE answer is:**
   A. Thyroid cancer.
   B. Renal cell carcinoma.
   C. Malignant melanoma.
   D. Breast cancer.
   E. Sarcoma.

✅ **Answer D**

▬ Breast cancer is moderately sensitive to WBXRT.

❓ 12. **Factors associated with better prognosis in brain metastases. The FALSE answer is:**
   A. Karnofsky score (KPS) > 70.
   B. Age < 60 years.
   C. Metastases to the brain only.
   D. Less than 1 year from the diagnosis of primary tumor.
   E. Absent or controlled primary disease.

✅ **Answer D**

- A diagnosis of the primary tumor more than 1 year ago is a good prognostic factor.
- The most important better prognostic factor is KPS >70.

❓ 13. **Carcinomatous meningitis. The FALSE answer is:**
   A. The most common primaries are breast, lung, and melanoma.
   B. Is the presenting finding in up to 48% of patients with cancer.
   C. Low glucose is the most common LP abnormality.
   D. LP is positive in 45% of cases in the first study, with 81% eventually testing positive after up to 6 LPs.
   E. The survival rate is less than 2 months if untreated.

✅ **Answer C**

- Elevated protein is the most common abnormality.
- Glucose levels may be as low as approximately 40 mg/dL in about a third of patients.

❓ 14. **Carcinomatous meningitis (CM). The FALSE answer is:**
   A. Caused by intracranial malignancies such as medulloblastoma, ependymomas, and gliomas.
   B. Among hematological malignancies, leukemia is the most common etiology.
   C. Posterior fossa involvement causes both cerebellar signs and cranial neuropathies.
   D. The most common presenting symptom is headache caused by meningeal irritation or raised ICP.
   E. Intrathecal chemotherapy is the mainstay of treatment for CM due to the selective BBB.

✅ **Answer B**

- Among hematological malignancies, B-cell lymphoma is the most common etiology.

❓ 15. **Gamma knife radiosurgery (GKRS) in large posterior fossa metastases. The FALSE answer is:**
   A. The major advantage of GKRS over surgery is that it is less invasive.
   B. GKRS monotherapy cannot be considered a treatment option.
   C. Associated with significant recovery time.

D. Used to treat multiple lesions in the same session and to treat deep-seated lesions.

E. Results in a reduction in peritumoral edema and tumor size.

✅ **Answer B**

▬ GKRS monotherapy can be considered a potential treatment option for patients with LPFMs, including lesions that are associated with marked peritumoral edema and compression/distortion of the fourth ventricle.

❓ 16. **Radiation Therapy Oncology Group (RTOG) recursive partitioning analysis (RPA) classification. The FALSE answer is:**

A. The specific tumor type is not as prognostically important as the Karnofsky Performance Scale score.

B. The applicability of RPA to melanoma metastases to the brain is controversial.

C. RPA Class 3 includes patients with a KPS of 70, with a median survival of 2 months.

D. RPA Class 1 has a median survival of 7 months.

E. RPA Class 2 has a median survival of 4 months.

✅ **Answer C**

▬ RPA Class 3 includes patients with a KPS of less than 70, and they have been shown to be unlikely to benefit from any of the numerous treatment modalities studied. Class 1 patients are more likely to benefit. Most patients fall into Class 2, and the benefit is unclear.

❓ 17. **Combination treatments for metastatic brain tumors. The FALSE answer is:**

A. Surgical resection + WBRT is superior in local control compared with surgical resection alone.

B. Evidence has consistently shown that a combination of SRS and WBRT is superior to WBRT alone.

C. SRS alone has shown equivalent survival rates compared with combined WBRT and SRS.

D. SRS alone has shown equivalent functional and survival outcomes compared to surgery + WBRT.

E. Surgical resection + WBRT shows a better survival rate than SRS + WBRT.

✅ **Answer E**

- A level 2 recommendation states that both combinations represent effective treatment strategies, resulting in equal survival rates.

❓ 18. **Medical management of metastatic brain tumors. The FALSE answer is:**
- A. Metastatic lesions cause seizures, but their epileptogenic potential is less than that of gliomas.
- B. Dexamethasone is the steroid of choice and should tapered over 2 months.
- C. The use of antiepileptic drugs is discouraged in patients without seizures.
- D. Dexamethasone reduces vasogenic edema by downregulating pro-inflammatory factors.
- E. Corticosteroids can provide temporary relief of symptoms related to increased ICP.

✅ **Answer B**

- According to a level 3 recommendation, dexamethasone is the steroid of choice and once started should be tapered off over 2 weeks.

❓ 19. **Chemotherapy in the management of newly diagnosed brain metastases. The FALSE answer is:**
- A. Chemotherapy is considered ineffective due to poor penetration of the blood-brain barrier.
- B. There is a level 1 recommendation against the routine use of chemotherapy in brain metastasis.
- C. Brain tumors resulting from metastatic breast cancer respond to chemotherapy.
- D. Germinomas metastatic to the brain are considered chemo-resistant tumors.
- E. The treatment of choice for multiple small-cell carcinomas is radiation plus chemotherapy.

✅ **Answer D**

- There is a level 1 recommendation against the routine use of chemotherapy in newly diagnosed brain metastases. However, this recommendation does not apply to exquisitely chemosensitive tumors, such as germinomas metastatic to the brain.

❓ 20. Whole-brain radiotherapy (WBRT) for metastatic brain tumors. The FALSE answer is:

A. WBRT is considered the standard treatment for patients with brain metastases.

B. Helps in the prevention of widely disseminated metastases throughout the brain outside of the tumor bed.

C. A dose of 54 Gy in 30 fractions is recommended.

D. WBRT is associated with the development of neurocognitive deficits.

E. Different doses/fractionations of WBRT do not result in significant differences in median survival.

✓ Answer C

— The usual dose is 30 Gy in 10 fractions given over 2 weeks. With this dose, 11% of 1-year survivors and 50% of 2-year survivors develop severe dementia.

Bibliography

1. Muhsen BEA, Joshi KC, Lee BS, Thapa B, Borghei-Razavi H, Jia X, et al. The effect of gamma knife radiosurgery on large posterior fossa metastases and the associated mass effect from peritumoral edema. J Neurosurg. 2020;134(2):466–74.

2. Nugent JL, Bunn PA, Matthews MJ, et al. CNS metastases in small-cell bronchogenic carcinoma: increasing frequency and changing pattern with lengthening survival. Cancer. 1979;44:1885–93.

3. Zakrzewski J, Geraghty LN, Rose AE, et al. Clinical variables and primary tumor characteristics predictive of the development of melanoma brain metastases and post-brain metastases survival. Cancer. 2011;117:1711–20.

4. Bryan P. CSF seeding of intra-cranial tumours: a study of 96 cases. Clin Radiol. 1974;25(3):355–60.

5. Davies MA, Liu P, McIntyre S, et al. Prognostic factors for survival in melanoma patients with brain metastases. Cancer. 2011;117:1687–96.

6. Ruderman NB, Hall TC. Use of glucocorticoids in the palliative treatment of metastatic brain tumors. Cancer. 1965;18:298–306.

7. Smalley SR, Laws ER, O'Fallon JR, et al. Resection for solitary brain metastasis: role of adjuvant radiation and prognostic variables in 229 patients. J Neurosurg. 1992;77:531–40.

8. Tobler WD, Sawaya R, Tew JM. Successful laser assisted excision of a metastatic midbrain tumor. Neurosurgery. 1986;18:795–7.

9. Patchell RA, Tibbs PA, Walsh JW, et al. A randomized trial of surgery in the treatment of single metastases to the brain. N Engl J Med. 1990;322(8):494–500.

10. Pollock BE. Management of patients with multiple brain metastases. Contemp Neurosurg. 1999;21:1–6.

11. Sze G, Soletsky S, Bronen R, et al. MR imaging of the cranial meninges with emphasis on contrast enhancement and meningeal carcinomatosis. AJNR. 1989;10:965–75.

12. Le Rhun E, Taillibert S, Chamberlain MC. Carcinomatous meningitis: leptomeningeal metastases in solid tumors. Surg Neurol Int. 2013;4:S265–88.

13. Gaspar L, Scott C, Rotman M, et al. Recursive partitioning analysis (RPA) of prognostic factors in three radiation therapy oncology group (RTOG) brain metastases trials. Int J Radiat Oncol Biol Phys. 1997;37:745–51.

14. Gaspar LE, Mehta MP, Patchell RA, et al. The role of whole brain radiation therapy in the management of newly diagnosed brain metastases: a systematic review and evidence-based clinical practice guideline. J Neuro-Oncol. 2010;96(1):17–32.

15. Ryken TC, McDermott M, Robinson PD, et al. The role of steroids in the management of brain metastases: a systematic review and evidence-based clinical practice guideline. J Neuro-Oncol. 2010;96(1):103–14.

16. Mehta MP, Paleologos NA, Mikkelsen T, et al. The role of chemotherapy in the management of newly diagnosed brain metastases: a systematic review and evidence-based clinical practice guideline. J Neuro-Oncol. 2010;96(1):71–83.

20

Orbital Tumors

Muhammad S. Umerani, Oday Atallah,
Ruqaya A. Kassim, Ahmed Muthana, Maliya Delawan,
and Samer S. Hoz

21

❓ 1. **Orbital tumors: common presenting symptoms. The FALSE answer is:**
   A. Pain.
   B. Diplopia.
   C. Enophthalmos.
   D. Blurred vision.
   E. Vision loss.

✅ **Answer C**
— Orbital tumors may present with exophthalmos, not enophthalmos. Exophthalmos is also seen in thyroid diseases, orbital varices, collagen vascular diseases, and congenital defects of the orbital wall.

❓ 2. **Orbital tumors: clinical manifestations. The FALSE answer is:**
   A. Diplopia is usually present if the tumor is within the orbital apex.
   B. May involve the optic nerve circumferentially.
   C. Orbital apex tumors do not interfere with orbital motility.
   D. If visual acuity is affected, it may suggest intrinsic disease of the optic nerve.
   E. Tumors within the optic canal do not usually affect visual acuity.

✅ **Answer E**
— Comprehensive tumors within the optic canal do affect visual acuity.

❓ 3. **Orbital tumors: location of the lesion. The FALSE answer is:**
   A. Proptosis is a late manifestation of extraconal tumors.
   B. With extraconal tumors, the orbit is displaced superiorly.
   C. Visual impairment depends on the involvement of individual muscles.
   D. The orbit is displaced medially with extraconal tumors.
   E. Extraconal tumors are located outside the muscle cone.

✅ **Answer A**
— Extraconal tumors have proptosis as an early manifestation due to the involvement of individual muscles and deformity of the globe.

❓ 4. **Intracanalicular tumors. The FALSE answer is:**
   A. Cause optic disk swelling.
   B. Proptosis may be present.
   C. Patients usually present with early loss of vision.

D. Associated with the appearance of optic ciliary shunts.

E. Are usually located within the muscle cone.

✅ **Answer E**

– As the name suggests, intracanalicular tumors are located within the optic canal.

❓ 5. **Intraconal tumors. The FALSE answer is:**

A. Cause direct pressure on the optic nerve.

B. Cause visual loss at later stages of the disease.

C. Cause direct pressure on the oculomotor nerve.

D. Axial proptosis is a prominent feature.

E. Orbital motility is usually affected due to direct pressure on the individual muscles.

✅ **Answer B**

– Intraconal orbital tumors are notorious for causing early visual loss due to their location.

❓ 6. **Intraconal tumors may cause compression of the following structures within their compartment. The FALSE answer is:**

A. Ciliary ganglion.

B. Ophthalmic artery.

C. Lacrimal gland.

D. Oculomotor nerve.

E. Abducens nerve.

✅ **Answer C**

– The lacrimal gland is in the extraconal compartment.

❓ 7. **Extraconal tumors may cause compression of the following structures within their compartment. The FALSE answer is:**

A. Trochlear nerve.

B. Ophthalmic artery.

C. Lacrimal gland.

D. Lacrimal and frontal branches of the ophthalmic nerve.

E. Fat.

✅ **Answer B**

– The ophthalmic artery is in the intraconal compartment.

8. Through annulus of Zinn, a tendinous ring at the orbital apex, the following structures pass. The FALSE answer is:
   A. Optic nerve.
   B. Ophthalmic artery.
   C. Superior and inferior divisions of the trigeminal nerve.
   D. Abducens nerve.
   E. Nasociliary branch of the ophthalmic nerve.

21

✓ **Answer C**
— The superior and inferior divisions of the oculomotor nerve enter through the annulus of Zinn, rather than those of the trigeminal nerve.

9. Miscellaneous. The FALSE answer is:
   A. Cavernous malformations, also known as cavernous hemangiomas, are the most common benign orbital tumors in infants.
   B. The most common primary adult ocular malignancy is choroidal melanoma.
   C. Lymphoma (primary or secondary) is the most prevalent orbital neoplasm in adults $\geq$60 years of age.
   D. The most common malignancy to metastasize to the orbit is breast cancer.
   E. Orbital pseudotumor is the most common orbital lesion in adults.

✓ **Answer A**
— Cavernous hemangiomas are the most common benign orbital tumors in adults, but not in infants.

10. Orbital schwannoma: clinical manifestations. The FALSE answer is:
   A. Visual disturbance is a common symptom.
   B. Optic disk edema may be present on physical examination.
   C. Proptosis is a predominant symptom in all patients.
   D. Patients may experience pain around the eye or brow.
   E. Changes in appearance such as eyelid fullness or bulging may occur.

✓ **Answer C**
— Symptoms can vary due to the location and size of the tumor.

? 11. **Orbital schwannoma: tumor characteristics. The FALSE answer is:**

A. Orbital schwannomas mostly arise from the intraorbital branch of the trigeminal nerve.

B. These tumors are mostly unilocular, well-defined, encapsulated, and benign.

C. They seldom infiltrate into the optic nerve.

D. These tumors are frequently slow-growing.

E. Schwannomas can invade the bony orbit, causing bone destruction.

✓ **Answer E**

— Schwannomas are generally noninvasive and do not usually cause bone destruction.

? 12. **Optic nerve sheath meningiomas: tumor characteristics. The FALSE answer is:**

A. Typically arises from arachnoid cap cells in the optic nerve sheath.

B. The tumor generally shows calcification on radiographic imaging.

C. The peak incidence occurs in the fifth and sixth decades of life.

D. Women are more frequently affected than men.

E. The tumor can extend along the optic nerve toward the brain.

✓ **Answer C**

— The peak incidence occurs in the third and fourth decades of life.

? 13. **Optic nerve glioma: treatment. The FALSE answer is:**

A. Chemotherapy is commonly used to treat optic nerve gliomas.

B. Surgery can lead to a complete cure in most cases.

C. Radiation therapy is employed sparingly due to its potential for long-term side effects.

D. Treatment strategies are individualized depending on factors such as patient age, tumor size, and symptoms.

E. Nonsurgical treatments are considered first-line in most cases to avoid surgical complications.

✓ **Answer B**

— Surgery can debulk the tumor and improve symptoms, but complete removal is often difficult.

? 14. **Optic nerve gliomas: tumor characteristics. The FALSE answer is:**
   A. Most commonly affect children.
   B. Typically present with painless, progressive loss of vision.
   C. Can cause proptosis.
   D. Can spread to the hypothalamus.
   E. Are aggressive, fast-growing tumors.

✓ **Answer E**
— They are usually slow-growing, and their progression is often indolent.

? 15. **Granular cell tumors: epidemiology. The FALSE answer is:**
   A. They can occur at any age but are commonly diagnosed in adulthood.
   B. Often affect the eyes and eyelids.
   C. They are typically benign tumors.
   D. Represent the majority of all granular cell tumors.
   E. Affect males and females almost equally.

✓ **Answer D**
— They are quite rare and represent a minority of all granular cell tumors.

? 16. **Apocrine hidrocystomas: epidemiology. The FALSE answer is:**
   A. Can occur at any age but are most common in adults.
   B. These cysts are usually harmless.
   C. They are most commonly found on the eyelids.
   D. There is no gender predisposition.
   E. Are potentially malignant and frequently metastasize.

✓ **Answer E**
— Apocrine hidrocystomas are usually benign and rarely, if ever, malignant or metastatic.

Bibliography

1. Winn HR. Youmans and Winn Neurological Surgery E-Book: 4-Volume Set. Elsevier Health Sciences; 2022 Jan 21. 3rd edition.
2. Orbital neoplasms in adults: clinical, radiological and pathologic review; Head and Neck Neoplasms RadioGraphics. 2013;33:1739–1758.

21

3. Farag A, Farag S, Daigle P. Orbital schwannoma with frontal bone lysis. J Craniofac Surg. 2023;34(3):e298–300.

4. Colas Q, Khanna RK, Arsène S, Fontaine A, Cohen C, Joly A, Laure B. Pediatric orbital schwannoma: case report and review of the literature. J Fr Ophtalmol. 2022;45(6): e291–5.

5. Kapur R, Mafee MF, Lamba R, Edward DP. Orbital schwannoma and neurofibroma: role of imaging. Neuroimaging Clin N Am. 2005;15(1):159–74.

6. Low CM, Stokken JK. Typical orbital pathologies: hemangioma. J Neurol Surg B Skull Base. 2021;82(1):20–6.

7. Zhou A, Hummel L, Pakravan M, Lee AG. Rapidly progressive optic neuropathy due to optic nerve sheath meningioma following hormonal fertility treatment. Can J Ophthalmol. 2023;58(6):e253–5.

8. Goodyear K, Roelofs KA, Chen AC, Goldberg RA. Visual outcomes following surgical debulking in exophytic optic nerve sheath meningiomas. Ophthalmic Plast Reconstr Surg. 2023; https://doi.org/10.1097/IOP.0000000000002497.

9. Hill CS, Khan M, Phipps K, Green K, Hargrave D, Aquilina K. Neurosurgical experience of managing optic pathway gliomas. Childs Nerv Syst. 2021;37(6):1917–29.

10. Hill CS, Devesa SC, Ince W, Borg A, Aquilina K. A systematic review of ongoing clinical trials in optic pathway gliomas. Childs Nerv Syst. 2020;36(9):1869–86.

11. Barrantes PC, Zhou P, MacDonald SM, Ioakeim-Ioannidou M, Lee NG. Granular cell tumor of the orbit: review of the literature and a proposed treatment modality. Ophthalmic Plast Reconstr Surg. 2022;38(2):122–31.

12. Li XF, Qian J, Yuan YF, Bi YW, Zhang R. Orbital granular cell tumours: clinical and pathologic characteristics of six cases and literature review. Eye (Lond). 2016;30(4): 529–37.

13. Epperson J, Bergfeld W. Apocrine papillary hidrocystoma with mucinous metaplasia (goblet cell type): a case report and review of the literature. Am J Dermatopathol. 2023;45(5):330–2.

14. Koumaki D, Papadakis M, Lagoudaki E, Manios GA, Kassotakis D, Doxastaki A, Krasagakis K, Manios A. Apocrine and eccrine hidrocystomas: a clinicopathological study. Acta Dermatovenerol Alp Pannonica Adriat. 2021;30(2):53–6.

15. Lacey H, Oliphant H, Smith C, Koenig M, Rajak S. Topographical anatomy of the annulus of Zinn. Sci Rep. 2022;12(1):1064.

16. Dailey RA, Saulny SM, Tower RN. Treatment of multiple apocrine hidrocystomas with trichloroacetic acid. Ophthalmic Plast Reconstr Surg. 2005;21(2):148–50.

Tumors and Tumor-like Lesions of the Skull

*Oday Atallah, Ali A. Dolachee, Wamedh E. Matti,
Mahmood F. Alzaidy, Ahmed Muthana,
Mohammed A. Alrawi, and Samer S. Hoz*

© The Author(s), under exclusive license to Springer Nature Switzerland AG 2024
S. S. Hoz et al. (eds.), *Surgical Neuro-Oncology*,
https://doi.org/10.1007/978-3-031-53642-7_22

? 1. **Tumors and TLL of the skull: types. The FALSE answer is:**
   A. Multiple myeloma.
   B. Fibrous dysplasia.
   C. Osteoma.
   D. Chondroma.
   E. Choriocarcinoma.

✓ Answer E
— Choriocarcinoma is a germ cell tumor, not a tumor of the skull.

22

? 2. **Tumors and TLL of the skull: associated syndromes. The FALSE answer is:**
   A. Neurofibromatosis type 2.
   B. McCune-Albright syndrome.
   C. Ollier syndrome.
   D. Gardner syndrome.
   E. Maffucci syndrome.

✓ Answer A
— Neurofibromatosis type 2 is associated with vestibular schwannomas. It is not associated with tumors or TLL of the skull.

? 3. **Tumors and TLL of the skull: imaging findings. The FALSE answer is:**
   A. Chondroma: well-defined lytic lesion.
   B. Plasmacytoma: hyperdense, uniformly enhancing lesion.
   C. Chondrosarcoma: onion skin appearance.
   D. Aneurysmal bone cyst: multiloculated expansile lesion.
   E. Osteosarcoma: sunburst appearance.

✓ Answer C
— The onion skin appearance is commonly associated with Ewing sarcoma.

? 4. **Tumors and TLL of the skull: differential diagnosis. The FALSE answer is:**
   A. Encephalocele.
   B. Choroid plexus carcinoma.
   C. Fractures.
   D. Osteomyelitis.
   E. Congenital hemolytic anemia.

✓ Answer B
— Choroid plexus carcinoma is found inside the ventricles, not close to the skull.

5. Tumors and TLL of the skull: treatment. The FALSE answer is:
A. Osteoid osteoma: NSAID.
B. Osteosarcoma: radiosurgery.
C. Plasmacytoma: chemotherapy.
D. Asymptomatic benign lesions: chemotherapy.
E. Angiosarcoma: preoperative embolization.

✅ **Answer D**
▬ Treatment is not necessary for asymptomatic benign lesions.

6. Chordoma: general information. The FALSE answer is:
A. It constitutes 1% of all intracranial tumors.
B. It is rather common among children.
C. There is no preference for any gender.
D. Of all primary bone tumors, it represents 4% of cases.
E. The clivus is the second most common site for this tumor.

✅ **Answer B**
▬ It often manifests between the age ranges of 20 and 60 years.

7. Chordoma: clinical manifestation. The FALSE answer is:
A. A chordoma situated in the upper clivus may cause oculomotor palsy.
B. It has the potential to transform into a sarcoma.
C. Lung and hepatic metastases are possible.
D. The recurrence rate is minimal.
E. Abducens palsy may be caused by a chordoma situated in the lower clivus.

✅ **Answer D**
▬ Chordoma exhibits a notable propensity for recurrence.

8. Chordoma: radiological finding. The FALSE answer is:
A. Homogenous contrast enhancement.
B. Skeletal destruction.
C. Hypointense lesion on T1-weighted imaging.
D. Low vascularity.
E. Hyperintense lesion on T2-weighted imaging.

✅ **Answer A**
— It has a heterogeneous enhancing pattern characterized by a honeycomb appearance.

❓ 9. **Chordoma: treatment. The FALSE answer is:**
   A. Surgical resection.
   B. Adjuvant radiotherapy.
   C. Proton beam radiation.
   D. Imatinib.
   E. Cabergoline.

22

✅ **Answer E**
— Cabergoline is used to treat prolactinoma.

❓ 10. **Chondrosarcoma: general information. The FALSE answer is:**
   A. It makes up around 0.2% of all intracranial tumors.
   B. Patients between the ages of 40 and 50 are particularly affected.
   C. It is more commonly observed in females.
   D. Accounts for approximately 25% of all primary malignant bone tumors.
   E. It originates from embryonic remnants.

✅ **Answer C**
— Males are more likely to be affected.

❓ 11. **Chondrosarcoma: radiological findings and treatment. The FALSE answer is:**
   A. Calcification is present.
   B. Heterogeneous contrast enhancement.
   C. Less commonly presents as a midline tumor compared to chordoma.
   D. The first line of treatment is chemotherapy.
   E. Local resection is considered the preferred therapeutic option.

✅ **Answer D**
— Chemotherapy typically has limited efficacy.

❓ 12. **Plasmacytoma: general information. The FALSE answer is:**
   A. It is composed of monoclonal plasma cells.
   B. It impacts individuals in the third decade of life.

C. It represents 2% of all plasma cell tumors.
D. Radiation therapy, surgery, and chemotherapy are used in its treatment.
E. The prevalence is higher in males.

✅ **Answer B**
▬ The majority of afflicted men are in their fifth and sixth decades of life.

❓ 13. **Hyperostosis frontalis interna: general information. The FALSE answer is:**
A. It is typically bilateral.
B. It is more prevalent among females.
C. The preferred treatment modality is surgical resection.
D. Paget's disease is a potential differential diagnosis.
E. Could exist without symptoms.

✅ **Answer C**
▬ There is considerable debate over the therapy.

❓ 14. **Fibrous dysplasia: general information. The FALSE answer is:**
A. It accounts for around 27% of all benign bone tumors.
B. Frequency is higher in women.
C. Malignant transformation can occur.
D. Skeletal lesions causing refractory pain might need to be surgically removed.
E. Radiation treatment is recommended.

✅ **Answer E**
▬ Radiotherapy is contraindicated in XRT-induced malignancies.

❓ 15. **Epidermoid and dermoid tumors: general information. The FALSE answer is:**
A. These lesions are considered to be benign.
B. Dermoid cysts have the potential to induce chemical meningitis.
C. They are hypodense on CT.
D. They resemble CSF in every signal.
E. Surgical resection is the preferred treatment.

✅ **Answer D**
▬ In contrast to the CSF, these entities exhibit a heightened signal intensity on DWI.

16. Hemangioma: general information. The FALSE answer is:
A. It comprises around 7% of all skull tumors.
B. The capillary type is the most prevalent.
C. X-ray demonstrates a honeycomb pattern.
D. Surgery is recommended for lesions that are easily accessible.
E. Radiation therapy is recommended for lesions that are difficult to approach.

Answer B
− The cavernous type is the most common.

22

Bibliography

1. Greenberg MS. Handbook of surgery, section 2023, 48. p. 804–12.
2. Iqbal QUA, Majid HJ. Plasmacytoma. In: StatPearls. Treasure Island, FL: StatPearls Publishing; 2023.
3. Kunimatsu A, Kunimatsu N. Skull base tumors and tumor-like lesions: a pictorial review. Pol J Radiol. 2017;82:398–409.
4. Georgalas C, Goudakos J, Fokkens WJ. Osteoma of the skull base and sinuses. Otolaryngol Clin N Am. 2011;44(4):875–90. vii
5. Gozzetti A, Cerase A, Defina M, Bocchia M. Plasmacytoma of the skull. Eur J Haematol. 2012;88(4):369.
6. Na'ara S, Amit M, Gil Z, Billan S. Plasmacytoma of the skull base: a meta-analysis. J Neurol Surg B Skull Base. 2016;77(1):61–5.
7. Burke AB, Collins MT, Boyce AM. Fibrous dysplasia of bone: craniofacial and dental implications. Oral Dis. 2017;23(6):697–708.
8. Wei YT, Jiang S, Cen Y. Fibrous dysplasia of skull. J Craniofac Surg. 2010;21(2):538–42.
9. Liu H, Chang X, Shang H, Li F, Zhou H, Xue X. Diffuse cavernous hemangioma of the skull misdiagnosed as skull metastasis in breast cancer patient: one case report and literature review. BMC Cancer. 2019;19(1):172.
10. Prior A, Anania P, Pacetti M, Secci F, Ravegnani M, Pavanello M, Piatelli G, Cama A, Consales A. Dermoid and epidermoid cysts of scalp: case series of 234 consecutive patients. World Neurosurg. 2018;120:119–24.
11. Ozgen T, Oge HK, Erbengi A, Bertan V. Cranial dermoid and epidermoid cysts. Neurochirurgia (Stuttg). 1990;33(1):16–9.
12. Patel V, Hwa TP, Kaufman AC, Kolster RA, Bigelow DC. Lateral skull base chordoma mimicking a paraganglioma. Otol Neurotol. 2022;43(2):e279–81.
13. Mendenhall WM, Mendenhall CM, Lewis SB, Villaret DB, Mendenhall NP. Skull base chordoma. Head Neck. 2005;27(2):159–65.
14. Kremenevski N, Schlaffer SM, Coras R, Kinfe TM, Graillon T, Buchfelder M. Skull base chordomas and chondrosarcomas. Neuroendocrinology. 2020;110(9–10):836–47.
15. Vuong HG, Dunn IF. Chondrosarcoma and chordoma of the skull base and spine: implication of tumor location on patient survival. World Neurosurg. 2022;162:e635–9.

16. Stiene JM, Frank PW. Hyperostosis frontalis Interna and a question on its pathology: a case report. Am J Case Rep. 2022;23:e937450.
17. She R, Szakacs J. Hyperostosis frontalis interna: case report and review of literature. Ann Clin Lab Sci. 2004;34(2):206–8.

Tumors of the Spine and Spinal Cord

Waeel O. Hamouda, Minaam Farooq,
Iman Mohamoud, and Samer S. Hoz

? 1.   **Primary vertebral column tumors. Malignant hematopoietic tumors that are usually initially located in the anterior vertebral elements (i.e., vertebral body). The FALSE answer is:**
   A. Plasmacytoma.
   B. Multiple myeloma.
   C. Non-Hodgkin's lymphoma (NHL).
   D. Leukemia.
   E. Eosinophilic granuloma.

✓ **Answer E**
   – Although eosinophilic granuloma is usually initially located within the anterior vertebral elements, it is a benign hematopoietic tumor.

23

? 2.   **Primary vertebral column tumors. Vascular tumors that are usually initially located in the anterior vertebral elements (i.e., vertebral body). The FALSE answer is:**
   A. Aneurysmal bone cyst (ABC)—benign tumor.
   B. Hemangioma—benign tumor.
   C. Lymphangioma—benign tumor.
   D. Hemangioendothelioma—malignant tumor.
   E. Hemangiopericytoma—malignant tumor.

✓ **Answer A**
   – Aneurysmal bone cyst (ABC) is a benign tumor that is usually initially located within the posterior vertebral elements.

? 3.   **Primary vertebral column tumors. Tumors that are usually initially located in the anterior vertebral elements (i.e., vertebral body). The FALSE answer is:**
   A. Eosinophilic granuloma—benign tumor.
   B. Ewing sarcoma—malignant tumor.
   C. Hemangioma—benign tumor.
   D. Chordoma—benign tumor.
   E. Giant cell tumor (GCT)—benign tumor.

✓ **Answer B**
   – Ewing sarcoma is usually initially located within the posterior vertebral elements in the sacrum.

4. **Primary vertebral column tumors. Benign osteogenic or chondrogenic tumors that are usually initially located in the posterior vertebral elements (i.e., pedicle, pars, lamina, and spinous process). The FALSE answer is:**
   A. Osteoid osteoma.
   B. Osteoblastoma.
   C. Osteosarcoma.
   D. Osteochondroma (chondroma).
   E. Chondromyxoid fibroma (CMF).

✅ **Answer C**
   − Similar to chondrosarcoma, osteosarcoma is usually initially located within the posterior vertebral elements, but it is a malignant osteogenic tumor.

5. **Primary vertebral column tumors. Tumors that most commonly occur in the thoracic region. The FALSE answer is:**
   A. Eosinophilic granuloma.
   B. Osteochondroma.
   C. Hemangioma.
   D. Plasmacytoma.
   E. Chondrosarcoma.

✅ **Answer B**
   − Osteochondroma is more common in the cervical region.

6. **Primary vertebral column tumors. Tumors that most commonly occur in the lumbar region. The FALSE answer is:**
   A. Chordoma.
   B. Osteoid osteoma and osteoblastoma.
   C. Osteosarcoma.
   D. Hemangioma.
   E. Aneurysmal bone cyst.

✅ **Answer A**
   − Chordoma is more common in the cervical and sacral regions.

7. **Primary vertebral column tumors. Tumors that most commonly occur in the sacral region. The FALSE answer is:**

A. Chordoma.
B. Giant cell tumor (GCT).
C. Ewing sarcoma.
D. Plasmacytoma.
E. Hemangioma.

Answer E

— Hemangioma is more common in the thoracic and lumbar regions.

8. **Primary vertebral column tumors. Benign tumors most common in pediatrics and adolescents (i.e., 0–20 years of age). The FALSE answer is:**

A. Eosinophilic granuloma.
B. Aneurysmal bone cyst.
C. Osteoid osteoma.
D. Osteoblastoma.
E. Osteosarcoma.

Answer E

— Osteosarcoma is the most common malignant primary vertebral column tumor in children, followed by Ewing sarcoma.

9. **Primary vertebral column tumors. Tumors that occur more commonly in adults (i.e., 30–60 years of age). The FALSE answer is:**

A. Hemangioma and lymphangioma.
B. Giant cell tumor (GCT).
C. Osteosarcoma.
D. Plasmacytoma and multiple myeloma.
E. Chordoma.

Answer C

— Osteosarcoma occurs most commonly in children and elderly people above 60 years, but not in middle-aged adults between 20 and 60 years of age.

10. **Primary vertebral column tumors. Tumors that are more common in males. The FALSE answer is:**

A. Hemangioma and lymphangioma.
B. Osteoid osteoma and osteoblastoma.

C. Osteochondroma and chondromyxoid fibroma.

D. Plasmacytoma and multiple myeloma.

E. Aneurysmal bone cyst (ABC) and giant cell tumor (GCT).

✔ **Answer E**

▬ Aneurysmal bone cyst (ABC) and giant cell tumor (GCT) are the only primary vertebral column tumors that tend to occur more commonly in females than males.

❓ 11. **Primary vertebral column tumors. Osteoid osteoma characteristics. The FALSE answer is:**

A. Mainly present with nocturnal spine aches.

B. Pain can lead to secondary scoliosis or torticollis.

C. Pain dramatically responds to muscle relaxants.

D. Characterized by a focal lytic nidus harboring a central sclerotic dot surrounded by reactive sclerosis or edema.

E. Usually circumscribed with a diameter of less than 15 mm.

✔ **Answer C**

▬ Pain dramatically responds to NSAIDs, especially acetylsalicylic acid (ASA, aspirin), as the nidus releases prostaglandins, which induce pain.

❓ 12. **Primary vertebral column tumors. Osteoblastoma characteristics. The FALSE answer is:**

A. Similar to osteoid osteoma, the neoplastic nidus contains vessels, osteoblasts, and woven bone.

B. Similar to osteoid osteoma, the nidus enhances after contrast administration.

C. Similar to osteoid osteoma, it usually arises from the posterior vertebral elements.

D. Similar to osteoid osteoma, it is circumscribed with a diameter of less than 15 mm.

E. It can rarely transform into malignant osteosarcoma and lead to metastasis.

✔ **Answer D**

▬ Osteoblastoma is more expansile than osteoid osteoma and is usually larger than 15 mm in diameter, which can result in an epidural mass effect and neurological symptoms and signs.

? 13. **Primary vertebral column tumors. Osteosarcoma characteristics. The FALSE answer is:**

   A. Can also grow near the ends of long bones, the mandible, and the pelvis.
   B. Always arises from the malignant transformation of an osteoblastoma.
   C. Destructive osteoblastic lesions are seen on radiology images.
   D. Has a poor prognosis with a median survival rate of less than 10 months.
   E. Can metastasize to other remote body locations.

✓ Answer B
   — Osteosarcoma can also arise from the malignant transformation of Paget's disease.

? 14. **Primary vertebral column tumors. Osteochondroma (chondroma) characteristics. The FALSE answer is:**

   A. Can show an expansile growth from within the medullary cavity, referred to as enchondroma.
   B. Can show an exophytic growth from the cortical surface, referred to as periosteal chondroma.
   C. Resembles lobules of firm mature cartilage well-circumscribed from adjacent bone.
   D. Appears hypointense in both T1 and T2 MRI images and enhances after contrast administration.
   E. Typically circumscribed with no surrounding reactive sclerosis.

✓ Answer D
   — Cartilage appears as low attenuation areas in CT due to its water content, so it appears hypointense in T1 and hyperintense in T2 MRI images with no post-contrast enhancement.

? 15. **Primary vertebral column tumors. Osteochondroma (chondroma) characteristics. The FALSE answer is:**

   A. Typically, a solitary small lesion and can be sessile or pedunculated.
   B. If multiple lesions are present, multiple chondromatosis syndrome (MCS) should be suspected.
   C. MCS is also called "hereditary multiple exostoses."

D. MCS is also called "Ollier disease" or "Maffucci syndrome."

E. MCS carries a lower risk of sarcomatous transformation than a solitary osteochondroma.

✅ **Answer E**

− Multiple chondromatosis syndrome (MCS) carries a higher risk than a solitary osteochondroma for malignant transformation, especially in large tumors with a diameter of more than 7 cm.

❓ **16. Primary vertebral column tumors. Chondrosarcoma characteristics. The FALSE answer is:**

A. According to the WHO classification, it is categorized into four grades: I, II, III, and IV.

B. The higher the grade, the more cellular, softer, and friable the tumor is.

C. The risk of metastasis with high grades (II–IV) is as high as 70–80%.

D. The histological subtypes are conventional, clear cell, mesenchymal, and dedifferentiated.

E. The mesenchymal type has the best prognosis with the highest 5-year survival rate.

✅ **Answer E**

− The conventional type, which represents 90% of diagnosed chondrosarcomas, has the best prognosis with a 5-year survival rate of 90% because only 10% of this type are high-grade tumors. This is followed by the clear cell type with a 5-year survival rate of 70%, the mesenchymal type with a 5-year survival rate of 50%, and the dedifferentiated type with a 5-year survival rate of only 10%.

❓ **17. Primary vertebral column tumors. Hemangioma characteristics. The FALSE answer is:**

A. Multiple in about 30% of cases.

B. Symptomatic in about 40% of cases.

C. Symptoms can be secondary congestion, compression fracture, or spontaneous epidural hemorrhage.

D. It can be treated with radiosurgery if symptomatic because it is radiosensitive.

E. Can be treated with vertebroplasty if symptomatic.

✓ Answer B
- Hemangiomas are rarely symptomatic; only 1% of cases are symptomatic.

❓ 18. Primary vertebral column tumors. Hemangioma characteristics. The FALSE answer is:
  A. Shows uptake in bone scan.
  B. Lytic lesion.
  C. Sagittal CT images show vertical lucencies separated by thick bone trabeculae, i.e., jail bars sign.
  D. Axial CT images show white dots representing thickened vertical trabeculae, i.e., polka-dot sign.
  E. Hyperintense lesion in T1 and T2 MRI images due to its fat content.

23

✓ Answer A
- Hemangioma shows no uptake in bone scan, which can differentiate it from metastasis.

❓ 19. Primary vertebral column tumors. Hemangioma in pregnancy. The FALSE answer is:
  A. Most often occurs during the third trimester of pregnancy.
  B. Most commonly affects the thoracic spinal levels.
  C. Most exhibit a benign course.
  D. Treatment options are induction of preterm delivery, expectant observation, or surgery.
  E. Although spontaneous postpartum improvement occurs in a few patients, future recurrence is frequent.

✓ Answer C
- Hemangiomas typically demonstrate an aggressive course during pregnancy, necessitating subtotal surgical decompression, especially in the absence of preoperative embolization. This is why many surgeons advocate for early postpartum adjuvant treatments such as re-surgery or radiotherapy.

❓ 20. Primary vertebral column tumors. Eosinophilic granuloma (EG) characteristics. The FALSE answer is:
  A. Solitary lesion in 50–75% of cases.
  B. Demonstrates expanding erosive accumulations of foamy and vacuolated histiocytes.

C. Occurs primarily in the skull (50% of cases), mandible, ribs, and femur.

D. Can metastasize to the lung (20% of cases), skin, pituitary, liver, and lymph nodes.

E. Can lead to strong dense vertebrae.

✅ **Answer E**

- Eosinophilic granuloma can lead to "vertebra plana," characterized by a markedly compressed vertebra without kyphosis due to weakening of the bone.

❓ 21. **Primary vertebral column tumors. Eosinophilic granuloma (EG) characteristics. The FALSE answer is:**

A. Lytic lesions.

B. If it occurs in multiple lesions, it is termed "Langerhans cell histiocytosis (LCH)."

C. It represents a subset of histiocytosis X.

D. In LCH, if a new solitary lesion appears after 4 years, the condition is still classified as LCH.

E. LCH is less common than EG and carries a poorer prognosis.

✅ **Answer D**

- In LCH, if a new osseous lesion appears within less than 2 years, the condition is still classified as LCH. In contrast, if a new osseous lesion appears after more than 4 years, the new lesion is classified as localized EG.

❓ 22. **Primary vertebral column tumors. Multiple myeloma WHO diagnostic criteria mandate one of the following two findings: bone marrow aspirate yielding more than 15% plasma cells present in the aspirate OR biopsy of the suspected lesion proving plasmacytoma, plus one of the following. The FALSE answer is:**

A. Anemia <10 mg/dL.

B. Decreased vitamin D serum level.

C. Creatinine >2 mg/dL.

D. Hypercalcemia >10 mg/dL.

E. Bone osteolytic lesion.

✅ **Answer B**

? **23.** **Primary vertebral column tumors. Multiple myeloma adjuvant laboratory findings. The FALSE answer is:**

A. High parathyroid hormone.

B. Blood electrophoresis showing hyper-gammaglobulinemia (mainly IgG spike).

C. Bence-Jones proteinuria, i.e., the light chain of immunoglobulins without the accompanying heavy chain.

D. Hyperuricemia.

E. High alkaline phosphatase.

✓ **Answer A**

? **24.** **Primary vertebral column tumors. Multiple myeloma characteristics. The FALSE answer is:**

A. The most common primary vertebral column malignant tumor (20% of vertebral malignant tumors).

B. Solitary lesions are called plasmacytoma.

C. Solitary lesions are not associated with M proteins in serum or urine.

D. Seen as lytic punched-out "moth-eaten" lesions in radiology images.

E. Radioresistant.

✓ **Answer E**

— Multiple myeloma is radiosensitive and responds to radiotherapy.

? **25.** **Primary vertebral column tumors. Multiple myeloma radiological differential diagnosis of "moth-eaten" bony lesions (multiple small bone marrow lucent holes) with poorly defined margins and sparing of the cortex. The FALSE answer is:**

A. Malignant fibrous histiocytoma.

B. Lymphoma.

C. Hemangioma.

D. Ewing sarcoma.

E. Eosinophilic granuloma.

✓ **Answer C**

— Hemangiomas are not classically associated with "moth-eaten" bony lesions with poorly defined margins and sparing of the cortex. They exhibit a "corduroy cloth" or "jail bar" appearance on sagittal imaging, which manifests as a "polka-dotted" or "salt and pepper" appearance on axial imaging.

26. Primary vertebral column tumors. Aneurysmal bone cyst (ABC) characteristics. The FALSE answer is:

A. Can also occur in long bones, e.g., femur, tibia, and humerus.
B. Arise from preexisting tumors (e.g., GCT, osteoblastoma, or sarcomas) in 5% of cases.
C. Can develop after acute fractures or from fibrous dysplasia.
D. Giant cell reparative granuloma is a solid variant of ABC that occurs in 5% of cases.
E. Radiological images show fluid level, trabeculations, cortical shell, and hemosiderin.

Answer B
— Almost 1/3 of the cases arise from preexisting tumors.

27. Primary vertebral column tumors. Ewing's sarcoma characteristics. The FALSE answer is:

A. Primary spine lesions are more common than secondary spine metastatic lesions.
B. Is a small round blue cell tumor.
C. Usually presents with nonspecific local pain.
D. Associated periosteal calcifications and invasion of surrounding soft tissue.
E. Is radiosensitive.

Answer A
— Secondary spine metastatic lesions are more common than primary spine lesions.

28. Primary vertebral column tumors. Giant cell tumor (GCT) characteristics. The FALSE answer is:

A. Also known as osteoclastoma, as the cells of origin are osteoclasts.
B. Results from RANK/RANKL signaling overexpression leading to osteoclast hyperproliferation.
C. Usually affects the upper sacrum (S1, S2) and can cross the sacroiliac joint.
D. Affects long bones near joints and the sphenoid bone of the skull.
E. Commonly metastasizes to the kidneys.

Answer E
— GCT commonly metastasizes to the lung; therefore, it is advisable to perform a chest CT before initiating any intervention.

? 29. Primary vertebral column tumors. Chordoma characteristics. The FALSE answer is:

A. Represents a remnant of the notochord.
B. 1/3 of the total cases occur in the clivus at the skull base.
C. The conventional type is the most common, while the chondroid type has the best prognosis.
D. The dedifferentiated type is the least common and carries the worst prognosis.
E. Is well-circumscribed with well-defined thick margins.

✔ Answer E

– The lesions are poorly marginated with microscopic distal extension of tumor cells, explaining the high recurrence rate after surgical excision.

? 30. Primary vertebral column tumors. Chordoma characteristics. The FALSE answer is:

A. Destructive lytic lesion.
B. Infiltrates the disk space.
C. Areas of necrosis or hemorrhage with intratumoral calcifications.
D. The soft-tissue mass is typically small relative to the amount of bony destruction.
E. Heterogeneous honeycomb enhancement.

✔ Answer D

– The soft-tissue mass is typically disproportionately large relative to the amount of bony destruction.

? 31. Primary vertebral column. Chordoma versus giant cell tumor characteristics. The FALSE answer is:

A. Both are considered benign tumors with locally aggressive behavior.
B. Both almost invariably (97–99%) occur when the growth plates have closed.
C. Both usually occur in career years, i.e., from the age of 25 to 60 years.
D. Chordoma tends to occur at a younger age than giant cell tumors.
E. Their most common location is the sacrum.

✔ Answer D

– Giant cell tumor tends to occur at a younger age than chordoma.

? 32. **Primary vertebral column tumors. Biopsy. The FALSE answer is:**
   A. Needle biopsy is the standard technique.
   B. If percutaneous biopsy revealed sarcoma, the needle tract must be excised in the subsequent surgery.
   C. ABC might bleed after percutaneous biopsy, so an open biopsy followed by excision in the same setting is preferred.
   D. Important to examine the entire biopsy; high-grade cell pockets may reside within a low-grade sample.
   E. Sampling error may lead to the mistaken identification of chondrosarcoma as osteochondroma.

✅ **Answer A**
   – Core biopsy is the standard technique as it reduces sampling errors in comparison with needle biopsy.

? 33. **Primary vertebral column tumors. Criteria for embolization. The FALSE answer is:**
   A. The diagnosis is certain.
   B. There is no neurological compromise.
   C. Stability is not of concern.
   D. Could be safely performed (i.e., the feeding artery does not also supply the anterior spinal artery).
   E. Can be done only once.

✅ **Answer E**
   – Some cases may need serial embolization (3–7 times), especially with GCT.

? 34. **Primary vertebral column tumors. Indications for embolization. The FALSE answer is:**
   A. To reduce pain, especially in symptomatic hemangiomas.
   B. May stop GCT growth for up to 10 years.
   C. Preoperatively to reduce bleeding during surgery.
   D. May be done as a curative treatment for eosinophilic granuloma.
   E. Can be used for treating ABC but recurrent neovascularization may occur.

✅ **Answer D**
   – Eosinophilic granuloma is not a highly vascular lesion.

❓ 35. Primary vertebral column tumors. Surgery. The FALSE answer is:
  A. Helps confirm the diagnosis if biopsies were nonconclusive.
  B. Simple curettage of the lesions has demonstrated similar outcomes as "en bloc" excision.
  C. Indicated to control refractory pain not responding to other measures.
  D. Indicated to reverse neurological deficits or preserve neurological functions.
  E. Indicated to fix pathological fractures.

✅ Answer B
  - Although en bloc excision is usually more technically demanding, it achieves a lower recurrence rate and is associated with less intraoperative bleeding.

23

❓ 36. Primary vertebral column tumors. Radiotherapy. The FALSE answer is:
  A. May be used for painful hemangioma as it is radiosensitive and undergoes sclerotic obliteration.
  B. May be used alone for painful inoperable eosinophilic granulomas.
  C. Preoperative as a surgical adjunct in hemangioma or eosinophilic granuloma.
  D. Post-op following residual/recurrence for all lesions.
  E. Proton beam therapy may be used for chordomas and sarcomas.

✅ Answer D
  - Re-surgery is preferable to radiotherapy for recurrent/residual cases, so radiotherapy is only used for inoperable symptomatic residual/recurrent lesions.

❓ 37. Primary spinal cord tumors (SCTs). General points. The FALSE answer is:
  A. Include tumors of the spinal cord, spinal meninges, and spinal nerve roots.
  B. Are 10 times less common than their cranial counterparts.
  C. Are classified into extradural, intradural extramedullary, and intradural intramedullary.
  D. Intradural intramedullary tumors (IDIM-SCT) are the most common type.
  E. Nerve sheath tumors are the most common type of SCTs.

✅ **Answer D**
- The most common type of SCT is intradural extramedullary (IDEM-SCT), which represents about 75% of SCTs, while intradural intramedullary tumors (IDIM-SCT) only represent about 15% of SCTs.

❓ **38. Primary spinal cord tumors (SCTs). Clinical presentation. The FALSE answer is:**
    A. Symptoms frequently precede the diagnosis by about 2 years due to the slow-growing nature of many of these tumors.
    B. Acute sudden deterioration has not been reported.
    C. Pain especially during recumbency ("nocturnal pain") is the most common complaint.
    D. Scoliosis is observed in one-third of patients, mostly affecting children, and is more notable with gangliogliomas.
    E. Weakness and gait disturbances are the second most common presenting symptoms following pain.

✅ **Answer B**
- Acute deterioration has been reported in some cases secondary to intratumoral hemorrhage, which can occur with hemangioblastoma and more commonly with ependymoma.

❓ **39. Primary spinal cord tumors (SCTs). Presentation of pain. The FALSE answer is:**
    A. Almost always present in filum tumors.
    B. Characteristically absent with lipomas.
    C. Schwannomas often start with myelopathic symptoms.
    D. Radicular pain increases with the Valsalva maneuver and spine movement.
    E. A spinal cord tumor should be suspected if the affected dermatome is unusual for disk herniation.

✅ **Answer C**
- Schwannomas often start with radicular symptoms including pain that later progresses to cord involvement.

❓ **40. Primary spinal cord tumors (SCTs). Presentation of sphincteric disturbances. The FALSE answer is:**
    A. Are the least common presenting symptoms and usually present late.

B. Usually anal with stool incontinence or constipation.

C. Early in lesions affecting the conus medullaris or cauda equina.

D. Lipomas usually present initially with sphincteric disturbances rather than pain.

E. Common with age less than 5 years due to frequency of lumbosacral lesions (e.g., dermoids).

✅ **Answer B**

— Usually urogenital and less commonly anal.

❓ 41. **Primary spinal cord tumors (SCTs). CT myelography. The FALSE answer is:**

A. Complete subarachnoid block cannot be detected by lumbar puncture alone without myelography.

B. Extradural tumors show hourglass deformity (with incomplete block) or paintbrush effect (with complete block).

C. Intradural extramedullary tumors show a capping effect with a sharp cutoff (meniscus sign).

D. Intramedullary tumors may show fusiform cord widening.

E. Elevated protein is seen in about 95% of concurrently obtained CSF samples.

✅ **Answer A**

— Although myelography in the pre-CT and MRI era was the gold standard to detect the presence of spinal cord tumors, some historical tests were described to be performed during lumbar puncture to detect complete subarachnoid block by a spinal cord tumor. Examples include Froin's sign, which is CSF clotting due to high level of fibrinogen and xanthochromia induced by the tumor presence, and Queckenstedt's test, which is failure of jugular vein compression to increase CSF pressure during lumbar puncture.

❓ 42. **Primary spinal cord tumors (SCTs). Intradural extramedullary tumors (IDEM-SCT). General points. The FALSE answer is:**

A. All IDEM-SCT are benign WHO grade I tumors.

B. Nerve sheath tumors (schwannomas and neurofibromas) constitute about 50–60% of IDEM-SCT.

C. Meningiomas are the second most common type of IDEM-SCT after nerve sheath tumors.

D. Spinal paragangliomas are considered IDEM-SCT.

E. Surgical excision of IDEM-SCT is the main treatment modality if feasible.

✓ **Answer A**

▬ About 5% of IDEM-SCT are high-grade tumors.

❓ 43. **Primary spinal cord tumors (SCTs). Intradural extramedullary tumors (IDEM-SCT). Spinal meningioma incidence. The FALSE answer is:**

A. IDEM-SCT meningiomas represent 3% of all CNS tumors.

B. IDEM-SCT meningiomas represent 10% of all CNS meningiomas.

C. Meningiomas represent about 30% of IDEM-SCT.

D. The peak age of diagnosis is 40–70 years.

E. There is no specific gender predilection.

✓ **Answer E**

▬ Spinal meningiomas demonstrate a strong female gender predilection with a female-to-male ratio of 4:1, showing stronger female predilection than cranial meningiomas. However, the ratio is 1:1 in the lumbar spine region and in pediatric cases.

❓ 44. **Primary spinal cord tumors (SCTs). Intradural extramedullary tumors (IDEM-SCT). Spinal meningioma locations. The FALSE answer is:**

A. 90% are intradural, 5% are extradural, 5% are both intra- and extradural, and less than 1% are intramedullary.

B. Meningiomas are most common in the cervical region.

C. 75% lie ventral to the denticulate ligament, with 35% being lateral, 30% anterolateral, and 10% anterior.

D. Cervical meningiomas are more common in males than females.

E. In the cervical region, meningiomas tend to be located anterior to the cord.

✓ **Answer B**

▬ The most common spine region for meningiomas is the thoracic region, which harbors 75% of the lesions. This is followed by the cervical region with 20%, and finally, the lumbar region with 5%.

❓ 45. **Primary spinal cord tumors (SCTs). Intradural extramedullary tumors (IDEM-SCT). Spinal meningioma pathology. The FALSE answer is:**

A. Arise from meningothelial arachnoid cells.

B. WHO grade I meningiomas represent more than 90%.

C. Are usually solitary.

D. WHO grade II clear cell meningiomas do not typically occur in the spine.

E. WHO grade III meningiomas represent less than 5% of IDEM-SCT meningiomas.

✅ **Answer D**

— WHO grade II clear cell meningiomas have a predilection for the spine and are believed to originate from the denticulate ligaments. They have a higher recurrence rate.

23

❓ 46. **Primary spinal cord tumors (SCTs). Intradural extramedullary tumors (IDEM-SCT). Spinal meningiomas in neurofibromatosis type 2 patients. The FALSE answer is:**

A. Represent 14% of all spinal tumors found in NF2 patients.

B. Are multiple.

C. Typically occur in elderly patients.

D. Have a more aggressive course.

E. May be associated with spine schwannomas.

✅ **Answer C**

— Spinal meningiomas are predominantly identified in younger patients, and diagnosis in the pediatric population is often linked to NF2.

❓ 47. **Primary spinal cord tumors (SCTs). Intradural extramedullary tumors (IDEM-SCT). Spinal meningioma features in MRI imaging. The FALSE answer is:**

A. Isointense to slightly hypointense in T1WI.

B. Isointense to slightly hyperintense in T2WI.

C. Usually shows homogeneous enhancement after contrast administration.

D. Dural tail sign (dural contrast enhancement beyond tumor attachment) is present in almost all cases.

E. Heterogeneous enhancement may occur due to calcifications, hemorrhage, or necrosis.

✅ **Answer D**

— Post-contrast dural tail sign can be detected in only 40–60% of spinal tumors, which is less frequent than with cranial tumors.

? 48. Primary spinal cord tumors (SCTs). Intradural extramedullary tumors (IDEM-SCT). "en plaque" spinal meningiomas in comparison with the more commonly encountered circumscribed lesions. The FALSE answer is:

A. Frequently associated with intramedullary signal changes on T2WI.

B. Only occurs intradurally.

C. Are larger in size at diagnosis as the diffuse growth pattern delays clinical manifestations.

D. Have higher surgical risk due to the large size and arachnoiditis which limit gross total excision.

E. Poorer prognosis due to recurrence after incomplete excision and worse clinical status at presentation.

✓ **Answer B**

− Can occur on the extradural surface extending to the foramen along the spinal nerve dural sleeves.

? 49. Primary spinal cord tumors (SCTs). Intradural extramedullary tumors (IDEM-SCT). Spinal meningioma management. The FALSE answer is:

A. For small and asymptomatic lesions, a wait-and-see strategy is employed with regular follow-up MRIs.

B. The recommended follow-up MRI schedule is once every year for the first 5 years and once every 2 years thereafter.

C. If the lesions are growing and symptomatic, opt for resection if feasible.

D. If multiple meningiomas are detected, surgery is recommended for the growing and symptomatic lesions only.

E. There is no need to follow an already diagnosed meningioma if the patient becomes pregnant.

✓ **Answer E**

− Some meningiomas show accelerated growth patterns in response to hormonal changes associated with pregnancy. If a female patient with a previously diagnosed nonsurgical meningioma gets pregnant, a very close observation of her clinical status should be planned during the pregnancy period for early detection of any subtle changes in her neurological status.

② 50. Primary spinal cord tumors (SCTs). Intradural extramedullary tumors (IDEM-SCT). Spinal meningioma surgical approaches. Although the posterior approach is usually sufficient to excise most spinal meningiomas, posterolateral, anterolateral, or anterior approaches for excision might be needed for anterior or anterolateral lesions in the following conditions. The FALSE answer is:

A. The presence of a large dural tail.
B. Extradural extension with dumbbell-shaped lesions extending paravertebrally.
C. Extradural extension infiltrating the vertebral body (intraosseous meningioma).
D. Massively calcified large meningioma.
E. Recurrent lesion with adhesions to the spinal cord.

23

✓ Answer A

— Simpson grade I surgical excision with removal of the tumor with all its enhancing dural base is rarely feasible, especially in patients with anterior dural attachment because of the risk of damaging the spinal cord during retraction or the difficulty of adequate dural repair after radical dural excision and the high risk of CSF leak. Therefore, Simpson grade II resection with complete removal of the exophytic tumor along with coagulation of suspicious dural attachment has been proposed as an acceptable option with a very low recurrence rate.

② 51. Primary spinal cord tumors (SCTs). Intradural extramedullary tumors (IDEM-SCT). Spinal meningioma: risk factors for poor surgical outcome. The FALSE answer is:

A. Ventral location of the tumor due to increased risk of cord traction during surgery.
B. Poor preoperative neurological status.
C. Lumbar location of the tumor due to the presence of the cauda equina.
D. Thoracic location of the tumor due to frail vascularization of the spinal cord.
E. Injury to the radiculomedullary arteries.

✓ Answer C

— The lumbar spinal canal provides a large space for low-risk surgical manipulation. In contrast, in the cervical or thoracic regions (especially at the conus and upper thoracic) the spinal canal is relatively narrow, and surgical risk is much higher.

52. Primary spinal cord tumors (SCTs). Intradural extramedullary tumors (IDEM-SCT). Spinal meningioma: risk factors for recurrence. The FALSE answer is:

A. Elderly patients.

B. Cervical location of the tumor (usually ventrally located tumors with difficult total excision).

C. High-grade meningioma (WHO grade III).

D. En plaque growth.

E. Extradural, foraminal, or interosseous extension.

Answer A

- Young patients less than 50 years of age usually show a higher rate of recurrence due to longer expected survival.

53. Primary spinal cord tumors (SCT). Intradural extramedullary tumors (IDEM-SCT). Spinal meningioma: indications of radiotherapy. The FALSE answer is:

A. WHO grade 1 with large residual components (Simpson IV-V grades) and a high risk of reoperation.

B. WHO grade 1 with recurrence after complete excision and a high risk of reoperation.

C. WHO grade 2 with recurrence after complete excision.

D. WHO grade 3.

E. WHO grade 1 after complete tumor excision without removal of affected dura (Simpson grade II).

Answer E

54. Primary spinal cord tumors (SCTs). Intradural extramedullary tumors (IDEM-SCT). Spinal schwannoma incidence. The FALSE answer is:

A. Contributes to 30% of intradural extramedullary spinal cord tumors.

B. Contributes to two-thirds of intradural extramedullary spinal nerve sheath tumors.

C. Peak age is 40 to 70 years of age.

D. More common in females.

E. Represent 2–3% of all CNS tumors.

Answer D

- There is no specific gender predilection.

? 55. **Primary spinal cord tumors (SCTs). Intradural extramedullary tumors (IDEM-SCT). Spinal schwannoma location. The FALSE answer is:**
  A. 65–70% are intradural, 12–15% are extradural, and 12–15% are both intra- and extradural.
  B. Less than 1% are intramedullary.
  C. The lumbar region tends to have a higher occurrence of lesions with extraforaminal tumor growth than the cervical region.
  D. The most common affected region is the cervical spine.
  E. The second most common region is the lumbar spine.

✓ Answer C
  ▬ The ratio of the intradural segment to the extradural segment of the spinal nerve root within the spinal canal gradually increases from the high cervical region to the lumbar region. Similarly, the length of the nerve root within the spinal canal gradually increases from the cervical region to the lumbar region. Hence, the cervical region tends to have a higher occurrence of lesions with extraforaminal tumor growth than the lumbar region.

? 56. **Primary spinal cord tumors (SCT). Intradural extramedullary tumors (IDEM-SCT). Spinal schwannoma pathology. The FALSE answer is:**
  A. Arise from neoplastic Schwann cells of ventral root motor fibers.
  B. Almost all are benign WHO grade I lesions.
  C. Can be either of the classic or the cellular type.
  D. The cellular type is formed exclusively of Antoni A regions (no Antoni B) with an absence of Verocay bodies.
  E. Usually solitary except if associated with neurofibromatosis type 2.

✓ Answer A
  ▬ Arise from neoplastic Schwann cells of dorsal root sensory fibers.

? 57. **Primary spinal cord tumors (SCTs). Intradural extramedullary tumors (IDEM-SCT). Spinal schwannoma radiological features. The FALSE answer is:**
  A. CT and X-ray do not usually show any significant findings.
  B. They are isointense to slightly hypointense in T1WI in about 25% of the lesions.
  C. They are isointense to slightly hyperintense in T2WI in about 95% of the lesions.

23

D. They usually show intense homogeneous post-contrast enhancement.

E. Images might show identifiable attachment to the nerve root from which they arise.

✅ **Answer A**
- CT and X-ray show enlarged neural foramina or pedicle erosion in spinal nerve sheath tumors.

❓ **58. Primary spinal cord tumors (SCTs). Intradural extramedullary tumors (IDEM-SCT). Spinal schwannomas of the malignant melanotic variant. The FALSE answer is:**

A. Show melanotic pigmentation of Schwann cell cytoplasm.

B. Differ from schwannomas on MRI as they appear hyperintense in T1WI and hypointense in T2WI.

C. The characteristic signal on MRI is due to the presence of melanin.

D. Usually part of neurofibromatosis type 2 syndrome.

E. Occurs most commonly in the lumbosacral region.

✅ **Answer D**
- Usually part of the Carney complex, which is characterized by skin pigmentation abnormalities, myxomas, endocrine tumors or overactivity, and schwannomas.

❓ **59. Primary spinal cord tumors (SCT). Intradural extramedullary tumors (IDEM-SCT). Spinal schwannoma of the dumbbell shape. The FALSE answer is:**

A. 10–20% of schwannomas.

B. The dumbbell appearance of tumors is specific to schwannomas.

C. Develop an "hourglass" shape due to an anatomic barrier encountered during growth.

D. The waist may be due to dural constriction or foraminal narrowing.

E. Some tumors might have two distinct waists at both the dura and the foramen.

✅ **Answer B**
- Although most are seen with schwannoma tumors, not all dumbbell tumors are schwannomas. Other tumors that may show a dumbbell-shaped growth in the spine are neuroblastoma, neurofibroma, ganglioneuroma, and meningioma.

60. Primary spinal cord tumors (SCTs). Intradural extramedullary tumors (IDEM-SCT). Spinal schwannoma: radiological differentiation from meningioma. The FALSE answer is:
  A. Wide neural exit foramina.
  B. Show cystic changes with areas of fatty degeneration.
  C. Frequently associated with hemorrhage and intrinsic vascular changes (sinusoidal dilatation).
  D. No dural base.
  E. Located anterolateral to the cord.

Answer E
  - Schwannomas are usually located posterolateral to the cord, while meningiomas are usually located anterolateral.

61. Primary spinal cord tumors (SCTs). Intradural extramedullary tumors (IDEM-SCT). Spinal schwannoma in the setting of schwannomatosis. The FALSE answer is:
  A. Is a condition characterized by multiple schwannomas and occasionally meningiomas (in 5%).
  B. Meningiomas are predominantly located along the falx cerebri.
  C. It is considered part of the neurofibromatosis type 2 syndrome.
  D. Most patients demonstrate schwannomas confined to one limb.
  E. Spinal lesions affect less than six contiguous spinal segments (segmental schwannomatosis).

Answer C
  - Schwannomatosis does not meet the criteria for neurofibromatosis type 2 (NF2), but some consider this condition as a variant of NF2.

62. Primary spinal cord tumors (SCT). Intradural extramedullary tumors (IDEM-SCT). Spinal schwannoma: criteria to diagnose schwannomatosis. The FALSE answer is:
  A. At least two non-intradermal schwannomas, including at least one with pathological confirmation, and evidence of bilateral vestibular schwannomas.
  B. Or a pathologically confirmed schwannoma or intracranial meningioma and an affected first-degree relative.
  C. Patients are excluded if there is a clinical diagnosis of neurofibromatosis type 2.

D. Patients are excluded if there is a first-degree relative with neurofibromatosis type 2.

E. Patients are excluded if schwannomas occur only within a radiation treatment field.

✅ **Answer A**

– At least two non-intradermal schwannomas, including at least one with pathological confirmation, and no evidence of bilateral vestibular schwannomas.

❓ 63. **Primary spinal cord tumors (SCTs). Intradural extramedullary tumors (IDEM-SCT). Spinal neurofibroma: incidence. The FALSE answer is:**
A. 15% of intradural extramedullary spinal cord tumors.
B. One-third of intradural extramedullary spinal nerve sheath tumors.
C. Peak age is 40–70 years of age.
D. More common in females.
E. Represent 1–2% of all CNS tumors.

✅ **Answer C**

– Peak age is 25–50 years, almost two decades younger than peak ages for schwannoma and meningiomas.

❓ 64. **Primary spinal cord tumors (SCT). Intradural extramedullary tumors (IDEM-SCT). Spinal neurofibromas: location. The FALSE answer is:**
A. Are typically extradural lesions that extend intradurally.
B. In general, they can be intradural, extradural, or both intra- and extradural.
C. Are most common in the cervical spine.
D. In juxta spinal areas, they can develop from the spinal root, neural plexus, peripheral nerve, or end organs.
E. Are usually solitary.

✅ **Answer E**

❓ 65. **Primary spinal cord tumors (SCTs). Intradural extramedullary tumors (IDEM-SCT). Spinal neurofibroma: pathology. The FALSE answer is:**
A. Develop from Schwann cells, similar to schwannoma.
B. WHO grade I tumors.

C. Unlike schwannomas, nerve axons are scattered in the neoplasm rather than eccentrically compressed.

D. Always almost associated with NF1 (rarely sporadical).

E. Malignant transformation can occur in 5–10% of the tumors.

Answer A
- Develops from all components of a nerve, including Schwann cells, collagen, and perineurial cells.

66. Primary spinal cord tumors (SCTs). Intradural extramedullary tumors (IDEM-SCT). Spinal neurofibroma: radiological features. The FALSE answer is:

A. Fusiform enlargement of the involved nerve.

B. Shows heterogeneous post-contrast enhancement.

C. Hyperintense in T2WI.

D. Hypointense in T1WI.

E. The "target sign" can rarely be detected.

Answer E
- The "target sign" is commonly seen in neurofibroma as a hyperintense rim and a hypointense central core in T2WI, which change after contrast administration to a hyperintense enhancing central core and a hypointense rim. This happens due to a dense central area of collagenous stroma. The "target sign" is highly suggestive of neurofibroma.

67. Primary spinal cord tumors (SCTs). Intradural extramedullary tumors (IDEM-SCT). Spinal paraganglioma: incidence. The FALSE answer is:

A. The peak age incidence is in the fourth to sixth decades of life.

B. Occurs more frequently in males.

C. Are usually located in the cervical spine.

D. The most common presenting complaints are lower back pain and leg pain.

E. Only a few extra-adrenal paragangliomas arise outside the carotid body and glomus jugulare.

Answer C
- They are mainly located in the lumbar and sacral regions, specifically the filum terminale.

❓ 68. **Primary spinal cord tumors (SCTs). Intradural extramedullary tumors (IDEM-SCT). Spinal paraganglioma: pathology. The FALSE answer is:**

A. Arises from extra-adrenal sympathetic ganglion cells.

B. Are secretory neoplasms.

C. Composed of chromaffin cells.

D. Represents extra-adrenal pheochromocytomas.

E. Are grade I neoplasms, although malignant transformation has been documented in about 5–10%.

✅ Answer B

– Spinal paragangliomas are non-secretory neoplasms, and they rarely produce catecholamine excess.

❓ 69. **Primary spinal cord tumors (SCTs). Intradural extramedullary tumors (IDEM-SCT). Spinal paraganglioma: radiology features. The FALSE answer is:**

A. Appears as a well-demarcated mass attached to the filum terminale.

B. Hypo- or isointense on T1WI and iso- or hyperintense on T2, in comparison with spinal cord tissue.

C. The tumor margin shows a hypointense rim indicative of the paramagnetic effects of hemosiderin.

D. The tumor core shows a uniform hyperintense matrix in T2WI.

E. Contrast produces intense heterogeneous enhancement, with multiple areas of signal void.

✅ Answer D

– The tumor exhibits a "salt and pepper" appearance on T2WI, characterized by hypointense areas of flow void within a hyperintense matrix of tumor cells.

❓ 70. **Primary spinal cord tumors (SCTs). Intradural extramedullary tumors (IDEM-SCT). Spinal paraganglioma: common differential diagnoses of filum terminale tumors. The FALSE answer is:**

A. Subependymoma.

B. Schwannoma.

C. Meningioma.

D. Metastasis.

E. Paraganglioma.

✅ **Answer A**

– Subependymomas do not commonly involve the filum terminale. Myxo-papillary ependymoma is the most common type of ependymoma that arises in the filum terminale.

❓ 71. **Primary spinal cord tumors (SCTs). Intradural extramedullary tumors (IDEM-SCT). Spinal ganglioneuroma: incidence. The FALSE answer is:**
   A. Is not a true intradural spinal tumor but resembles large schwan-nomas.
   B. Most commonly occurs in the neck.
   C. Tends to occur in the pediatric population.
   D. Most cases are diagnosed before the age of 20 years.
   E. Shows a slight male predominance.

✅ **Answer B**

– The most common locations, in descending order, are as follows: posterior mediastinum (42%) or retroperitoneum (38%), adrenal gland (21%), and neck (8%).

❓ 72. **Primary spinal cord tumors (SCTs). Intradural extramedullary tumors (IDEM-SCT). Spinal ganglioneuroma: pathology. The FALSE answer is:**
   A. Arise in the paravertebral sympathetic chains at ganglion sites.
   B. Arise from primordial neural crest cells.
   C. Are always solitary.
   D. Can occur de novo.
   E. Can arise in neuroblastomas and ganglioneuroblastomas that have been treated with chemotherapy.

✅ **Answer C**

– Multiple ganglioneuromas are often associated with NF and multiple endocrine neoplasia syndrome type IIB.

❓ 73. **Primary spinal cord tumors (SCTs). Intradural extramedullary tumors (IDEM-SCT). Spinal ganglioneuroma: radiological features. The FALSE answer is:**
   A. Are well-circumscribed masses.
   B. May appear encapsulated, although a true capsule is infrequent.

23

C. Frequently extends through the neural foramina to involve the epidural space of the spinal canal.

D. Patients typically become symptomatic early, even with small tumors.

E. Scoliosis may be present.

✅ **Answer D**

– The lesions can be quite large when discovered, but only a few are symptomatic.

❓ **74. Primary spinal cord tumors (SCTs). Intradural extramedullary tumors (IDEM-SCT). Spinal ganglioneuroma: radiological features. The FALSE answer is:**

A. Calcifications are very rare.

B. Sometimes causes rib spreading and foraminal erosion.

C. Are homogenously hypointense in T1WI.

D. Are heterogeneously hyperintense in T2WI.

E. Post-contrast enhancement varies from mild to marked heterogeneous enhancement.

✅ **Answer A**

– Calcifications are seen in 33% of cases and are typically fine and speckled but may be coarse.

❓ **75. Primary spinal cord tumors (SCTs). Intradural extramedullary tumors (IDIM-SCT). Lipoma (without dysraphism). The FALSE answer is:**

A. The peak age of occurrence is the second and third decades of life with no sex predilection.

B. Most common in cervicothoracic region with frequent overlying local subcutaneous masses or dimples.

C. Are hyperintense in T1-weighted images and hyperintense in T2-weighted images show no enhancement post-contrast and appear hypointense in fat-suppressed sequences.

D. The most common symptom is ascending mono- or paraparesis rather than pain.

E. Are all intradural extramedullary.

✅ **Answer E**

– Usually, these lesions are intradural extramedullary, but a reported subtype is truly intramedullary and essentially replaces the cord.

? 76. Primary spinal cord tumors (SCTs). Intradural extramedullary tumors (IDIM-SCT). Dermoids and epidermoids. The FALSE answer is:

A. Usually develop before late childhood.
B. Show slight female predominance.
C. The most common location is the conus and they rarely occur in the cervical and upper thoracic regions.
D. Are usually intradural extramedullary, but lesions in the conus/cauda equina region may exhibit an intramedullary component.
E. The recommended management is radical excision.

✓ Answer E
- They can be quite adherent to the spinal cord. Hence, given the slow growth rates of these tumors, the role of radical surgery to remove all traces of the tumor is not advocated by most surgeons.

? 77. Primary spinal cord tumors (SCTs). Intradural intramedullary tumors (IDIM-SCT). Incidence. The FALSE answer is:

A. 2–4% of all CNS tumors.
B. Most common at the thoracic spine.
C. 5–10% of all spinal tumors in adults.
D. 25% of all spinal cord tumors.
E. Most common spinal tumor in children.

✓ Answer B
- Most common at the cervical (33%), followed by thoracic (26%) and lumbar (24%) levels. The higher incidence of IDIM-SCTs at the cervical level may be related to the higher volume of gray matter present at that level.

? 78. Primary spinal cord tumors (SCTs). Intradural intramedullary tumors (IDIM-SCT). X-ray features. The FALSE answer is:

A. Early in the course of the disease, X-ray shows typical and atypical scoliotic curvatures.
B. Late in the course of the disease, X-ray shows widening of interpedicular distance and scalloping of dorsal aspects of vertebral bodies.
C. Widening of the neural foramina.
D. Intratumoral calcification can be seen in extremely rare cases.
E. Postoperative findings might include progressive scoliosis, kyphotic deformities, or spinal instability.

✓ Answer C

23

? 79. **Primary spinal cord tumors (SCTs). Intradural intramedullary tumors (IDIM-SCT). Advantages of using intraoperative ultrasonography. The FALSE answer is:**

A. Confirm adequate laminectomy exposure over the whole length of the tumor.

B. Define superior and inferior margins of the mass for planning the extent of dural opening.

C. Locate any associated cysts to be drained initially to reduce cord swelling.

D. Evaluate the extent of resection at the end of the surgery.

E. Can be used before laminectomy for tumor localization.

✓ **Answer E**

− Ultrasonography cannot provide imaging through bone.

? 80. **Primary spinal cord tumors (SCTs). Intradural intramedullary tumors (IDIM-SCT). Role of postoperative radiotherapy. The FALSE answer is:**

A. Can be given without tissue diagnosis for the treatment of intramedullary lesions in patients unfit for surgery.

B. Not done routinely after gross total resection of ependymoma.

C. Can be added after subtotal resection of ependymoma.

D. Not routinely done after surgery for low-grade astrocytoma even if subtotal resection only was achieved.

E. Can be used before laminectomy for tumor localization.

✓ **Answer A**

− No lesion should undergo radiotherapy without a tissue diagnosis.

? 81. **Primary spinal cord tumors (SCTs). Intradural intramedullary tumors (IDIM-SCT). Postoperative: recurrence. The FALSE answer is:**

A. 5–10% with ependymoma.

B. 50% with astrocytoma.

C. Hemangioblastoma in patients with VHL has a low rate of recurrence after complete lesion excision.

D. A risk factor for recurrence is histologic anaplasia and high-grade tumors.

E. A risk factor for ependymoma recurrence is piecemeal resection.

✅ **Answer C**

- Hemangioblastoma in patients with VHL has a significant risk of recurrence even after completely resecting the index lesion due to the possible development of new lesions in other locations within the spine after excising the first one. Therefore, these patients must have their entire neuroaxis imaged periodically postoperatively.

❓ 82. **Primary spinal cord tumors (SCTs). Intradural intramedullary tumors (IDIM-SCT). Ependymoma: incidence. The FALSE answer is:**
   A. Is the most common intramedullary spinal cord tumor (60–70%).
   B. Has approximately twice the incidence of intramedullary astrocytoma.
   C. Peak age is at 30–60 years.
   D. Is the most common intramedullary spinal cord tumor in pediatrics.
   E. Has a slight male predominance.

✅ **Answer D**

- Ependymoma is the most common intramedullary spinal cord tumor in adults. In contrast, astrocytoma is the most common intramedullary spinal cord tumor in the pediatric group.

❓ 83. **Primary spinal cord tumors (SCTs). Intradural intramedullary tumors (IDIM-SCT). Ependymoma: location. The FALSE answer is:**
   A. 50% are located in the filum terminale.
   B. Most of the filum terminale lesions are of the myxopapillary type.
   C. 50% are distributed in the cervical and thoracic regions.
   D. Is more common in the cervical region than the thoracic region.
   E. Usually occupies an eccentric location within the cord.

✅ **Answer E**

- Spinal ependymoma usually occupies a central position within the spinal cord as it arises from the central canal of the spinal cord.

❓ 84. **Primary spinal cord tumors (SCTs). Intradural intramedullary tumors (IDIM-SCT). Ependymoma: pathology. The FALSE answer is:**
   A. It arises from ependymal cells lining the central canal of the spinal cord.
   B. WHO grade 1 ependymomas encompass myxopapillary ependymoma and subependymoma.

23

C. WHO grade 2 tumors are referred to as ependymoma, while grade 3 is anaplastic ependymoma.

D. Ependymoma can be of either the papillary, cellular, epithelial, or mixed type.

E. Patients with the NF2 gene are predisposed to develop schwannomas but not ependymomas.

✅ **Answer E**

- NF2 patients are predisposed to develop schwannomas and/or ependymomas.

❓ **85. Primary spinal cord tumors (SCTs). Intradural intramedullary tumors (IDIM-SCT). Ependymoma: MRI features. The FALSE answer is:**

A. Intratumoral hemorrhage, especially at the cranial or caudal margins, exhibits a high signal on T1WI.

B. A low-signal intensity rim around some tumors in T2WI represents hemosiderin.

C. All ependymomas look hypo- or isointense on T1WI.

D. Post-contrast homogeneous enhancement is seen.

E. The tumor has a well-defined border.

✅ **Answer C**

- Although most ependymomas look hypo- or isointense on T1WI, the myxopapillary type may appear hyperintense on T1WI.

❓ **86. Primary spinal cord tumors (SCTs). Intradural intramedullary tumors (IDIM-SCT). Ependymoma: MRI features. The FALSE answer is:**

A. Associated syrinx is sometimes seen.

B. Tumor-reactive cysts are rarely seen.

C. Cord enlargement secondary to the tumor growth is symmetrical due to the central position of the tumor.

D. The average tumor length spans four vertebral levels.

E. Subarachnoid or intratumoral hemorrhage usually occurs with the papillary type, which is highly vascular.

✅ **Answer B**

- Cysts are seen in more than 50% of spinal ependymomas. Most of these cysts are reactive CSF-filled cysts with non-enhancing walls that develop at both rostral and caudal poles of the tumor rather than true intratumoral cysts with enhancing walls.

❓ 87. Primary spinal cord tumors (SCTs). Intradural intramedullary tumors (IDIM-SCT). MRI differentiation of myxopapillary ependymoma from schwannoma of the filum. The FALSE answer is:

A. Schwannoma appears multilobulated.

B. Schwannoma assumes a dumbbell configuration.

C. Schwannoma can result in the enlargement of adjacent neural foramina.

D. Schwannoma's periphery is strongly enhancing, while its central areas might show poor enhancement.

E. Schwannoma pushes nerve roots circumferentially to the periphery of the thecal sac while ependymoma pushes nerve roots in an eccentric fashion.

23

✅ Answer E

- Schwannoma pushes nerve roots as one group in an eccentric fashion toward one side of the thecal sac, while ependymoma of the filum pushes nerve roots circumferentially to the periphery of the thecal sac.

❓ 88. Primary spinal cord tumors (SCTs). Intradural intramedullary tumors (IDIM-SCT). Ependymoma: surgical notes. The FALSE answer is:

A. The main goal is gross total resection.

B. Attempting gross total resection depends on the presence of a good separation plan and IONM.

C. In cases where only a subtotal resection is achieved, it is recommended to add postoperative radiotherapy.

D. The filum is first cut below the myxopapillary ependymoma lesion.

E. Intraoperatively, an initial biopsy with immediate frozen section analysis can differentiate ependymoma from astrocytoma and guide further surgical planning.

✅ Answer D

- Surgical removal of filum tumors consists of coagulating and dividing the filum terminale just above and below the lesion before excising it in total. The filum is first cut above the lesion to prevent retraction of the rostral filum with the tumor upward away from the level of the dural opening.

❓ 89. Primary spinal cord tumors (SCTs). Intradural intramedullary tumors (IDIM-SCT). Ependymoma: postoperative good prognosis indices. The FALSE answer is:

A. Modest initial deficits.

B. Symptoms for less than 2 years before surgery.

C. Absence of associated syrinx.

D. Total surgical removal.

E. Myxopapillary type.

✓ **Answer C**

— The presence of syrinx suggests a non-infiltrative lesion.

❓ **90. Primary spinal cord tumors (SCTs). Intradural intramedullary tumors (IDIM-SCT). Ependymoma: postoperative poor prognosis indices. The FALSE answer is:**

A. Mid-thoracic lesions.

B. Intraoperative finding of arachnoid scarring.

C. Preoperative cord atrophy evident on imaging.

D. Elderly patients with an age of more than 60 years.

E. High-grade lesions.

✓ **Answer A**

— Poorer functional outcome is associated with surgeries on upper thoracic and conus lesions due to the relative narrowing of the spinal canal at these two regions.

❓ **91. Primary spinal cord tumors (SCTs). Intradural intramedullary tumors (IDIM-SCT). Astrocytoma: incidence. The FALSE answer is:**

A. Is the second most common intramedullary spinal cord tumor (30–40%).

B. Has half the incidence of intramedullary ependymoma.

C. Peak age is at 30–50 years.

D. Is the most common intramedullary spinal cord tumor in pediatrics and adolescents (60%).

E. Has a slight male predominance.

✓ **Answer C**

— Peak age is at 5–10 years.

❓ **92. Primary spinal cord tumors (SCTs). Intradural intramedullary tumors (IDIM-SCT). Astrocytoma: location. The FALSE answer is:**

A. Usually causes asymmetrical cord swelling.

B. Does not occur in the filum terminale.

C. 100% are distributed in the cervical and thoracic regions.

D. More common in the cervical region than the thoracic region.

E. Usually occupies an eccentric location within the cord.

✅ **Answer D**
- Astrocytoma is more commonly found in the thoracic region than the cervical region.

❓ **93. Primary spinal cord tumors (SCTs). Intradural intramedullary tumors (IDIM-SCT). Astrocytoma: pathology. The FALSE answer is:**
   A. WHO grade 1 (usually pilocytic astrocytoma) represents 25%.
   B. WHO grade 2 represents 50% (most common).
   C. WHO grades 3 and 4 represent 25%.
   D. The tumor length may span several vertebral levels with an average number of seven levels.
   E. Patients with the NF2 gene are predisposed to develop astrocytomas.

23

✅ **Answer E**
- Patients with the NF1 gene are predisposed to develop astrocytomas.

❓ **94. Primary spinal cord tumors (SCTs). Intradural intramedullary tumors (IDIM-SCT). Astrocytoma: MRI features. The FALSE answer is:**
   A. All spinal astrocytomas show post-contrast heterogeneous enhancement.
   B. They have ill-defined borders on MRI.
   C. Development of syrinx is common.
   D. Only one-third (33%) of the lesions are associated with cysts.
   E. Cord enlargement is usually asymmetrical due to the eccentric growth of the tumor.

✅ **Answer A**
- Some spinal astrocytoma lesions do not show enhancement in post-contrast images.

❓ **95. Primary spinal cord tumors (SCTs). Intradural intramedullary tumors (IDIM-SCT). Astrocytoma: MRI differentiating features from demyelinating diseases. The FALSE answer is:**
   A. Demyelinating lesions extend along a large part of the cord.
   B. Demyelinating lesions are most common in the cervical region (vs thoracic region).
   C. Demyelinating lesions are not associated with cord enlargement.
   D. Demyelinating lesions are not associated with syrinx or cysts.
   E. Demyelinating lesions do not usually enhance unless they are at an acute stage (vs 90% of astrocytomas).

✓ Answer A

- Demyelinating lesions do not usually extend more than two vertebral levels, while the average length of intramedullary astrocytoma is seven vertebral levels.

❓ 96. Primary spinal cord tumors (SCTs). Intradural intramedullary tumors (IDIM-SCT). Astrocytoma: management plan. The FALSE answer is:

A. For low-grade lesions (grades 1 or 2) with a discernible plane of separation, it is advisable to attempt total excision.

B. Radiotherapy should be routinely performed following surgery for low-grade astrocytomas.

C. For low-grade lesions without a plane of separation, biopsy and limited excision are recommended.

D. For high-grade lesions (grades 3 and 4), biopsy and limited excision are recommended.

E. For high-grade lesions, surgery is followed by postoperative radiotherapy and chemotherapy.

✓ Answer B

- Radiotherapy is not recommended following surgery for low-grade astrocytoma even if there is a residual lesion and gross total resection has not been achieved.

❓ 97. Primary spinal cord tumors (SCTs). Intradural intramedullary tumors (IDIM-SCT). Astrocytoma: postoperative outcomes. The FALSE answer is:

A. Regrowth or recurrence occurs in about 50% of cases.

B. Gross total resection can be achieved in 0% of grade 3 and 4 lesions.

C. Gross total resection can be achieved in about 50% of grade 2 lesions.

D. There is a risk of rapid progression of spinal gliomas in pregnant patients.

E. Intraoperative frozen section histopathological analysis can determine the extent of attempted resection.

✓ Answer C

- Gross total resection can be achieved in not more than 10% of grade 2 lesions.

? 98. **Primary spinal cord tumors (SCTs). Intradural intramedullary tumors (IDIM-SCT). Hemangioblastoma: incidence. The FALSE answer is:**

A. Is the third most common intramedullary spinal cord tumor (3–4%).

B. Represents 15% of hemangioblastoma tumors within the whole CNS.

C. Peak age is at 40–50 years.

D. Sporadic solitary hemangioblastomas commonly occur in children.

E. Has no gender predilection.

✓ Answer D

— Sporadic solitary hemangioblastomas rarely occur in children. Spinal hemangioblastomas in children are usually associated with VHL disease and are frequently multiple.

? 99. **Primary spinal cord tumors (SCTs). Intradural intramedullary tumors (IDIM-SCT). Hemangioblastoma: location. The FALSE answer is:**

A. Usually causes asymmetrical cord swelling.

B. Is usually located at the ventral portion of the cord.

C. Is more common in the thoracic region than the cervical region.

D. 75% of spinal hemangioblastomas have an exophytic component extending to the extramedullary region.

E. Occupies an eccentric location within the cord.

✓ Answer B

— Spinal hemangioblastomas usually occupy the dorsal portion of the cord and thus usually present with progressive sensory deficits, particularly proprioceptive.

? 100. **Primary spinal cord tumors (SCTs). Intradural intramedullary tumors (IDIM-SCT). Hemangioblastoma: pathology. The FALSE answer is:**

A. Is WHO grade 1.

B. Histologically, they consist of large pale neoplastic stromal cells packed between blood vessels.

C. Has a high risk for malignant transformation.

D. 25% of cases of spinal hemangioblastoma are associated with Von Hippel-Lindau (VHL) disease.

E. Patients with VHL usually develop hemangioblastomas at an earlier age and commonly have multiple lesions.

✅ **Answer C**

━ Hemangioblastomas are not known to undergo malignant transformation.

❓ **101. Primary spinal cord tumors (SCTs). Intradural intramedullary tumors (IDIM-SCT). Hemangioblastoma: MRI features. The FALSE answer is:**

A. Non-enhanced T1WI images show hyperintense cord signals.

B. Sometimes signal voids can be detected on the dorsal surface of the spinal cord.

C. Hemosiderin capping may be present and seen as a hypointense rim in T2WI.

D. Has well-defined borders.

E. The tumor nodule shows homogenous vivid enhancement in post-contrast images.

✅ **Answer A**

━ Non-enhanced T1WI images show hypointense cord signals mostly representing cord edema, which is seen as hyperintense in T2WI. Edema develops from altered cord vasculature.

❓ **102. Primary spinal cord tumors (SCTs). Intradural intramedullary tumors (IDIM-SCT). Hemangioblastoma: MRI features. The FALSE answer is:**

A. Associated syrinx is very common.

B. Reactive cysts are seen in 98% of the lesions (much more common than ependymoma or astrocytoma).

C. The mural nodule is situated on the deep central surface within the cyst.

D. Only 25% of the lesions are entirely intramedullary.

E. High risk of associated subarachnoid (75%) or intramedullary hemorrhage (25%).

✅ **Answer C**

━ The mural nodule is classically situated on the superficial pial surface of the cyst.

? 103. **Primary spinal cord tumors (SCTs). Intradural intramedullary tumors (IDIM-SCT). Hemangioblastoma: angiographical features. The FALSE answer is:**

A. Most lesions commonly receive blood supply from lateral or posterior spinal arteries.

B. The anterior spinal artery mainly supplies neoplasms that abut the ventral pial surface.

C. Venous drainage follows the arterial supply.

D. More edema appears to be present when drainage predominantly occurs via the anterior surface veins.

E. No arteriovenous shunting occurs in these tumors.

✓ Answer C

– In contrast to arterial supply, the venous drainage pattern of spinal hemangioblastomas is unpredictable on MRI. Venous drainage may be through the anterior or posterior surface veins and in a rostral or caudal direction.

? 104. **Primary spinal cord tumors (SCTs). Intradural intramedullary tumors (IDIM-SCT). Hemangioblastoma: surgical management. The FALSE answer is:**

A. A very good separation plane can usually be identified during surgery.

B. Gross total resection should be attempted based on the plane of dissection and IONM.

C. Embolization is usually not feasible because of the small caliber of feeding vessels.

D. Pre-op angiogram might be important to define the vascular anatomy of large tumors for early surgical control.

E. Piecemeal removal can be safely done.

✓ Answer E

– Cannot incise through the core of the hemangioblastoma because of high vascularity. Requires microsurgical approach similar to AVM circumferential resection.

? 105. **Primary spinal cord tumors (SCTs). Intradural intramedullary tumors (IDIM-SCT). Germ cell tumors. The FALSE answer is:**

A. Often occurs at the lower thoracic level.

B. Radiotherapy alone is sufficient to treat all germ cell tumors.

23

    C. Post-contrast enhancement can vary.

    D. Focal spinal cord atrophy may be an important radiological sign.

    E. Tumor markers in the serum and CSF can help with diagnosis.

✅ **Answer B**

▬ Germinomas are sensitive to radiotherapy, so treatment with radiation usually yields good results. In contrast, non-germinomatous germ cell tumors show little sensitivity to radiotherapy alone and are often treated in combination with chemotherapy.

❓ **106. Primary spinal cord tumors (SCTs). Intradural intramedullary tumors (IDIM-SCT). Primary spinal lymphoma: incidence. The FALSE answer is:**

    A. 3.3% of all CNS lymphomas.

    B. Peak age at presentation is 40–50 years.

    C. Females are more commonly affected than males.

    D. The most common intramedullary location is the cervical cord, followed by the thoracic cord.

    E. Risk factors include diabetes mellitus.

✅ **Answer E**

▬ Risk factors include immunosuppression (HIV or EBV, congenital immunodeficiency, and transplant recipients).

❓ **107. Primary spinal cord tumors (SCTs). Intradural intramedullary tumors (IDIM-SCT). Primary spinal lymphoma: MRI features. The FALSE answer is:**

    A. It is recommended to administer steroids before MRI imaging.

    B. T2WI demonstrates high signal (in contrast to T2 low signals seen in intracranial lymphoma).

    C. DWI shows restriction.

    D. Is not usually associated with cord enlargement, cysts, syrinx, or a hemorrhagic component.

    E. Most are solitary lesions; multifocal lesions are more common in immunocompromised patients.

✅ **Answer A**

▬ There is a rapid decrease in tumor size with steroid administration, and some small lesions may become undetectable on MRI.

? 108. Primary spinal cord tumors (SCTs). Intradural intramedullary tumors (IDIM-SCT). Primary spinal lymphoma: management. The FALSE answer is:

    A. There is a rapid decrease in tumor size and improvement of symptoms on steroid administration.

    B. Its diffuse nature makes resection and radiotherapy more challenging.

    C. High-dose intravenous chemotherapy appears to be the most effective treatment.

    D. Oral chemotherapy is as effective as high-dose intravenous chemotherapy.

    E. Radiotherapy is usually reserved for cases refractory to or who cannot tolerate chemotherapy.

✓ Answer D

    — Oral chemotherapy does not appear to be effective in treating these tumors, and patients who fail to receive high-dose intravenous chemotherapy suffer from a high rate of recurrence.

? 109. Secondary spinal tumors. Incidence. The FALSE answer is:

    A. 90% of all spinal neoplasms are considered metastatic in origin.

    B. 10% of newly diagnosed cancer patients already have vertebral mets.

    C. Bone is the most common site for metastatic disease.

    D. 50% of cancer patients will develop secondary spinal tumors at some time.

    E. 70% of osseous metastasis occurs in the spine.

✓ Answer C

    — Bone is the third most common site for metastatic disease behind lung and liver.

? 110. Secondary spinal tumors. Osseous destructive lesions. The FALSE answer is:

    A. Metastatic lesions are the second most common reason for a destructive spine lesion in adults after spondylitis.

    B. Lytic vertebral lesions are caused by tumors inducing osteoclast activation.

    C. Osteoclast activation occurs through the RANK-RANK ligand (RANKL)-osteoprotegerin pathway.

23

D. Sclerotic vertebral lesions are caused by tumors inducing osteoblast activation.

E. Osteoblast activation occurs through the endothelin 1 (ET-1)-endothelin A receptor (ETAR) pathway.

✅ **Answer A**

− Metastatic tumors are the most common reason for a destructive spine lesion in adults.

❓ **111. Secondary spinal tumors. Source of primary tumor. The FALSE answer is:**

A. Lung—50% of secondary spinal tumors.

B. Breast—15% of secondary spinal tumors.

C. Prostate—12% of secondary spinal tumors.

D. GI tract—10% of secondary spinal tumors.

E. Kidney, lymphoma, and melanoma—each represent 5% of secondary spinal tumors.

✅ **Answer A**

− Lung represents 1/5 (20%) of secondary spinal tumors.

❓ **112. Secondary spinal tumors. Epidural location characteristics. The FALSE answer is:**

A. The most common site for secondary spinal tumors (95%).

B. 50–60% are located at the vertebral body.

C. 20–30% are located at the pedicle or lamina.

D. 10–15% are located at both posterior and anterior elements of the vertebral column.

E. None are located solely in the epidural space.

✅ **Answer E**

− 2–5% are located in the epidural space with no vertebral osseous involvement. This is particularly common in lymphoma and renal cell carcinoma.

❓ **113. Secondary spinal tumors. Intradural location characteristics. The FALSE answer is:**

A. Usually detected in the lumbosacral region and are commonly multiple.

B. Lung, breast, and prostate are the most common primary sources in both adults and pediatrics.

C. Only in 2–4% of secondary spinal tumor cases.

D. Enhancing tumor nodules can be seen on MRI images of the spinal cord and nerve roots.

E. "Sugar coating/icing" of the spinal cord refers to diffuse sheet-like leptomeningeal contrast enhancement.

✅ **Answer B**
- Although in adults intradural secondary spinal tumors are mainly from non-CNS tumors like lungs and breasts, in pediatrics, leptomeningeal metastases are mainly from primary brain tumors, e.g., GBM, PNET, ependymoma, medulloblastoma, pineal germ cell tumors, and choroid plexus papilloma.

23

❓ **114. Secondary spinal tumors. Intramedullary location characteristics. The FALSE answer is:**

A. Is the least common site for secondary spinal tumors (in less than 2%).

B. Most frequently involves the cervical region.

C. Arise from hematogenous dissemination of neoplastic cells that grow along Virchow-Robin spaces.

D. Associated cysts and syrinx are common.

E. 50% are metastases from lung cancer.

✅ **Answer D**
- In contrast to primary intramedullary neoplasms, associated cysts and syrinx are rare.

❓ **115. Secondary spinal tumors. Location according to spinal level. The FALSE answer is:**

A. The thoracic spine harbors 50–60%, particularly at the middle third (T5-T8).

B. The lumbar spine harbors 20–30%.

C. The cervical spine harbors 10–20%.

D. 50% of patients with spinal metastasis have several levels of involvement.

E. Only 10% of patients have involvement of noncontiguous segments.

✅ **Answer E**

- Almost a little more than 50% of patients have involvement of noncontiguous segments, which makes radiological screening of the whole spine mandatory.

❓ **116. Secondary spinal tumors. Clinical presentation: pain. The FALSE answer is:**
  A. The most common initial symptom (90% of patients).
  B. Local pain is caused by periosteal stretching from the growing lesion and increased local vascularity.
  C. Local pain is usually sharp, decreases with recumbency, and is more in the daytime.
  D. Radicular shooting pain from nerve root infiltration.
  E. Mechanical pain from pathological fracture instability increases with movements.

✅ **Answer C**

- Local pain is usually dull aching and associated with tenderness at the level of involvement. The pain increases by recumbency and is more at night (nocturnal pain) due to congestion induced by the increased local vascularity.

❓ **117. Secondary spinal tumors. Clinical presentation: neurological deficits. The FALSE answer is:**
  A. 50% of diagnosed cancer patients have paraparesis on presentation with spinal metastasis.
  B. 10% of undiagnosed cancer patients initially present with cord compression.
  C. 25% of paraparetic patients have total paraplegia.
  D. 50% of paraplegic patients may ambulate after surgery.
  E. Sphincteric disturbances are mainly bladder dysfunction.

✅ **Answer D**

- Unfortunately, only 15–20% of patients presenting with paraplegia may ambulate again after surgical decompression.

❓ **118. Secondary spinal tumors. Clinical presentation: hypercalcemic crisis. The FALSE answer is:**
  A. Occurs with marked elevation of serum calcium, usually more than 14 mg/dL.

B. Clinical features include constipation, flank pain, fatigue, polyuria, polydipsia, confusion, and coma.

C. Measured by corrected total calcium serum level or by ionized calcium serum level.

D. Other causes of hypercalcemia are hyperparathyroidism and hyperthyroidism.

E. The initial treatment should be by administering bisphosphates.

Answer E

- Initial treatment is by hydration using NaCl 0.9% and forced calciuresis using furosemide. Although bisphosphates can inhibit osteoclast activity for up to a month, it may take 48–72 h before reaching the full therapeutic effect.

23

119. Secondary spinal tumors. Investigations: radiology. The FALSE answer is:

A. X-ray can be used effectively for screening as it can detect early small metastatic lesions.

B. Myeloma and thyroid carcinoma are often cold on bone scans.

C. PET-CT is used for whole-body workup as its sensitivity is high for bone metastasis.

D. MRI with contrast and fat suppression differentiates metastasis from degenerative bone marrow changes.

E. DWI differentiates osteoporotic fracture with no restriction from pathologic fracture with restriction.

Answer A

- Usually, at least 1/3 of the vertebral body has to be affected by the tumor before it can be detected on X-ray. Hence, in 20% of the patients, the initial X-ray may be falsely negative.

120. Secondary spinal tumors. Investigations: radiology. The following are lytic metastatic lesions. The FALSE answer is:

A. Lung cancer.

B. GIT cancers.

C. Renal cell carcinoma.

D. Prostatic cancer.

E. Multiple myeloma.

✔ **Answer D**

 ▬ Prostatic cancer and medullary thyroid carcinoma are both sclerotic metastatic lesions.

❓ **121. Secondary spinal tumors. Investigations: radiology. The following are non-metastatic sclerotic lesions. The FALSE answer is:**
 A. Brown tumor.
 B. Paget's disease.
 C. Post-radiotherapy sclerosis.
 D. Bone island (incidental enostosis).
 E. Osteoid osteoma and osteoblastoma.

✔ **Answer A**

 ▬ Brown tumor is a lytic lesion associated with hyperparathyroidism.

❓ **122. Secondary spinal tumors. Investigations: radiology. Signs favoring the diagnosis of pathological fracture over osteoporotic fractures in the spine of the elderly. The FALSE answer is:**
 A. Bony destruction rather than a hypointense fracture line.
 B. Presence of the "fluid sign."
 C. Replaced signal of the vertebral body, especially extending into the pedicles or posterior elements.
 D. Convex bulging (not retropulsion of fragment) of the posterior vertebral cortex into the spinal canal.
 E. Associated epidural or paraspinal mass.

✔ **Answer B**

 ▬ "Fluid sign" is an area of T2 hyperintensity, best seen with fat suppression, on a background of diffuse hyperintensity (edema) in the vertebral body. It is thought to develop when fluid from bone marrow edema collects in an area of ischemic osteonecrosis after an acute fracture.

❓ **123. Secondary spinal tumors. Investigations: radiology. Criteria for assessing tumor response after radiotherapy according to the SPINO group. The FALSE answer is:**
 A. Post-radiation follow-up imaging should include 2–3 MRI examinations performed 6–8 weeks apart.
 B. Local control is defined as the absence of progression within the treated area at serial imaging.

   C. Local progression is defined as a gross increase in tumor volume or linear dimension.

   D. Local progression is defined as any new or progressive tumor within the epidural space.

   E. Local progression is defined as neurologic decline attributable to an enlarging preexisting epidural lesion.

✅ **Answer E**

– Local progression is defined as neurologic deterioration attributable to a preexisting epidural disease even if the changes in dimensions of the epidural disease at MRI are equivocal.

❓ **124. Secondary spinal tumors. NOMS management framework. The FALSE answer is:**

   A. NOMS stands for neurological, oncological, mechanical instability, and systemic illness.

   B. Neurological is determined using the American Spinal Injury Association (ASIA) grading scale.

   C. Oncological is determined using the responsiveness of the tumor to radiotherapy.

   D. Mechanical is determined using the Spinal Instability Neoplastic Score (SINS).

   E. Systemic illness is determined using different prognostic scales.

✅ **Answer B**

– Neurological is determined using the Epidural Spinal Cord Compression (ESCC) grading scale.

❓ **125. Secondary spinal tumors. NOMS management framework. Neurological factors. The FALSE answer is:**

   A. The Epidural Spinal Cord Compression (ESCC) grading scale is also called the Bilsky scale.

   B. ESCC consists of six grades in total.

   C. ESCC grades 0 and 1 are considered low, while grades 2 and 3 are considered high compression grades.

   D. ESCC grades 2 and 3 describe spinal cord deformation with no CSF visible around the cord.

   E. ESCC grade 1 is divided into subgrades A, B, and C according to dura deformation and cord abutment.

23

✅ **Answer D**

- Although ESCC grades 2 and 3 describe spinal cord deformation, in grade 2 there is still some CSF visible around some parts of the cord while in grade 3 there is no CSF visible around any part of the cord denoting a higher degree of compression.

❓ **126. Secondary spinal tumors. NOMS management framework. Oncological factors. The FALSE answer is:**

A. Radiosensitivity is based on tumors' response to stereotactic radiotherapy (SRT).

B. Radiosensitive tumors include lymphoma, multiple myeloma, seminoma, and small-cell lung carcinoma.

C. Moderately radiosensitive tumors include breast, prostate, ovarian, and neuroendocrine carcinomas.

D. Moderately radioresistant tumors include colon and non-small-cell lung carcinoma.

E. Radioresistant tumors include renal, thyroid, melanoma, hepatocellular, and sarcoma.

✅ **Answer A**

- Radiosensitivity is historically based on tumors' response to conventional external beam radiotherapy (cEBRT), which delivers lower tumoricidal doses, applies less focused radiation, and necessitates a higher number of sessions in comparison with stereotactic radiotherapy (SRT).

❓ **127. Secondary spinal tumors. NOMS management framework. Mechanical instability factors. The FALSE answer is:**

A. The Spinal Instability Neoplastic Score (SINS) is composed of six components.

B. All SINS components are radiological parameters.

C. The total SINS score varies from 0 to 18.

D. A total score of 7–12 indicates potential instability with a possible need for surgical fixation.

E. A total score of 13–18 indicates high instability with a strong recommendation for surgical fixation.

✅ **Answer B**

- There are five radiological parameters for the SINS: location of the lesion within the vertebral column, status of the spinal alignment, involvement of the posterolateral vertebral elements, degree of involved vertebral body collapse, and lytic or sclerotic nature of the lesion. The only clinical parameter of the SINS is the presence or absence of mechanical pain, which increases with movement and upright posture but decreases by recumbence.

128. **Secondary spinal tumors. NOMS management framework. Assessing the pain component of mechanical instability. The FALSE answer is:**
   A. Mechanical pain increases with movement/upright posture but decreases with recumbence.
   B. Instability pain must be distinguished from biological and neurogenic pains.
   C. Biologic pain is present in the evenings and responds to steroids and radiation.
   D. Neurogenic pain is usually secondary to nerve root compression and responds to decompression.
   E. Tender aching lesions without mechanical pains are given a score of 0.

✅ **Answer E**
   - Tender aching lesions without mechanical pains are given a score of 1.

129. **Secondary spinal tumors. NOMS management framework. Systemic illness factors. Commonly used prognostic scores. The FALSE answer is:**
   A. Tomita and the revised Tokuhashi scores are commonly cited in the literature.
   B. The modified Bauer score provides high predictive accuracy.
   C. The Oswestry Risk Index (ORI) is the most complex score to calculate.
   D. Skeletal Oncology Research Group (SORG) scores are the most recently published in 2016 and 2019.
   E. The revised Katagiri and SORG ML scores depend heavily on laboratory markers.

✅ **Answer C**
   - Oswestry Risk Index (ORI) is the simplest as it scores only two items: primary tumor pathology (PTP) rate of growth and Karnofsky performance status for general condition (GC).

130. Secondary spinal tumors. NOMS management framework. Systemic illness factors. Commonly reported risk factors that negatively impact outcomes and are associated with complications. The FALSE answer is:
   A. Demographic factors such as being young, obese, and female.
   B. Motor weakness and limited ambulation measured by the ASIA scale and Frankel scale.
   C. Performance status indicated by high ASA status, low KPS, and high ECOG.
   D. Laboratory markers such as anemia, low albumin, elevated neutrophil count, and elevated monocytes.
   E. Systemic disease burden assessed by a number of visceral metastases and uncontrolled systemic diseases.

✅ **Answer A**
   ▬ Demographic factors that are associated with worse outcomes and complications include age older than 60 years, male gender, low BMI, and smoking.

131. Secondary spinal tumors. NOMS management framework. Systemic illness factors. Performance status scores. The FALSE answer is:
   A. The Eastern Cooperative Oncology Group (ECOG) performance status score is a 5 grade scale.
   B. ECOG grade 0 is a fully active patient able to carry out all pre-disease activities without restrictions.
   C. ECOG grade 4 is a disabled patient confined to a bed or chair who cannot carry on any self-care.
   D. ECOG grade 0 is equivalent to Karnofsky Performance Status (KPS) 80–100%.
   E. Each ECOG grade is equal to 30% of the Karnofsky Performance Status (KPS).

✅ **Answer E**
   ▬ Each ECOG grade is equal to 20% of the Karnofsky Performance Status (KPS). Therefore, ECOG 3 is equivalent to Karnofsky Performance Status (KPS) 20–40%.

132. Secondary spinal tumors. NOMS management framework. General management outlines. The FALSE answer is:
   A. Patients with low-grade ESCC do not need decompression.

B. Patients with high-grade ESCC with soft radiosensitive tumors do not need decompression.

C. Patients with high-grade ESCC with solid or radioresistant tumors do not need decompression.

D. Patients with radioresistant tumors will receive SRT rather than conventional external beam radiotherapy (cEBRT).

E. Patients with SINS above 12 will need stabilization.

✅ **Answer C**

— Patients with high-grade ESCC with radioresistant tumors need "separation" decompression surgery. Separation surgeries are operations where minimal tumor resection is carried out to separate the tumor margin from the spinal cord by at least 2 mm leaving the bulk of the tumor mass to be treated with SRT radiation. This allows the delivery of high tumoricidal radiation doses to the entire tumor margin without risking spinal cord toxicity.

23

❓ **133. Secondary spinal tumors. NOMS management framework. General management pathways. The FALSE answer is:**

A. Low-grade ESCC/radiosensitive tumor/stable spine: cEBRT.

B. Low-grade ESCC/radiosensitive tumor/unstable spine: stabilization followed by cEBRT.

C. Low-grade ESCC/radioresistant tumor/stable spine: SRT.

D. Low-grade ESCC/radioresistant tumor/unstable spine: SRT.

E. High-grade ESCC/radiosensitive tumor/stable spine: cEBRT.

✅ **Answer D**

— For low-grade ESCC by a radioresistant tumor in an unstable spine, the suggested approach is stabilization followed by SRT. Spinal instability is an independent indication for intervention regardless of the radiosensitivity of the tumor, the degree of spinal cord compression, or the type of radiotherapy used. Radiotherapy does not restore spinal stability. Stabilization can be achieved with minimally invasive percutaneous kyphoplasty under local anesthesia (or percutaneous pedicle screw fixation) in surgically unfit patients.

❓ **134. Secondary spinal tumors. NOMS management framework. General management pathways. The FALSE answer is:**

A. High-grade ESCC/radiosensitive tumor/unstable spine: stabilization followed by cEBRT.

B. High-grade ESCC/radioresistant tumor/stable spine/good systemic condition: decompression and stabilization followed by SRT.
C. High-grade ESCC/radioresistant tumor/stable spine/bad systemic condition: SRT.
D. High-grade ESCC/radioresistant tumor/unstable spine/good systemic condition: decompression and stabilization followed by SRT.
E. High-grade ESCC/radioresistant tumor/unstable spine/bad systemic condition: stabilization followed by cEBRT.

✅ **Answer C**
- High-grade ESCC by a radioresistant tumor cannot be treated with SRT except after performing a "separation" decompression surgery in which a minimal tumor resection is carried out to separate the tumor margin from the spinal cord by at least 2 mm allowing delivery of the high-dose SRT to the tumor without inducing post-radiation myelitis and worsening of the neurological functions. If the patient's systemic condition prevents undergoing decompression surgery, cEBRT (although less tumoricidal in cases of radioresistant tumors) is used instead of SRT because it delivers less radiation dose, which can be tolerated by the spinal cord.

❓ **135. Secondary spinal tumors. Management modalities. Corticosteroids. The FALSE answer is:**
A. Should be only started if there is evidence of neurological function deterioration.
B. Control pain within 24–48 h in about 75% of patients.
C. Improve motor function in about 55% of patients.
D. Should be continued until any planned surgery has been executed.
E. Should be continued until any planned radiotherapy has been started.

✅ **Answer A**
- Corticosteroid administration should be started as soon as a spinal metastasis with cord compression has been diagnosed.

❓ **136. Secondary spinal tumors. Management modalities. Medications. The FALSE answer is:**
A. Bisphosphonates reduce the risk of vertebral compression fractures (VCF) by about 50%.
B. RANK ligand (RANKL) inhibitors counteract RANKL overexpression by lytic bony metastases.

C. Chemotherapy is effective for treating spinal metastasis.

D. Blood glucose levels should be monitored while administering corticosteroids.

E. Treatment of metastatic hypercalcemia includes hydration, loop diuretics, and bisphosphonate.

✅ **Answer C**
  − Chemotherapy is ineffective for osseous spinal metastasis but may help to control primary tumors.

❓ **137. Secondary spinal tumors. Management modalities. Biopsy. The FALSE answer is:**

A. Treatment of a bone lesion should not proceed without tissue diagnosis of the lesion.

B. If a primary neoplasm is not identified, obtaining a biopsy is necessary to rule out a primary bone lesion.

C. The diagnostic yield of a fine-needle biopsy in blastic vertebral lesions is typically high.

D. A true cut needle biopsy is preferred whenever possible.

E. An open biopsy should be carried out if a needle biopsy is nonconclusive.

✅ **Answer C**
  − The diagnostic yield of fine-needle biopsy in blastic sclerotic vertebral lesions is typically low.

❓ **138. Secondary spinal tumors. Management modalities. Vertebroplasty and kyphoplasty. The FALSE answer is:**

A. Indicated for painful pathologic compression fractures in the absence of gross spinal instability.

B. There is a reduction in the safety or efficacy of SRT application after interventions utilizing polymethyl methacrylate (PMMA).

C. Effective in reducing pain in 75% of patients.

D. Can obtain biopsy concomitantly through the transpedicular approach.

E. The exothermic reaction of PMMA may help to partially ablate the lesion.

✅ **Answer B**

- Studies show no reduction either in the safety or the efficacy of using SRS postoperatively after interventions utilizing PMMA (e.g., vertebroplasty, kyphoplasty, and cement-augmented screws).

❓ **139.** **Secondary spinal tumors. Management modalities. Vascular metastases that would benefit from preoperative embolization. The FALSE answer is:**
  A. Follicular thyroid carcinoma.
  B. Renal cell carcinoma and hepatocellular carcinoma.
  C. Multiple myeloma.
  D. Paraganglioma and neuroendocrine tumor.
  E. Leiomyosarcoma and angiosarcoma.

✅ **Answer C**

❓ **140.** **Secondary spinal tumors. Management modalities. Non-vascular metastases that do not require preoperative embolization. The FALSE answer is:**
  A. Colon carcinoma.
  B. Melanoma.
  C. Non-small-cell lung carcinoma.
  D. Breast carcinoma.
  E. Sarcomas.

✅ **Answer B**

❓ **141.** **Secondary spinal tumors. Management modalities. Indications for surgery in the absence of neurological deficits. The FALSE answer is:**
  A. Pathology identification if needle biopsies were nonconclusive.
  B. Spinal instability.
  C. Separation surgery for radioresistant tumors with high-grade ESCC before radiotherapy.
  D. Palliative if radiotherapy is ineffective.
  E. Tumor debulking before radiotherapy.

✅ **Answer E**

- Debulking surgery for the mere reduction of the tumor volume before radiotherapy is not indicated.

? 142. Secondary spinal tumors. Management modalities. Indications for surgery in the presence of neurological deficits. The FALSE answer is:

A. If the neurological deficit is rapidly progressing.

B. If the neurological deficit is due to spinal cord compression by fractured bone rather than by tumor.

C. If the neurological deficit is due to spinal cord compression by a soft tumor.

D. If the primary tumor is unknown, the metastasis is considered radioresistant until proven otherwise.

E. If there is associated instability.

✓ **Answer C**

— If the neurological deficit is due to spinal cord compression by a solid tumor (except germ cell tumors), immediate surgical intervention is mandated even if the tumor is radiosensitive, because of the potential to achieve rapid decompression by inducing tumor shrinkage with cEBRT to maximize neurological recovery is limited and usually delayed for few weeks.

? 143. Secondary spinal tumors. Management modalities. Relative contraindication to surgery. The FALSE answer is:

A. Total paraplegia (Brice and McKissock group 4) of any duration.

B. Very radiosensitive tumors (multiple myeloma, lymphoma, etc.) that are not previously radiated.

C. Expected survival of less than 3 months.

D. Multiple lesions at multiple levels.

E. Patients who are unable to tolerate surgery.

✓ **Answer A**

— Some surgeons advocate that patients presenting with total paralysis (Brice and McKissock group 4) of less than 8-h duration or inability to walk (Brice and McKissock group 2) for less than 24-h duration are still candidates for emergency decompression with good postoperative functional outcomes.

? 144. Secondary spinal tumors. Management modalities. Separation surgery. The FALSE answer is:

A. Also coined as "hybrid therapy," i.e., separation surgery followed by SRT.

23

B. Total tumor resection must be carried out to separate the tumor margin from the spinal cord.

C. The targeted separation distance is at least 2 mm between the cord and the lesion.

D. It is done via a posterolateral approach that allows for stabilization and circumferential decompression.

E. Postoperative confirmation of thecal sac reconstitution can be done by CT myelogram or MRI T2.

✅ **Answer B**

— Only minimal tumor resection is carried out to separate the tumor margin from the spinal cord, leaving the bulk of the remaining tumor mass to be treated with SRT.

❓ **145.** **Secondary spinal tumors. Management modalities. Separation surgery. The FALSE answer is:**

A. The assumed maximal safe radiation dose to a single voxel on the spinal cord is 14 Gy.

B. Failures reported in SRT treatments occurred when the radiation dose to specific portions of the target tumor volume was below 15 Gy.

C. In ESCC grade 0 and 1, the targeted tumor and the spinal cord are in close proximity.

D. In ESCC grade 2 and 3, 15 Gy cannot be delivered to the entire tumor without risking cord toxicity.

E. To avoid underdosing any portion of the tumor, the tumor has to be separated from the cord.

✅ **Answer C**

— In grades 2 and 3 of ESCC, the targeted tumor and the spinal cord are in close proximity.

❓ **146.** **Secondary spinal tumors. Management modalities. Spine radiotherapy EBRT vs SRT. The FALSE answer is:**

A. cEBRT is delivered in one or two radiation beams without precise conformal techniques.

B. SRT delivers high doses of focused radiation relying on image-guided radiotherapy platforms.

C. Both SRT and EBRT deliver the same amount of radiation dose in a similar number of sessions.

D. SRT creates more lethal double-stranded DNA breaks in the tumor cells than cEBRT.

E. SRT induces damage to tumor vasculature via the acid sphingomyelinase pathway.

✅ **Answer C**

– In comparison with cEBRT, SRT delivers a higher dose of radiation (up to 24Gy) in only 1–5 fractions. Therefore, SRT provides good durable clinical response (pain and myelopathy) and high local control rates independent of both tumor histology and prior radiation, but these responses appear to be dose dependent.

23

❓ **147. Secondary spinal tumors. Management modalities. Spine radiotherapy complications. The FALSE answer is:**
   A. Mucositis, esophagitis, and dysphagia.
   B. Hair loss.
   C. Radiculitis and paresthesias.
   D. Vertebral compression fractures.
   E. Radiation-induced myelitis.

✅ **Answer B**

❓ **148. Secondary spinal tumors. Management modalities. Spine radiotherapy benefits. The FALSE answer is:**
   A. Reduce pain.
   B. Improve motor function.
   C. Control local recurrence.
   D. Decrease cord compression.
   E. Increase stability.

✅ **Answer E**

❓ **149. Secondary spinal tumors. Management modalities. Spine radiotherapy-induced delayed vertebral compression fractures. The FALSE answer is:**
   A. Radiologically, it is more frequently detected in patients who receive cEBRT compared to those who undergo SRT.
   B. Symptomatic fractures requiring intervention occur in only about 5–8% of cases at the 5-year follow-up.
   C. More likely to occur following treatment with high doses of more than 20 Gy per fraction.

D. High-risk factors are old age, lytic lesions, spinal malalignment, and previous compression fractures.

E. Some experts recommend pre-treatment kyphoplasty in selected patients.

✅ **Answer A**

– Delayed vertebral compression fractures are detected in up to 40% of SRS patients compared with less than 5% of cEBRT patients.

❓ 150. **Secondary spinal tumors. Management modalities. Pain management for biological pain in the absence of instability. The FALSE answer is:**
A. Dexamethasone.
B. Radiotherapy.
C. Tumor ablation procedures including radiofrequency, cryoablation, and laser interstitial thermal therapy.
D. Intrathecal drug delivery pump (e.g., morphine).
E. Kyphoplasty and vertebroplasty.

✅ **Answer E**

– Kyphoplasty and vertebroplasty are more commonly used for painful compression fractures with minimal gross instability causing mechanical pain.

Bibliography

1. Aboulafia AJ, Levine AM. Musculoskeletal and metastatic tumors. In: Fardon DF, Garfin SR, et al., editors. OKU: Spine 2, rosemont. American Academy of Orthopaedic Surgeons; 2002. p. 411–31.
2. Abul-Kasim K, Thurnher MM, McKeever P, Sundgren PC. Intradural spinal tumors: current classification and MRI features. Neuroradiology. 2008;50(4):301–14.
3. Aebi M. Spinal metastasis in the elderly. In: Aebi M, Gunzburg R, Szpalski M, et al., editors. Aging spine. Berlin: Springer-Verlag; 2005. p. 120–31.
4. Akhaddar A, Zyani M, Rharrassi I. Multiple hereditary exostoses with Tetraparesis due to cervical spine Osteochondroma. World Neurosurg. 2018;116:247–8. https://doi.org/10.1016/j.wneu.2018.05.078.
5. Albrecht S, Crutchfield JS, SeGall GK. On spinal osteochondromas. J Neurosurg. 1992;77:247–52. https://doi.org/10.3171/jns.1992.77.2.0247.
6. Altaf F, Movlik H, Brew S, Rezajooi K, Casey A. Osteochondroma of C1 causing vertebral artery occlusion. Br J Neurosurg. 2013;27:130–1. https://doi.org/10.3109/026 88697.2012.707701.

7. Amelot A, et al. Spinal metastases from lung cancer: survival depends only on geno-type, neurological and personal status, scarcely of surgical resection. Surg Oncol. 2020;34:51–6.

8. Amendola L, Simonetti L, Simoes CE, Bandiera S, De Iure F, Boriani S. Aneurysmal bone cyst of the mobile spine: the therapeutic role of embolization. Eur Spine J. 2013;22:533–41. https://doi.org/10.1007/s00586-012-2566-7.

9. Amer HZ, Hameed M. Intraosseous benign notochordal cell tumor. Arch Pathol Lab Med. 2010;134:283–8. https://doi.org/10.5858/134.2.283.

10. Atesok KI, Alman BA, Schemitsch EH, Peyser A, Mankin H. Osteoid osteoma and osteoblastoma. J Am Acad Orthop Surg. 2011;19:678–89. https://doi.org/10.5435/00124635-201111000-00004.

11. Barcena A, et al. Spinal metastatic disease: analysis of factors determining functional prognosis and the choice of treatment. Neurosurgery. 1984;15:820–7.

12. Bartels RH, van der Linden YM, van der Graaf WT. Spinal extradural metastasis: review of current treatment options. CA Cancer J Clin. 2008;58(4):245–59.

13. Barzilai O, et al. Predictors of quality of life improvement after surgery for metastatic tumors of the spine: prospective cohort study. Spine J. 2018;18:1109–15.

14. Bernard SA, Murphey MD, Flemming DJ, Kransdorf MJ. Improved differentiation of benign osteochondromas from secondary chondrosarcomas with standardized measurement of cartilage cap at CT and MR imaging. Radiology. 2010;255:857–65. https://doi.org/10.1148/radiol.10082120.

15. Bhojraj SY, Nene A, Mohite S, Varma R. Giant cell tumor of the spine: a review of 9 surgical interventions in 6 cases. Indian J Orthop. 2007;41:146–50. https://doi.org/10.4103/0019-5413.32047.

16. Bilsky M, Smith M. Surgical approach to epidural spinal cord compression. Hematol Oncol Clin N Am. 2006;20:1307–17.

17. Bjornsson J, Wold LE, Ebersold MJ, Laws ER. Chordoma of the mobile spine. A clinicopathologic analysis of 40 patients. Cancer. 1993;71(3):735–40.

18. Bollen L, et al. Predictive value of six prognostic scoring systems for spinal bone metastases: an analysis based on 1379 patients. Spine. 2016;41:E155–62.

19. Boos N, Fuchs B. Primary tumors of the spine. In: Boos N, Aebi M, et al., editors. Spinal disorders: fundamentals of diagnosis and treatment. Berlin: Springer-Verlag; 2008. p. 951–76.

20. Boriani S, Bandiera S, Biagini R, Bacchini P, Boriani L, Cappuccio M, Chevalley F, Gasbarrini A, Picci P, Weinstein JN. Chordoma of the mobile spine: fifty years of experience. Spine (Phila Pa 1976). 2006;31:493–503.

21. Boriani S, De Iure F, Bandiera S, et al. Chondrosarcoma of the mobile spine: report on 22 cases. Spine (Phila Pa 1976). 2000;25(7):804–12.

22. Boriani S, Weinstein JN, Biagini R. Primary bone tumors of the spine. Terminology and surgical staging. Spine (Phila Pa 1976). 1997;22:1036–44.

23. Boude AB, Vásquez LG, Alvarado-Gomez F, Bedoya MC, Rodríguez-Múnera A, Morales-Saenz LC. A simple bone cyst in cervical vertebrae of an adolescent patient. Case Rep Orthop. 2017;2017:8908216. https://doi.org/10.1155/2017/8908216.

24. Bush LA, Gayle RB, Berkey BD. Multicentric osteoid osteoma presenting a diagnostic dilemma. Radiol Case Rep. 2008;3:217–25. https://doi.org/10.2484/rcr.v3i3.217.

25. Campanacci M. Bone and soft tissue tumors. 2nd ed. Padova: Piccin Nuova Libraria; 1999. p. 46–52.

23

26. Caruso JP, Cohen-Inbar O, Bilsky MH, Gerszten PC, Sheehan JP. Stereotactic radiosurgery and immunotherapy for metastatic spinal melanoma. Neurosurg Focus. 2015;38:E6.

27. Cassidy JT, Baker JF, Lenehan B. The role of prognostic scoring systems in assessing surgical candidacy for patients with vertebral metastasis: a narrative review. Global Spine J. 2018;8:638–51.

28. Chan MS, Wong YC, Yuen MK, Lam D. Spinal aneurysmal bone cyst causing acute cord compression without vertebral collapse: CT and MRI findings. Pediatr Radiol. 2002;32:601–4. https://doi.org/10.1007/s00247-001-0648-5.

29. Chang EL, Brown P, Lo SS, Sahgal A, Suh J, editors. Adult CNS radiation oncology: principles and practice. Cham: Springer International Publishing; 2018.

30. Chen C, Lee I, Tatsui C, Elder T, Sloan AE. Laser interstitial thermotherapy (LITT) for the treatment of tumors of the brain and spine: a brief review. J Neuro-Oncol. 2021;151:429–42.

31. Choi D, et al. Prediction accuracy of common prognostic scoring systems for metastatic spine disease: results of a prospective international multicentre study of 1469 patients. Spine. 2018;43:1678–84.

32. Choi D, Crockard A, Bunger C, Harms J, Kawahara N, Mazel C, Melcher R, Tomita K. Review of metastatic spine tumour classification and indications for surgery: the consensus statement of the global spine tumour study group. Eur Spine J. 2010;19:215–22.

33. Ciftdemir M, Kaya M, Selcuk E, Yalniz E. Tumors of the spine. World J Orthop. 2016;7:109–16. https://doi.org/10.5312/wjo.v7.i2.109.

34. Cloran FJ, Pukenas BA, Loevner LA, Aquino C, Schuster J, Mohan S. Aggressive spinal haemangiomas: imaging correlates to clinical presentation with analysis of treatment algorithm and clinical outcomes. Br J Radiol. 2015;88:20140771. https://doi.org/10.1259/bjr.20140771.

35. Cohen-Gadol AA, Zikel OM, Koch CA, Scheithauer BW, Krauss WE. Spinal meningiomas in patients younger than 50 years of age: a 21-year experience. J Neurosurg. 2003;98(3 Suppl):258–63.

36. Copuroglu C, Yalniz E. Spinal oncologic reconstruction. World Spinal Column J. 2010;1:176–83.

37. Crapanzano JP, Ali SZ, Ginsberg MS, Zakowski MF. Chordoma: a cytologic study with histologic and radiologic correlation. Cancer. 2001;93(1):40–51.

38. Criscitiello C, et al. Clinical outcomes of patients with metastatic breast cancer enrolled in phase I clinical trials. Eur J Cancer. 2021;157:40–9.

39. Crist BD, Lenke LG, Lewis S. Osteoid osteoma of the lumbar spine. A case report highlighting a novel reconstruction technique. J Bone Joint Surg Am. 2005;87:414–8.

40. Cui Y, Lei M, Pan Y, Lin Y, Shi X. Scoring algorithms for predicting survival prognosis in patients with metastatic spinal disease: the current status and future directions. Clin Spine Surg. 2020;33:296–306.

41. Dang L, Liu X, Dang G, et al. Primary tumors of the spine: a review of clinical features in 438 patients. J Neuro-Oncol. 2015;121(3):513–20.

42. Davies AM, Cassar-Pullicino VN. Principles of detection and diagnosis. In: Davies AM, Sundaram M, James SLJ, et al., editors. Imaging of bone tumors and tumor-like lesions. Berlin: Springer-Verlag; 2009. p. 111–35.

43. De Filippo M, Russo U, Papapietro VR, Ceccarelli F, Pogliacomi F, Vaienti E, Piccolo C, Capasso R, Sica A, Cioce F, et al. Radiofrequency ablation of osteoid osteoma. Acta Biomed. 2018;89:175–85. https://doi.org/10.23750/abm.v89i1-S.7021.

44. Deol GS, Haydol R, Phillips FM. Tumors of the spine. In: Vaccaro AR, editor. OKU 8, Rosemont. American Academy of Orthopaedic Surgeons; 2005. p. 587–99.

45. Dorfman HD, Vanel D, Czerniak B, et al. WHO classification of tumours of bone: introduction. World Health Organization classification of tumours: pathology and genetics of tumours of soft tissue and bone. Lyon: International Agency for Research on Cancer (IARC) Press; 2002. p. 277–32.

46. Douglas S, Schild SE, Rades D. A new score predicting the survival of patients with spinal cord compression from myeloma. BMC Cancer. 2012;12:425.

47. Eleraky M, et al. Balloon kyphoplasty in the treatment of metastatic tumors of the upper thoracic spine. J Neurosurg Spine. 2011;14:372–6.

48. Enneking WF, Spanier SS, Goodman MA. A system for the surgical staging of musculoskeletal sarcoma. Clin Orthop Relat Res. 1980;153:106–20.

49. Fletcher CDM. Diagnostic histopathology of tumors, vol. 1. 1st ed. Edinburgh, Scotland: Churchill Livingstone; 1995.

50. Fourney DR, et al. Spinal instability neoplastic score: an analysis of reliability and validity from the spine oncology study group. J Clin Oncol. 2011;29:3072–7.

51. Galgano MA, Goulart CR, Iwenofu H, Chin LS, Lavelle W, Mendel E. Osteoblastomas of the spine: a comprehensive review. Neurosurg Focus. 2016;41:E4. https://doi.org/10.3171/2016.5.FOCUS16122.

52. Garg B, Batra S, Dixit V. Solitary anterior osteochondroma of cervical spine: an unusual cause of dysphagia and review of literature. J Clin Orthop Trauma. 2018;9:S5–7. https://doi.org/10.1016/j.jcot.2017.12.010.

53. Geirnaerdt MJ, Bloem JL, Eulderink F, Hogendoorn PC, Taminiau AH. Cartilaginous tumors: correlation of gadolinium-enhanced MR imaging and histopathologic findings. Radiology. 1993;186:813–7. https://doi.org/10.1148/radiology.186.3.8430192.

54. Gerszten PC, Burton SA, Quinn AE, Agarwala SS, Kirkwood JM. Radiosurgery for the treatment of spinal melanoma metastases. Stereotact Funct Neurosurg. 2005;83:213–21.

55. Girolami M, Caravelli S, Persiani V, Ghermandi R, Gasbarrini A. Do multiple fluid-fluid levels on MRI always reveal primary benign aneurysmal bone cyst? J Neurosurg Sci. 2018;62:234–6. https://doi.org/10.23736/S0390-5616.16.03794-2.

56. Gokaslan ZL, Aladag MA, Ellerhorst JA. Melanoma metastatic to the spine: a review of 133 cases. Melanoma Res. 2000;10:78–80.

57. Goodwin CR, et al. The challenges of renal cell carcinoma metastatic to the spine: a systematic review of survival and treatment. Global Spine J. 2018;8:517–26.

58. Grossman RI, Yousem DM. Neuroradiology: the requisites. 2nd ed. St Louis, MO: Mosby Inc.; 2003.

59. Hadzipasic M, Giantini-Larsen AM, Tatsui CE, Shin JH. Emerging percutaneous ablative and radiosurgical techniques for treatment of spinal metastases. Neurosurg Clin N Am. 2020;31:141–50.

60. Harel R, et al. Spine instrumentation failure after spine tumor resection and radiation: comparing conventional radiotherapy with stereotactic radiosurgery outcomes. World Neurosurg. 2010;74:517–22.

23

61. Hegde G, Azzopardi C, Davies AM, Patel A, James SL, Botchu R. Spinal collision lesions. J Clin Orthop Trauma. 2021;19:21–5. https://doi.org/10.1016/j.jcot.2021.05.003.

62. Held G, Zeynalova S, Murawski N, et al. Impact of rituximab and radiotherapy on outcome of patients with aggressive B-cell lymphoma and skeletal involvement. J Clin Oncol. 2013;31(32):4115–22.

63. Ilaslan H, Sundaram M, Unni KK, Dekutoski MB. Primary Ewing's sarcoma of the vertebral column. Skeletal Radiol. 2004;33(9):506–13.

64. Ilaslan H, Sundaram M, Unni KK, Shives TC. Primary vertebral osteosarcoma: imaging findings. Radiology. 2004;230(3):697–702.

65. Ilaslan H, Sundaram M, Unni KK. Vertebral chondroblastoma. Skeletal Radiol. 2003;32:66–71. https://doi.org/10.1007/s00256-002-0599-4.

66. Inwards CY, Krishnan UK. Dahlin's bone tumors: general aspects and data on 10,165 cases. 6th ed. Philadelphia, PA: Lippincott Williams & Wilkins; 2010.

67. Itshayek E, et al. Timing of surgery and radiotherapy in the management of metastatic spine disease: a systematic review. Int J Oncol. 2010;36:533–44.

68. Jackson RP, Reckling FW, Mants FA. Osteoid osteoma and osteoblastoma. Similar histologic lesions with different natural histories. Clin Orthop Relat Res. 1977;128:303–13.

69. Jackson TJ, Shah AS, Arkader A. Is routine spine MRI necessary in skeletally immature patients with MHE? Identifying patients at risk for spinal osteochondromas. J Pediatr Orthop. 2019;39:e147–52. https://doi.org/10.1097/BPO.0000000000001084.

70. Jawad MS, et al. Vertebral compression fractures after stereotactic body radiation therapy: a large, multi-institutional, multinational evaluation. J Neurosurg Spine. 2016;24:928–36.

71. Kashab M, Böker DK. Indication for surgery of spinal metastases within the cervical region. Neurosurg Rev. 1988;11:95–7.

72. Katonis P, Datsis G, Karantanas A, et al. Spinal osteosarcoma. Clin Med Insights Oncologia. 2013;7:199–208.

73. Katsoulakis E, Kumar K, Laufer I, Yamada Y. Stereotactic body radiotherapy in the treatment of spinal metastases. Semin Radiat Oncol. 2017;27:209–17.

74. Kelley SP, Ashford RU, Rao AS, Dickson RA. Primary bone tumours of the spine: a 42-year survey from the Leeds regional bone tumour Registry. Eur Spine J. 2007;16:405–9. https://doi.org/10.1007/s00586-006-0188-7.

75. Koeller KK, Shih RY. Intradural extramedullary spinal neoplasms: radiologic-pathologic correlation. Radiographics. 2019;39(2):468–90.

76. Konig MA, et al. Kyphoplasty for lytic tumour lesions of the spine: prospective follow-up of 11 cases from procedure to death. Eur Spine J. 2012;21:1873–9.

77. Kransdorf MJ, Stull MA, Gilkey FW, Moser RP Jr. Osteoid osteoma. Radiographics. 1991;11(4):671–96.

78. Krueger EG, Sobel GL, Weinstein C. Vertebral hemangioma with compression of spinal cord. J Neurosurg. 1961;18(3):331–8.

79. Kshettry VR, Hsieh JK, Ostrom QT, Kruchko C, Benzel EC, Barnholtz-Sloan JS. Descriptive epidemiology of spinal meningiomas in the United States. Spine (Phila Pa 1976). 2015;40(15):E886–9.

80. Kumar N, Malhotra R, Zaw AS, et al. Evolution in treatment strategy for metastatic spine disease: presently evolving modalities. Eur J Surg Oncol. 2017;43(9):1784–801.

81. Kyriakos M. Benign notochordal lesions of the axial skeleton: a review and current appraisal. Skeletal Radiol. 2011;40:1141–52. https://doi.org/10.1007/s00256-011-1167-6.

82. Laufer I, et al. Local disease control for spinal metastases following 'separation surgery' and adjuvant hypofractionated or high-dose single-fraction stereotactic radiosurgery: outcome analysis in 186 patients. J Neurosurg Spine. 2013;18:207–14.

83. Laufer I, et al. The NOMS framework: approach to the treatment of spinal metastatic tumors. Oncologist. 2013;18:744–51.

84. Lessnick SL, Ladanyi M. Molecular pathogenesis of Ewing sarcoma: new therapeutic and transcriptional targets. Annu Rev. Pathol. 2012;7:145–59.

85. Lewandrowski KU, Anderson ME, McLain RF. In: Herkowitz HN, Garfin SR, Eismont FJ, Bell GR, Balderston RA, et al., editors. Tumors of the spine. Philadelphia, PA: Elsevier Saunders; 2011. p. 1480–512.

86. Lin H-H, et al. Functional outcomes and survival after surgical stabilization for inoperable non-small-cell lung cancer with spinal metastasis of the thoracic and lumbar spines: a retrospective comparison between epidermal growth factor receptor-tyrosine kinase inhibitor and platinum-based chemotherapy groups. Spinal Cord. 2020;58:194–202.

87. Ling DC, et al. Long-term outcomes after stereotactic radiosurgery for spine metastases: radiation dose-response for late toxicity. Int J Radiat Oncol Biol Phys. 2018;101:602–9.

88. Lockney DT, et al. Spinal stereotactic body radiotherapy following intralesional curettage with separation surgery for initial or salvage chordoma treatment. Neurosurg Focus. 2017;42:E4.

89. Mallepally AR, Mahajan R, Pacha S, Rustagi T, Marathe N, Chhabra HS. Spinal osteoid osteoma: surgical resection and review of literature. Surg Neurol Int. 2020;11:308. https://doi.org/10.25259/SNI_510_2020.

90. Mankin HJ, Hornicek FJ, Ortiz-Cruz E, Villafuerte J, Gebhardt MC. Aneurysmal bone cyst: a review of 150 patients. J Clin Oncol. 2005;23:6756–62. https://doi.org/10.1200/JCO.2005.15.255.

91. Mavrogenis AF, Papagelopoulos PJ, Soucacos PN. Skeletal osteochondromas revisited. Orthopedics. 2008;31:1018.

92. Meyer S, Reinhard H, Graf N, Kramann B, Schneider G. Arterial embolization of a secondary aneurysmatic bone cyst of the thoracic spine prior to surgical excision in a 15-year-old girl. Eur J Radiol. 2002;43:79–81. https://doi.org/10.1016/S0720-048X(01)00406-5.

93. Moussazadeh N, Laufer I, Yamada Y, Bilsky MH. Separation surgery for spinal metastases: effect of spinal radiosurgery on surgical treatment goals. Cancer Control. 2014;21:168–74.

94. Murphey M, Nomikos G, Flemming D, Gannon F, Temple T, Kransdorf M. Imaging of giant cell tumor and giant cell reparative granuloma of bone: radiologic-pathologic correlation. Radiographics. 2001;21:1283–309. https://doi.org/10.1148/radiographics.21.5.g01se251283.

95. Murphey MD, Choi JJ, Kransdorf MJ, Flemming DJ, Gannon FH. Imaging of osteochondroma: variants and complications with radiologic-pathologic correlation. Radiographics. 2000;20(5):1407–34.

23

96. Nasrallah H, Yamada Y, Laufer I, Bilsky MH. A NOMS framework solution. Int J Radiat Oncol Biol Phys. 2019;103:17–8.

97. Nishida J, Kato S, Murakami H, Ehara S, Satoh T, Okada K, Shimamura T. Tetraparesis caused by chondroblastoma of the cervical spine: a case report. Spine. 2003;28:E173–8. https://doi.org/10.1097/01.BRS.0000058731.83977.61.

98. Noordin S, Allana S, Umer M, Jamil M, Hilal K, Uddin N. Unicameral bone cysts: current concepts. Ann Med Surg. 2018;34:43–9. https://doi.org/10.1016/j.amsu.2018.06.005.

99. O'Neil J, Gardner V, Armstrong G. Treatment of tumors of the thoracic and lumbar spinal column. Clin Orthop Relat Res. 1988;227:103–12.

100. Ofluoglu O, Boriani S, Gasbarrini A, De Iure F, Donthineni R. Diagnosis and planning in the management of musculoskeletal tumors: surgical perspective. Semin Intervent Radiol. 2010;27:185–90.

101. Oliveira AM, Chou MM. USP6-induced neoplasms: the biologic spectrum of aneurysmal bone cyst and nodular fasciitis. Hum Pathol. 2014;45:1–11. https://doi.org/10.1016/j.humpath.2013.03.005.

102. Onimus M, Schraub S, Bertin D, Bosset JF, Guidet M. Surgical treatment of vertebral metastasis. Spine. 1986;11:883–91.

103. Osawa T, et al. Overview of current and future systemic therapy for metastatic renal cell carcinoma. Jpn J Clin Oncol. 2019;49:395–403.

104. Ostrom QT, Gittleman H, Fulop J, et al. CBTRUS statistical report: primary brain and central nervous system tumors diagnosed in the United States in 2008-2012. Neuro-Oncology. 2015;17(Suppl 4):iv1–iv62.

105. Ottaviani G, Jaffe N. The epidemiology of osteosarcoma. Cancer Treat Res. 2009;152:3–13.

106. Pastushyn AI, Slin'ko EI, Mirzoyeva GM. Vertebral hemangiomas: diagnosis, management, natural history and clinicopathological correlates in 86 patients. Surg Neurol. 1998;50(6):535–47.

107. Patchell RA, et al. Direct decompressive surgical resection in the treatment of spinal cord compression caused by metastatic cancer: a randomised trial. Lancet. 2005;366:643–8.

108. Patel A, James SL, Davies AM, Botchu R. Spinal imaging update: an introduction to techniques for advanced MRI. Bone Jt J. 2015;97:1683–92. https://doi.org/10.1302/0301-620X.97B12.36164.

109. Patnaik S, Jyotsnarani Y, Uppin SG, Susarla R. Imaging features of primary tumors of the spine: a pictorial essay. Indian J Radiol Imaging. 2016;26:279–89. https://doi.org/10.4103/0971-3026.184413.

110. Perrin RG. Symptomatic spinal metastases. Am Fam Phys. 1989;39:165–72.

111. Pizzo P, Poplack D. Principles and practice of pediatric oncology. Philadelphia, PA: Lippincott Williams & Wilkins; 2006.

112. Plotkin SR, O'Donnell CC, Curry WT, Bove CM, MacCollin M, Nunes FP. Spinal ependymomas in neurofibromatosis type 2: a retrospective analysis of 55 patients. J Neurosurg Spine. 2011;14(4):543–7.

113. Posner JB. Neurologic complications of systemic cancer. Dis Mon. 1978;25(2):1–60.

114. Qian Z, et al. Kyphoplasty for the treatment of malignant vertebral compression fractures caused by metastases. J Clin Neurosci. 2011;18:763–7.

115. Rades D, et al. Prognostic factors in a series of 504 breast cancer patients with metastatic spinal cord compression. Strahlenther Onkol. 2012;188:340–5.

116. Rajakulasingam R, Murphy J, Botchu R, James SL. Osteochondromas of the cervical spine-case series and review. J Clin Orthop Trauma. 2020;11:905–9. https://doi.org/10.1016/j.jcot.2019.12.014.

117. Redmond KJ, et al. Consensus guidelines for postoperative stereotactic body radiation therapy for spinal metastases: results of an international survey. J Neurosurg Spine. 2017;26:299–306.

118. Rodallec MH, Feydy A, Larousserie F, et al. Diagnostic imaging of solitary tumors of the spine: what to do and say. Radiographics. 2008;28(4):1019–41.

119. Roesch J, et al. Risk for surgical complications after previous stereotactic body radiotherapy of the spine. Radiat Oncol. 2017;12:153.

120. Roodman GD. Mechanisms of bone metastasis. N Engl J Med. 2004;350(16):1655–64.

121. Sahgal A, et al. Probabilities of radiation myelopathy specific to stereotactic body radiation therapy to guide safe practice. Int J Radiat Oncol Biol Phys. 2013;85:341–7.

122. Saifuddin A, Tyler P, Hargunani R. Musculoskeletal MRI. 2nd ed. Boca Raton, FL: CRC Press; 2016.

123. Salgia NJ, Dara Y, Bergerot P, Salgia M, Pal SK. The changing landscape of management of metastatic renal cell carcinoma: current treatment options and future directions. Curr Treat Options in Oncol. 2019;20:41.

124. Sciubba DM, Petteys RJ, Dekutoski MB, et al. Diagnosis and management of metastatic spine disease. A review. J Neurosurg Spine. 2010;13(1):94–108.

125. Scottish Bone Tumor Registry, Sharma H, Mehdi SA, MacDuff E, Reece AT, Jane MJ, Reid R. Paget sarcoma of the spine: Scottish bone Tumor Registry experience. Spine (Phila Pa 1976). 2006;31(12):1344–50.

126. Shah LM, Salzman KL. Imaging of spinal metastatic disease. Int J Surg Oncol. 2011;2011:–769753.

127. Shaw B, Mansfield FL, Borges L. One-stage posterolateral decompression and stabilization for primary and metastatic vertebral tumors in the thoracic and lumbar spine. J Neurosurg. 1989;70:405–10.

128. Shrivastava RK, Epstein FJ, Perin NI, Post KD, Jallo GI. Intramedullary spinal cord tumors in patients older than 50 years of age: management and outcome analysis. J Neurosurg Spine. 2005;2(3):249–55.

129. Siker ML, Bovi J, Alexander B. Chapter 30—spinal cord tumors. In: Gunderson LL, Tepper JE, editors. Clinical radiation oncology. 4th ed. Philadelphia, PA: Elsevier; 2016. p. 521–540.e525.

130. Smith AB, Soderlund KA, Rushing EJ, Smirniotopolous JG. Radiologic-pathologic correlation of pediatric and adolescent spinal neoplasms: part 1, intramedullary spinal neoplasms. AJR Am J Roentgenol. 2012;198(1):34–43.

131. Smolders D, Wang X, Drevelengas A, Vanhoenacker F, De Schepper AM. Value of MRI in the diagnosis of non-clival, non-sacral chordoma. Skeletal Radiol. 2003;32(6):343–50.

132. Sundaresan N, Digiacinto GV, Hughes JE. Surgical treatment of spinal metastases. Clin Neurosurg. 1986;33:503–22.

133. Sundaresan N, Galicich JH, Bains MS, Martini N, Beattie EJJ. Vertebral body resection in the treatment of cancer involving the spine. Cancer. 1984;53:1393–6.

23

134. Suzuki M, Satoh T, Nishida J, Kato S, Toba T, Honda T, Masuda T. Solid variant of aneurysmal bone cyst of the cervical spine. Spine. 2004;29:E376–81. https://doi.org/10.1097/01.brs.0000137053.08152.a6.

135. Tafti D, Cecava N. Spinal hemangioma. Treasure Island, FL: StatPearls Publishing; 2022.

136. Tateda S, Hashimoto K, Aizawa T, Kanno H, Hitachi S, Itoi E, Ozawa H. Diagnosis of benign notochordal cell tumor of the spine: is a biopsy necessary? Clin Case Rep. 2018;6:63–7. https://doi.org/10.1002/ccr3.1287.

137. Tepelenis K, Papathanakos G, Kitsouli A, Troupis T, Barbouti A, Vlachos K, Kanavaros P, Kitsoulis P. Osteochondromas: an updated review of epidemiology, pathogenesis, clinical presentation, radiological features and treatment options. In Vivo. 2021;35:681–91. https://doi.org/10.21873/invivo.12308.

138. Thakur N, Daniels A, Schiller J, et al. Benign tumors of the spine. J Am Acad Orthop Surg. 2012;20(11):715–24.

139. Thomas JG, et al. A novel use of the intraoperative MRI for metastatic spine tumors: laser interstitial thermal therapy for percutaneous treatment of epidural metastatic spine disease. Neurosurg Clin N Am. 2017;28:513–24.

140. Todd B. Management of painful unstable spinal metastases. Br J Hosp Med. 1990;43:328.

141. Tokuhashi Y, Matsuzaki H, Oda H, Oshima M, Ryu J. A revised scoring system for preoperative evaluation of metastatic spine tumor prognosis. Spine (Phila Pa 1976). 2005;30(19):2186–91.

142. Tokuhashi Y, Matsuzaki H, Toriyama S, Kawano H, Ohsaka S. Scoring system for the preoperative evaluation of metastatic spine tumor prognosis. Spine. 1990;15:1110–3.

143. Tomita K, Kawahara N, Baba H, Tsuchiya H, Fujita T, Toribatake Y. Total en bloc spondylectomy. A new surgical technique for primary malignant vertebral tumors. Spine (Phila Pa 1976). 1997;22:324–33.

144. Tomita K, Kawahara N, Kobayashi T, Yoshida A, Murakami H, Akamaru T. Surgical strategy for spinal metastases. Spine (Phila Pa 1976). 2001;26:298–306.

145. Tomita Y, et al. Efficacy and safety of subsequent molecular targeted therapy after immuno-checkpoint therapy, retrospective study of Japanese patients with metastatic renal cell carcinoma (AFTER I-O study). Jpn J Clin Oncol. 2021;51:966–75.

146. Truong VT, et al. Surgical intervention for patients with spinal metastasis from lung cancer: a retrospective study of 87 cases. Clin Spine Surg. 2021;34:E133–40.

147. Ulano A, Bredella MA, Burke P, Chebib I, Simeone FJ, Huang AJ, Torriani M, Chang CY. Distinguishing untreated osteoblastic metastases from enostoses using CT attenuation measurements. Am J Roentgenol. 2016;207:362–8. https://doi.org/10.2214/AJR.15.15559.

148. Vega RA, Ghia AJ, Tatsui CE. Percutaneous hybrid therapy for spinal metastatic disease: laser interstitial thermal therapy and spinal stereotactic radiosurgery. Neurosurg Clin N Am. 2020;31:211–9.

149. Venkatasamy A, Chenard MP, Massard G, Steib JP, Bierry G. Chondroblastoma of the thoracic spine: a rare location. Case report with radiologic-pathologic correlation. Skeletal Radiol. 2017;46:367–72. https://doi.org/10.1007/s00256-016-2550-0.

150. Vialle R, Feydy A, Rillardon L, Tohme-Noun C, Anract P, Colombat M, De Pinieux G, Drapé JL, Guigui P. Chondroblastoma of the lumbar spine. Report of two cases and

review of the literature. J Neurosurg Spine. 2005;2:596–600. https://doi.org/10.3171/spi.2005.2.5.0596.

151. Vidoni A, Grainger M, James S. Experience of neuroprotective air injection during radiofrequency ablation (RFA) of spinal osteoid osteoma. Eur Radiol. 2018;28:4146–50. https://doi.org/10.1007/s00330-018-5406-2.

152. Wang V, Chou D. Anterior C1-2 osteochondroma presenting with dysphagia and sleep apnea. J Clin Neurosci. 2009;16:581–2. https://doi.org/10.1016/j.jocn.2008.05.024.

23

Familial Tumor Syndromes

Issa A. M. Lahirish, Abdullah H. Al Ramadan,
Younus M. Al-Khazaali, Abdullah K. Al-Qaraghuli,
and Samer S. Hoz

© The Author(s), under exclusive license to Springer Nature Switzerland AG 2024
S. S. Hoz et al. (eds.), *Surgical Neuro-Oncology*,
https://doi.org/10.1007/978-3-031-53642-7_24

? 1. **Neurofibromatosis type I: genetics. The FALSE answer is:**
   A. It is an autosomal dominant disease.
   B. Is due to a mutation in *NF1* tumor suppressor gene on chromo-
      some 22.
   C. Can be associated with pheochromocytomas.
   D. Can be associated with iris hamartomas.
   E. Has 100% penetrance.

✅ **Answer B**
— The NF1 tumor suppressor gene normally codes for neurofibromin, a
negative regulator of RAS. This gene is located on chromosome 17.

? 2. **Neurofibromatosis type I: clinical manifestations. A child with epilepsy
and struggling academically at school presented with multiple freckles
in the axillary and inguinal folds, along with numerous pigmented
macules on the chest and back. The patient can also present with fea-
tures of the following. The FALSE answer is:**
   A. Peripheral nerve tumors.
   B. Strong family history of the same illness.
   C. Multiple meningiomas.
   D. Optic pathway gliomas.
   E. Epilepsy.

✅ **Answer C**
— Multiple meningiomas are characteristic of NF2 but not typically associated with NF1.

? 3. **Neurofibromatosis type I: clinical manifestations. A 15-year-old girl has
pigmented lesions on her trunk and a dark lesion in the iris. The patient
is at risk of the following. The FALSE answer is:**
   A. Decreased vision.
   B. Thinning of the long bone cortex.
   C. Cardiac rhabdomyoma.
   D. Peripheral nerve tumors.

✅ **Answer C**
— NF1 is an autosomal dominant genetic condition associated with axillary
and inguinal freckles, Lisch nodules, café au lait spots, peripheral nerve
tumors, thinning of long bone, and optic pathway gliomas. NF1 is not
associated with cardiac rhabdomyomas.

24

? 4. **Neurofibromatosis type I: diagnostic criteria. The FALSE answer is:**
   A. Can be associated with bone abnormality.
   B. Intracranial tumors can occur.
   C. There is a strong family history.
   D. Is associated with hypopigmented skin lesions.
   E. Is associated with Lisch nodules.

✅ **Answer D**
— *NF1* is not associated with hypopigmented skin lesions.
   Current NF1 diagnostic criteria
   Developed in 1987 at NIH
   Two or more of the following manifestations:
   1. Six or more café-au-lait macules over 5 mm in diameter in prepubertal individuals and over 15 mm in greatest diameter in postpubertal individuals.
   2. Axillary or inguinal freckling (armpit or groin freckling).
   3. ≥2 neurofibromas of any type or 1 plexiform neurofibroma.
   4. Optic glioma.
   5. ≥2 Lisch nodules.
   6. Distinctive osseous lesions such as sphenoid dysplasia or thinning of long bone cortex with/without pseudarthrosis.
   7. Affected first-degree relative by 1–6.

? 5. **Neurofibromatosis type I: associations and diagnosis. The FALSE answer is:**
   A. Is associated with an increased risk of seizures.
   B. There is a risk of developing precocious puberty.
   C. NF1 patients with mental retardation are at even higher risk for seizures.
   D. Positron emission tomography is of great value in monitoring lesions with the potential for malignant transformation in NF1.
   E. Individuals with NF1 usually present with IQ levels in the normal range.

✅ **Answer E**
— Individuals with NF1 are usually present with IQ levels in the low-average normal range (~90 IQ points), with an increased incidence of intellectual disability (6–7%) and learning disabilities (50–70%).

6. Neurofibromatosis type I: optic pathway glioma (OPG). The FALSE answer is:
A. The most common CNS NF1 tumor.
B. Affects 15–30% of patients.
C. OPG in NF1 has a worse prognosis than OPG in non-NF1 individuals.
D. Carboplatin and vincristine are the chemotherapy of choice.
E. Treatment should be started if the patient presents with progressive visual loss.

Answer C
- Most OPGs in NF1 have a benign course and a better prognosis than OPGs in non-NF1 individuals.

7. Neurofibromatosis type I: neurofibromas. The FALSE answer is:
A. Neurofibromas occur in almost all cases of NF1.
B. Often arises in late childhood.
C. Spinal neurofibromas have a risk of malignant transformation.
D. Surgery is the treatment of choice for symptomatic plexiform neurofibromas.
E. Adjuvant radiotherapy has no role in the management of malignant peripheral sheath tumors.

Answer E
- Adjuvant radiotherapy provides local control and may delay the onset of recurrence but has little effect on long-term survival.

8. Neurofibromatosis type I: oral manifestations of NF1. The FALSE answer is:
A. Oral manifestations are very common in NF1.
B. Intraoral neurofibromas should not undergo surgical removal.
C. Associated with oral hygiene difficulties.
D. The most common findings are enlarged fungiform papillae of the tongue.
E. Jaw malformations are usually ipsilateral to facial plexiform neurofibromas.

Answer B
- Whenever possible, intraoral neurofibromas should undergo surgical removal (and subsequent histopathological analysis), especially those that are troubling or located in areas of trauma.

? 9. **Neurofibromatosis type II: ocular manifestations. The FALSE answer is:**
   A. A periodical ophthalmological examination is recommended.
   B. Juvenile posterior subcapsular opacities.
   C. Retinal hamartomas.
   D. Early detection of specific eye abnormality is associated with a worse prognosis.
   E. Bilateral optic gliomas are characteristic.

✅ **Answer E**
▬ NF2 presents as a spectrum of specific ocular abnormalities: juvenile posterior subcapsular/capsular or cortical lenticular opacities, disk gliomas, combined pigment epithelial and retinal hamartomas, epiretinal membrane, and optic nerve sheath meningiomas (ONSM). NF2 is not associated with an increased incidence of bilateral optic gliomas.

? 10. **Neurofibromatosis type II: genetics. The FALSE answer is:**
   A. Is due to mutations in NF2 tumor suppressor gene on chromosome 22.
   B. Can be associated with spinal meningioma.
   C. Can be associated with bilateral acoustic schwannomas.
   D. Can be associated with cataracts.
   E. Is an autosomal recessive disease.

✅ **Answer E**
▬ The inheritance in *NF* type II is autosomal dominant.

? 11. **Neurofibromatosis type II: diagnostic criteria. The FALSE answer is:**
   A. Can cause high-frequency hearing loss.
   B. Associated with bilateral vestibular schwannomas.
   C. Associated with meningiomas and nonvestibular schwannomas.
   D. A definite diagnosis can be made in a patient with a spinal schwannoma in addition to a family history of NF II.
   E. A definite diagnosis can be made in a patient with bilateral vestibular schwannomas.

✅ **Answer D**
▬ Diagnostic criteria for neurofibromatosis type **II**:
   Confirmed (definite) diagnosis of NF2:
   – Bilateral vestibular schwannomas.

A probable diagnosis of NF2:
- Family history of NF2.
- Unilateral vestibular schwannomas or any 2 of the following tumor types: meningioma, glioma, schwannoma, juvenile posterior subcapsular lenticular opacity, juvenile cortical cataract.

? 12. **Neurofibromatosis type II: diagnosis. All of the following may have essential roles in the evaluation. The FALSE answer is:**
   A. MRI of the brain.
   B. Auditory testing.
   C. Visual testing.
   D. EEG.

✓ **Answer D**
- There is no essential role of EEG in NF2 evaluation.

24

? 13. **Neurofibromatosis type II: clinical manifestations. The FALSE answer is:**
   A. Clinical manifestations of NF2 arise predominantly during early adulthood.
   B. Hearing loss and/or tinnitus are the most frequent symptoms.
   C. Bilateral vestibular schwannomas.
   D. After resection of a vestibular schwannoma, patients should undergo training for auditory abilities and lip reading training.
   E. Associated with non-progressive sensorineural hearing loss.

✓ **Answer E**
- Hearing loss and/or tinnitus are the most frequent symptoms in NF2 patients. They develop bilateral vestibular schwannomas that eventually lead to progressive sensorineural hearing loss, tinnitus, and loss of balance.

? 14. **Von Hippel-Lindau disease: associations. The FALSE answer is:**
   A. Deletion of *VHL* gene on chromosome 3p.
   B. Cerebellar and spinal hemangioblastomas.
   C. Pheochromocytoma.
   D. Renal angiomyolipomas.
   E. Anemia.

✓ **Answer D**
- Von Hippel-Lindau disease is associated with bilateral renal cell carcinoma, not renal angiomyolipoma.

? 15. **Von Hippel-Lindau disease: presentation. For a man with a recent history of dark-rusty colored urine, cytologic renal evaluation reveals malignant cells with chromosome 3p deletion. The FALSE answer is:**
   A. Can present with subarachnoid hemorrhage.
   B. Can have a high erythropoietin level.
   C. Can present with paroxysmal hypertension.
   D. Chromosomal deletion involving the *VHL* gene.
   E. Craniospinal MRI is essential.

✅ **Answer A**
— Von Hippel-Lindau disease is not associated with intracranial aneurysms and is instead associated with craniospinal hemangioblastomas.

? 16. **Von Hippel-Lindau disease: associations. The FALSE answer is:**
   A. Pancreatic islet tumors.
   B. Clear cell renal cell carcinoma.
   C. Endolymphatic sac tumors.
   D. Pancreatic cystadenomas.
   E. Pancreatic adenocarcinoma.

✅ **Answer E**
— VHL can be associated with central nervous system hemangioblastoma, clear cell renal cell carcinoma, pheochromocytomas, pancreatic islet tumors, and endolymphatic sac tumors. Additionally, renal and pancreatic cystadenomas and epididymal cystadenomas have been diagnosed in males and cystadenomas of the broad ligament of the uterus have been diagnosed in females. VHL is not known to be associated with pancreatic adenocarcinoma.

? 17. **Von Hippel-Lindau disease. The FALSE answer is:**
   A. Characterized by the development of multiple neoplasms.
   B. Associated tumors are typically bilateral and multifocal but rarely malignant.
   C. An autosomal recessive disease.
   D. Can present with episodic headaches and tachycardia.
   E. Screening of family members is essential.

✅ **Answer C**
— Von Hippel-Lindau syndrome is a rare autosomal dominant disorder.

18. Von Hippel-Lindau disease: genetics. Genetic tests should be carried out in the following. The FALSE answer is:

A. Any individual with two VHL-associated lesions.
B. Any individual with one or more CNS hemangioblastoma(s).
C. Any individual with > RCC diagnosed <20 years.
D. Any individual with paraganglioma and endolymphatic sac tumors.
E. Any individual with bilateral renal cysts.

Answer E

- In the case of diagnosis of VHL syndrome components, genetic tests should be performed on the patient and family members. Qualification can be based on criteria specified by Massachusetts General Hospital.
- Genetic tests should be carried out in:

1. Any individual with two VHL-associated lesions:
   HB, RCC, pheochromocytoma, endolymphatic sac tumor, epididymal or adnexal papillary cystadenoma, pancreatic cystadenomas, and neuroendocrine tumors.
2. Any individual with one or more of the following: CNS HB, pheochromocytoma or paraganglioma, endolymphatic sac tumor, and epididymal papillary cystadenoma.
3. Any individuals with > RCC diagnosed <20 years, bilateral or multiple RCC, in multiple pancreatic serous cystadenoma and neuroendocrine tumor, pancreatic cyst, and any VHL-associated lesion.

19. Tuberous sclerosis: pathogenesis and associations. The FALSE answer is:

A. *TSC1* mutation on chromosome 9 or *TSC2* mutation on chromosome 16.
B. Autosomal dominant.
C. Variable expression.
D. Mental retardation.
E. Increased incidence of subependymoma.

Answer E

- Tuberous sclerosis is associated with an increased incidence of subependymal giant cell astrocytomas and ungual fibromas.

? 20. **Tuberous sclerosis: clinical manifestations. A child presenting with refractory epilepsy and developmental delay. Physical examination showed multiple hypopigmented macules. This patient's presentation is most likely associated with the following. The FALSE answer is:**
  A. Optic nerve glioma.
  B. Intellectual disabilities.
  C. Cardiac rhabdomyoma.
  D. Calcified cortical lesions.
  E. Subependymal nodules.

✅ **Answer A**
− Tuberous sclerosis is not typically associated with optic nerve gliomas.

? 21. **Tuberous sclerosis: clinical manifestations. A child presented with abnormal movement, with a physical examination revealing hypopigmented macules. The child's mother also has similar lesions. The following is most likely to be associated with this patient's underlying condition. The FALSE answer is:**
  A. Subependymal giant cell tumor.
  B. Developmental delay.
  C. Intellectual disability.
  D. Epilepsy.
  E. Bilateral acoustic schwannomas.

✅ **Answer E**
− Tuberous sclerosis is an autosomal dominant condition that should be suspected in children with infantile spasms and ash leaf spots. It is not associated with bilateral acoustic schwannomas.

? 22. **Li-Fraumeni syndrome: genetics and associations. The FALSE answer is:**
  A. Family history of LFS-associated cancers.
  B. Associated with medulloblastoma.
  C. Associated with glioma.
  D. RB tumor suppressor gene mutation.
  E. Females have nearly a 100% risk of developing cancer in their lifetime.

✅ **Answer D**
− Li-Fraumeni syndrome (LFS) is an inherited genetic condition that increases the risk of various cancers. It results from mutations in the TP53 tumor suppressor gene.

? 23. **Li-Fraumeni syndrome: genetics and associations. The FALSE answer is:**
  A. Characterized by early-onset breast cancer.
  B. Associated with sarcomas.
  C. Autosomal recessive condition.
  D. Due to a mutation in the TP53 tumor suppressor gene.

✅ **Answer C**
— Li-Fraumeni syndrome is an inherited autosomal dominant disorder characterized by early-onset breast cancer, sarcomas, and other cancers in children and young adults.

? 24. **Cowden syndrome: genetics and associations. The FALSE answer is:**
  A. Autosomal dominant condition.
  B. Almost all patients with Cowden syndrome develop hamartomas.
  C. Associated with macrocephaly.
  D. Can develop malignant brain tumors like glioblastoma multiforme
  E. Is associated with an increased risk of developing breast cancer.

✅ **Answer D**
— Cowden syndrome is associated with an increased incidence of a benign brain tumor known as Lhermitte-Duclos disease.

? 25. **Cowden syndrome: genetics. The FALSE answer is:**
  A. Is an X-linked recessive condition.
  B. Is a genetic disease characterized by multiple noncancerous and tumor-like growths.
  C. Is associated with an increased risk of developing several types of cancer.
  D. Changes in the PTEN, KLLN, or WWP1 gene are most commonly identified.
  E. Also called multiple hamartoma syndrome.

✅ **Answer A**
— Cowden syndrome is inherited in an autosomal dominant pattern.

? 26. **Turcot Syndrome: clinical manifestations. The FALSE answer is:**
  A. Associated with adenomatous polyps in the gastrointestinal tract.
  B. Can present with fatigue and weight loss.

C. Associated with brain gliomas and medulloblastomas.
D. Increased risk of developing skull base meningiomas.
E. The patient may develop cafe-au-lait spots.

✅ **Answer D**

▬ Turcot Syndrome is not associated with an increased risk of meningiomas.

❓ 27. **Turcot Syndrome: clinical manifestations and inheritance. The FALSE answer is:**
A. Can be inherited in an autosomal recessive pattern.
B. Associated with basal cell carcinoma.
C. Characterized by the association of benign growths in the mucous lining of the gastrointestinal tract with tumors of the central nervous system.
D. Not associated with café au lait spots.
E. Males and females are affected equally.

✅ **Answer D**

▬ Turcot syndrome can be associated with café au lait spots, lipomas, and basal cell carcinomas.

❓ 28. **Schwannomatosis: diagnostic criteria. The FALSE answer is:**
A. Mutation of a tumor suppressor gene located on chromosome 22.
B. Can present with chronic pain, numbness, and weakness.
C. Does not cause hearing loss.
D. Associated with bilateral vestibular schwannomas.
E. The presence of a nonvestibular schwannoma in addition to a first-degree relative with schwannomatosis is one of the diagnostic criteria.

✅ **Answer D**

▬ Schwannomatosis is not typically associated with bilateral vestibular schwannomas. Bilateral vestibular schwannomas are more commonly associated with NF2. The diagnostic criteria for Schwannomatosis are as follows:

- **Definite**
  - Age >30 years and ≥2 non-intradermal schwannomas, at least one with histologic confirmation and no evidence of vestibular tumor on MRI scan and no known NF mutation.
  - One nonvestibular schwannoma plus a first-degree relative with schwannomatosis.
- **Possible**
  - Age <30 and ≥2 non-intradermal schwannomas, at least one with histologic confirmation and no evidence of vestibular tumor on MRI scan and no known NF mutation.
  - Age >45 and ≥2 non-intradermal schwannomas, at least one with histologic confirmation and no symptoms of eighth nerve dysfunction and no NF2.
  - Nonvestibular schwannoma and a first-degree relative with schwannomatosis.
- **Segmental**
  - Diagnosed as definite or possible but limited to one limb or ≤5 contiguous segments of the spine.

24

❓ 29. **Schwannomatosis. The FALSE answer is:**
   A. Characterized by the development of multiple schwannomas.
   B. Patients should undergo yearly follow-up.
   C. Special attention should be directed to new onset or worsening of pain.
   D. Whole-body MRI is particularly useful in this patient population.
   E. Not associated with intracranial schwannomas.

✅ **Answer E**
- Schwannomatosis is characterized by the development of multiple schwannomas (spinal, peripheral, intracranial) in the absence of vestibular schwannomas.

❓ 30. **Gorlin syndrome. The FALSE answer is:**
   A. Is an autosomal dominant disease.
   B. Associated with rib anomalies.
   C. Associated with an increased risk of ependymoma.
   D. Basal cell carcinoma.
   E. Palmar pits.

✅ **Answer C**

▬ Gorlin syndrome is an autosomal dominant neurocutaneous disease characterized by developmental anomalies such as palmar pits and rib anomalies, and tumors such as medulloblastoma and basal cell carcinoma. Gorlin syndrome is not associated with an increased incidence of ependymoma.

Bibliography

1. Abramowicz A, Gos M. Neurofibromin in neurofibromatosis type 1—mutations in NF1gene as a cause of disease. Med Wieku Rozwoj. 2014;18(3):297–306.
2. Stamenkovic I, Yu Q. Merlin, a "magic" linker between extracellular cues and intracellular signaling pathways that regulate cell motility, proliferation, and survival. Curr Protein Pept Sci. 2010;11(6):471–84. https://doi.org/10.2174/138920310791824011. PMC 2946555
3. Glenn PL, Walther GM, Parronas MM, Linehan NJ, Zbar WM, von Hippel-Lindau B. Disease: genetic, clinical, and imaging features [published correction appears in radiology. 1995; 196:582]. Radiology. 1995;194:629–42.
4. Tuberous sclerosis. National Organization for Rare Disorders. https://rarediseases.org/rare-diseases/tuberous-sclerosis/. Accessed 18 Sept 2017.
5. Hisada M, Garber JE, Li FP, Fung CY, Fraumeni JF. Multiple primary cancers in families with Li-Fraumeni syndrome. J Natl Cancer Inst. 1998;90(8):606–11. https://doi.org/10.1093/jnci/90.8.606.
6. Bennett KL, Mester J, Eng C. Germline epigenetic regulation of KILLIN in Cowden and Cowden-like syndrome. JAMA. 2010;304(24):2724–31. https://doi.org/10.1001/jama.2010.1877. Citation on PubMed or Free article on PubMed Central
7. Hobert JA, Eng C. PTEN hamartoma tumor syndrome: an overview. Genet Med. 2009;11(10):687–94. https://doi.org/10.1097/GIM.0b013e3181ac9aea. Review. Citation on PubMed
8. McLaughlin MR, et al. Medulloblastoma and glioblastoma multiforme in a patient with Turcot syndrome. Surg Neurol. 1998;49:295–301.
9. Yamada T, et al. Textbook of gastroenterology. 2nd ed. J.B. Lippincott Company; 1995. p. 1944–54.
10. Ferner RE, Huson SM, Gareth D, Evans R. Neurofibromatoses in clinical practice. Springer; 2011.
11. Neurofibromatosis, National Institutes of Health Consensus Development Conference. Neurofibromatosis: Conference Statement. Arch Neurol. 1988;45:575–578.
12. Beres SJ, Avery RA. Optic pathway gliomas secondary to neurofibromatosis type 1. Semin Pediatr Neurol. 2017;24(2):92–9. https://doi.org/10.1016/j.spen.2017.04.006. Epub 2017 Apr 10
13. Nabbout R, Belousova E, Benedik MP, Carter T, Cottin V, Curatolo P, Dahlin M, D'Amato L, d'Augères GB, de Vries PJ, Ferreira JC, Feucht M, Fladrowski C, Hertzberg C, Jozwiak S, Lawson JA, Macaya A, Marques R, O'Callaghan F, Qin J, Sander V, Sauter M, Shah S, Takahashi Y, Touraine R, Youroukos S, Zonnenberg B, Jansen A,

Kingswood JC, TOSCA Consortium and TOSCA Investigators. Epilepsy in tuberous sclerosis complex: findings from the TOSCA study. Epilepsia Open. 2018;4(1):73–84. https://doi.org/10.1002/epi4.12286. PMID: 30868117; PMCID: PMC6398114

14. Bernier A, Larbrisseau A, Perreault S. Café-au-lait macules and neurofibromatosis type 1: a review of the literature. Pediatr Neurol. 2016;60:24–29.e1. https://doi.org/10.1016/j. pediatrneurol.2016.03.003. Epub 2016 Mar 19

15. Kozaczuk S, Ben-Skowronek I. From arterial hypertension complications to von Hippel-Lindau syndrome diagnosis. Ital J Pediatr. 2015;41:56. https://doi.org/10.1186/s13052-015-0158-y.

16. Blumenthal GM, Dennis PA. PTEN hamartoma tumor syndromes. Eur J Hum Genet. 2008;16(11):1289–300. https://doi.org/10.1038/ejhg.2008.162. Epub 2008 Sep 10. Review

17. Neurofibromatosis. Conference statement. National Institutes of Health Consensus Development Conference. Arch Neurol. 1988;45(5):575–578.

18. Khattab A, Monga DK. Turcot syndrome. [Updated 2020 Jun 29]. In: StatPearls [Internet]. Treasure Island, FL: StatPearls Publishing; 2020. https://www.ncbi.nlm.nih. gov/books/NBK534782/.

19. Batista PB, Bertollo EM, Costa Dde S, Eliam L, Cunha KS, Cunha-Melo JR, Darrigo Junior LG, Geller M, Gianordoli-Nascimento IF, Madeira LG, Mendes HM, Miranda DM, Mata-Machado NA, Morato EG, Pavarino ÉC, Pereira LB, Rezende NA, Rodrigues Lde O, Sette JB. Neurofibromatosis: part 2—clinical management. Arq Neuropsiquiatr. 2015;73(6):531–43. https://doi.org/10.1590/0004-282X20150042.

20. Fujii K, Miyashita T. Gorlin syndrome (nevoid basal cell carcinoma syndrome): update and literature review. Pediatr Int. 2014;56(5):667–74. https://doi.org/10.1111/ped.12461.

21. Ferner RE. Neurofibromatosis 1. In: Ferner RE, Huson SM, Evans DG, editors. Neurofibromatosis in clinical practice. London: Springer; 2011. p. 162.

22. Chittiboina P, Lonser RR. von Hippel–Lindau disease. Handb Clin Neurol. 2015;132:139–56.

23. Nielsen SM, Rhodes L, Blanco IG, Chung WK, Eng C, Maher ER, Richard S, Giles RH. Von Hippel-Lindau disease: genetics and role of genetic counseling in a multiple neoplasia syndrome. Proc Am Soc Clin Oncol.

24. Gutmann DH, Ferner RE, Listernick RH, Korf BR, Wolters PL, Johnson KJ. Neurofibromatosis type 1. Nat Rev. Dis Primers. 2017;3(1):1–7.

25. Javed F, Ramalingam S, Ahmed HB, Gupta B, Sundar C, Qadri T, Al-Hezaimi K, Romanos GE. Oral manifestations in patients with neurofibromatosis type-1: a comprehensive literature review. Crit Rev. Oncol Hematol. 2014;91(2):123–9.

26. Schraepen C, Donkersloot P, Duyvendak W, Plazier M, Put E, Roosen G, Vanvolsem S, Wissels M, Bamps S. What to know about schwannomatosis: a literature review. Br J Neurosurg. 2022;36(2):171–4.

27. Asthagiri AR, Parry DM, Butman JA, Kim HJ, Tsilou ET, Zhuang Z, Lonser RR. Neurofibromatosis type 2. Lancet. 2009;373(9679):1974–86.

24

High Yield Facts on CNS Tumors

Contents

High Yield Facts on CNS Tumors

*Muthanna N. Abdulqader, Awfa Aktham,
Ammar S. Al-Adhami, Mahmood F. Alzaidy,
Ahmed Muthana, Zahraa A. Alsubaihawi,
and Samer S. Hoz*

1. Venous air embolism (VAE) is the most common complication in posterior fossa procedures in the sitting position.

2. Temporary postoperative DI is the most common complication in the trans-sphenoidal approach, occurring in 10–60% of patients, while permanent DI is much less common, affecting 0.5–5% of patients.

3. Hypothalamic injury is the most common cause of death in patients undergoing trans-sphenoidal operations.

4. Fifty percent of patients with optic nerve gliomas have neurofibromatosis type 1 (NF1). Fifteen percent of patients with NF1 harbor an optic nerve glioma.

5. Gliomas are the most common primary brain neoplasms in adults and children and represent half to two-thirds, respectively, of all brain tumors in these populations. Meningiomas are the second most common primary brain neoplasm.

6. Astrocytomas are the largest subgroup of gliomas, accounting for about 20–30% of all gliomas.

7. Glioblastoma multiforme (GBM) is considered both the most common glioma and the most malignant primary brain tumor in adults.

8. A dural tail is not unique to meningiomas and can be observed in other neoplastic and non-neoplastic processes, including exophytic gliomas, gliosarcoma, dural metastases, lymphoma, and granulomatous infections.

9. Vestibular schwannoma is the most common posterior fossa tumor resulting in vertigo in less than 20% of patients.

10. Vestibular schwannoma is the most common cerebellopontine angle lesion, contributing to around 75% of all CPA masses. The next most common CPA mass is meningioma.

11. The most common neoplasms in the spinal extradural space are metastatic lesions.

12. The most common location of chordoma is the sacral coccygeal region (50%), followed by the spheno-occipital region (35%), with the remaining involving vertebral bodies in other locations (15%).

13. The most common location of spinal meningiomas is the thoracic spine, in the lateral or posterolateral location.

14. There are three types of spinal arachnoid cysts: Type I is an extradural meningeal cyst that has no neural tissue; type II is an extradural meningeal cyst that has neural tissue; and type III is an intradural meningeal cyst. Type II (perineural or Tarlov) cysts are the most common and contain nerve roots that mostly adhere to the cyst's wall.

15. Complete tumor resection using an endoscope is typically performed for colloid cysts.

16. The most common mass lesions that cause secondary non-communicating hydrocephalus in both adults and children are pineal region tumors, tectal gliomas, and posterior fossa tumors.

17. The most common cause of vasogenic edema is primary or secondary brain tumors.

18. The most common tumors associated with epilepsy in young adults and children are dysembryoplastic neuroepithelial tumors (DNETs) and gangliogliomas, 70% of which are located in the temporal lobe.

19. The most common seizure type associated with brain tumors is secondary generalized tonic-clonic seizure (50%), followed by focal motor seizures (25%).

20. The most common appearance of ganglioglioma is a circumscribed cyst with a mural nodule. The next most common is a solid tumor expanding the cortex. In half of the cases, calcification and enhancement are present.

21. Asymptomatic meningiomas are the most common primary brain tumors found incidentally.

22. Pilomyxoid astrocytoma (WHO grade II), which is a variant of pilocytic astrocytoma but clinically more aggressive, occurs most commonly in the hypothalamic or chiasmatic region.

23. The histologic hallmark of ependymoma is the perivascular pseudorosette, characterized by perivascular collars of radiating tumor cell cytoplasmic processes.

24. The choroid plexus may be involved in neoplastic and non-neoplastic mass lesions other than choroid plexus tumors, most prominently intraventricular meningioma, metastatic carcinoma (especially renal cell carcinoma), and xanthogranuloma (reactive mass lesion with cholesterol clefts and multinucleated giant cell reaction).

25. The most common tumor associated with chronic temporal lobe epilepsy, found in 40% of the cases, is ganglioglioma.

26. Meningiomas are the most common intracranial extra-axial neoplasm in adults, accounting for about 25% of all adult intracranial neoplasms. Schwannomas are the second most common intracranial extra-axial tumor.

27. Germ cell tumors, lymphoma, Langerhans cell histiocytosis, and inflammatory lesions such as sarcoidosis, Wegener's granulomatosis, and lymphocytic hypophysitis are the most common causes of pituitary stalk dilatation.

28. The most common location of choroid plexus papilloma is at the glomus of the lateral ventricle in children (80% of childhood CPP) and the fourth ventricle in adults.

29. In pediatric patients, ependymomas are most commonly seen near the fourth ventricle, while in young adults they commonly arise in the supratentorial compartment extending to near the ventricles but usually appear as an intra-axial mass.

30. The most common locations of subependymoma are the fourth ventricle floor, along the septum pellucidum and along the lateral ventricular ependyma.

31. The molecular subtypes of medulloblastoma (MB) exhibit varying prognoses: Tumors in the cerebral peduncle and cerebellopontine angle (WNT-activated MB) have the best prognosis, tumors in the cerebellar hemisphere (SHH-activated MB) have intermediate prognosis, and midline tumors (group 3 and group 4 MB) near ventricles carry the worst prognosis.

32. The radiological finding of a multicystic or bubbly appearance is a characteristic feature of DNETs.

33. In adults, metastasis is the most common posterior fossa tumor in adults, followed by hemangioblastoma as the second most common.

34. The most common sites of supratentorial PCNSL are the frontal lobes, deep nuclei, and periventricular region. Infratentorially, the cerebellum is the most common location. Secondary lymphoma tends to involve meningeal surfaces and exhibits enhancing thickening of the dura.

35. Hemorrhagic metastases are most commonly seen in patients with melanoma, renal cell carcinoma, and thyroid carcinoma.

36. Meningiomas represent by far the most common indication for endovascular tumor embolization for preoperative devascularization.

37. Pituitary adenomas are the most common intrasellar lesions, constituting 5–8% of all intracranial tumors.

38. The most common genetically inherited neurological disorder affecting nearly 1 in 3000–4000 individuals is NF1. Tuberous sclerosis complex (TSC) is the second most common affecting approximately 1 in 6000–10,000 individuals.

39. Pilocytic astrocytomas are the most frequently encountered CNS neoplasms in NF1 patients, accounting for approximately 15% of cases. The most prevalent location for these tumors is within the optic pathway (optic pathway gliomas).

25

40. The most common CNS neoplastic process associated with Cowden's disease is dysplastic gangliocytoma of the cerebellum, known as *Lhermitte-Duclos disease* (LDD), which is pathognomonic for Cowden's disease.

41. The most common complication of stereotactic biopsy is intracranial hemorrhage, and the second most common complication is a new neurological deficit.

42. Somatosensory evoked potential (SSEP) is the most common neurophysiologic monitoring used in brain tumor surgeries.

43. The most common systemic complication of craniotomy for brain tumors is deep venous thrombosis, which affects 4–30% of patients during their disease.

44. The most common location of LGGs is the frontal lobe (44%), followed by the temporal lobe (28%) and parietal lobe (14%).

45. The most common histologic subtype of LGG is astrocytoma (69.3%), followed by oligodendroglioma (21.1%) and mixed glioma (9.6%).

46. The most common clinical presentation of patients with LGGs is seizure (65–95%), followed by headache (40%).

47. The most common genetic mutation found in oligodendrogliomas is loss of heterozygosity at chromosomes 1p and 19q (50–80%) and is associated with increased responsiveness to combined PCV (procarbazine, CCNU/lomustine, and vincristine) and radiation treatment with improved prognosis.

48. Mutations in the *TP53* tumor suppressor gene have been found in two-thirds of low-grade astrocytomas and are typically associated with progression to secondary glioblastoma.

49. Mutations such as *PTEN* and *PDGFR* increase the incidence of LGG transformation into high-grade glioma and are associated with a poor prognosis.

50. The most common post-radiation side effects were dermatitis, alopecia, and lethargy.

51. The most common primary location of gliosarcoma is the temporal lobe.

52. The most common symptoms of gliosarcoma are headache and hemiparesis. The most common signs are focal weakness, visual field defects, papilledema, and dysphasia.

53. The most common presenting clinical feature in ganglioglioma is seizure. It is the most common tumor found in temporal lobe epilepsy.

54. The most common site for pleomorphic xanthoastrocytoma (PXA) is in the temporal lobe.

55. The most common embryonal tumor in children is medulloblastoma.
56. The most common initial symptom in pineal region tumors is headache, which is associated with obstructive hydrocephalus.
57. Parinaud's syndrome is characterized by upgaze paralysis, convergence or retraction nystagmus, and pupillary light-near dissociation. The Sylvian aqueduct syndrome is characterized by paralysis of downgaze or horizontal gaze from further midbrain compression. Dorsal midbrain compression or infiltration can lead to lid retraction (Collier's sign) or ptosis.
58. Germinoma is the most common pineal region tumor, most commonly found in adolescent boys and young men.
59. Germinomas are the most common type of germ cell tumor (65%).
60. Medulloblastoma is the most common malignant brain neoplasm in children. Glioblastoma multiforme is the most common malignant brain neoplasm in adults.
61. In adults, the predominant molecular subgroup of medulloblastoma, constituting approximately 84% of cases, is the SHH subgroup. In contrast, among children, the most frequent molecular subgroup is group 4. The most common histological subtype of medulloblastoma is the classic type in both adults and children.
62. The most common sites of hemangioblastomas are the cerebellum, brainstem (posterior medulla), and posterior spinal cord.
63. The most common manifestation of VHL disease is CNS hemangioblastomas.
64. The most common cause of VHL disease-related death is renal cell carcinoma or CNS hemangioblastoma.
65. The most common cause of PCNSL (approximately 90% of cases) is diffuse large B-cell lymphomas (DLBCLs). The remaining 10% include T-cell lymphomas, poorly characterized low-grade lymphomas, and Burkitt's lymphomas.
66. The most common intracranial tumor in adults is metastasis.
67. The most common sources of brain metastasis in adults are cancers of the lung and breast, followed by melanoma.
68. The most common cause of brain metastasis in children is leukemia, followed by lymphoma.
69. The most common causes of solid brain metastasis among children younger than 15 years of age are osteogenic sarcoma and rhabdomyosarcoma, whereas germ cell tumors are the most common in patients that are between 15 and 21 years of age.

25

70. The most common causes of solid tumor-related leptomeningeal metastasis are breast and lung cancers.
71. The most common site of intracranial meningiomas is convexity (35%).
72. A histological distinctive feature of meningioma is the presence of the so-called Orphan Annie's eye nuclei (target-like nuclei) that have central clearing and a peripheral margin of chromatin.
73. Hyperintensity of meningiomas on T2 WI reflects higher water content, a meningothelial meningioma, a vascular meningioma, or an aggressive meningioma. It suggests that the tumor can be easily aspirated during surgery.
74. The highest recurrence rates (>20%) in meningiomas are found in sphenoid wing meningiomas, followed by parasagittal meningiomas (8–24%). The recurrence rate for convexity and suprasellar meningiomas is 5–10%.
75. Indications for radiation therapy in meningiomas include: (1) following surgery for a malignant meningioma, (2) for patients with multiple recurrent tumors for whom repeating surgery is too risky, and (3) as a sole therapy for patients with a meningioma that is inoperable. However, the adjuvant role of stereotactic radiotherapy has also been gaining ground.
76. The most common clinical presentations for convexity meningiomas are seizures and incidental findings on imaging.
77. The most common location of intraventricular meningioma (90% of cases) is the trigone of the lateral ventricles.
78. The most common clinical presentation of tuberculum sellae meningiomas is chiasmal syndrome, which is characterized by primary optic atrophy, bitemporal field defects, and an essentially normal sellae.
79. The most common funduscopic finding in tuberculum sellae meningioma is primary optic atrophy, which is asymmetrical between the two eyes with varying degrees of severity.
80. The most common symptoms of orbital meningioma are progressive painless visual loss and proptosis.
81. The most common type of posterior fossa meningiomas are cerebellopontine angle (CPA) meningiomas (approximately 50%).
82. The most common clinical findings in clival, petroclival, and sphenopetroclival meningiomas are headache and ataxia from cerebellar compression. Other findings include long-tract signs, spastic paresis, and cranial nerve palsy.

83. The most common clinical presentation in patients with foramen magnum meningioma is the clinical triad of cervical pain (usually unilateral), motor and sensory deficits (more in the upper extremities), and cold clumsy hands with intrinsic hand atrophy.

84. The most common complications of surgeries for foramen magnum meningiomas are cranial nerve IX and X palsy.

85. The most common intracranial sarcoma is fibrosarcoma, more frequently seen in adults.

86. The most common soft-tissue sarcoma in children is rhabdomyosarcoma. Intracranial rhabdomyosarcomas are rare, and primary types are even rarer.

87. The most common site of Ewing's sarcoma involving the nervous system is the spinal epidural space.

88. Radiological characteristics that help differentiate between hemangiopericytomas and meningiomas include a narrow-based dural attachment is seen more frequently in hemangiopericytomas. Hyperostosis of adjacent bone is seen in meningiomas, while hemangiopericytomas never show calcification or hyperostosis and instead may display features of bone erosion. Additionally, the mushroom-like appearance, although not diagnostic, is more commonly associated with hemangiopericytomas.

89. The most common sites of meningeal hemangiopericytoma metastasis are the bone, lung, and liver.

90. Vestibular schwannomas most commonly arise from the inferior division of the vestibular nerve (over 90%). They typically develop near the transition point between glial and Schwann cells, referred to as the Obersteiner-Redlich zone.

91. The earliest and most common symptom in VS is progressive unilateral hearing loss (85%).

92. The most common location of the facial nerve in relation to vestibular schwannomas is anterosuperiorly, followed by anteroinferiorly, and least commonly, posteriorly.

93. Pituitary tumors are the third most common primary intracranial tumor following gliomas and meningiomas.

94. The most common tumors to metastasize to the pituitary region include germ cell tumors (mainly germinomas) and cancers of the breast, lung, and GIT. Metastasis is mainly found in the posterior pituitary because of its high vascularity.

95. In cases of pituitary insufficiency due to large tumors compressing the pituitary gland or the stalk, gonadotrophs are the first to be affected as they are the most vulnerable, followed by thyrotrophs, somatotrophs, and, lastly, corticotrophs.
96. The most common complications after trans-sphenoidal include sinusitis, septal perforation, crusting, and epistaxis.
97. The most common site of subependymoma is within the fourth ventricle.
98. Histologic examination of central neurocytomas shows a perinuclear halo ("fried egg" appearance), perivascular pseudorosettes, and a honeycomb appearance that mimics the histological pattern of oligodendrogliomas and ependymomas.
99. The most common site of CPP in children is the atrium of the lateral ventricle (approximately 50%).
100. The most common non-neuroepithelial intracranial tumor seen in the pediatric population is craniopharyngioma.
101. The most common fourth ventricle tumor in adults is ependymoma, while in children it is medulloblastoma.
102. Germinomas are the most common type of germ cell tumor, accounting for up to 65%.
103. The most common benign tumors of the skull base are meningiomas, followed by pituitary tumors and vestibular schwannomas, whereas chordomas and chondrosarcomas are the most common malignant tumors.
104. Among metastatic brain tumors, prostate cancer and breast cancer are the most common cancers that metastasize to the skull base, followed by lung cancer and lymphoma.
105. The most common pituitary adenomas are prolactin-secreting tumors (prolactinomas) and represent about 50%.
106. Nonfunctioning pituitary adenomas are the second most common pituitary adenoma after prolactinoma representing about 20% of all pituitary adenomas; 80% of them are of gonadotroph cell origin.
107. The adamantinomatous type of craniopharyngioma represents the most common form in pediatric cases (up to 95%), while the papillary squamous epithelium type is the most common in adults.
108. Growth hormone deficiency is the most prevalent endocrine dysfunction in pediatric craniopharyngioma patients (up to 75%), followed by FSH and LH deficiency (40%), and ACTH and TSH deficiency (25%).

109. Vestibular schwannomas are the most common intracranial schwannomas (90%), followed by trigeminal schwannomas (1–8%), facial schwannomas (2.5%), and lower cranial nerve schwannomas (2%).
110. The most common initial symptom of trigeminal nerve schwannoma is facial hypoesthesia rather than facial pain.
111. Facial nerve schwannomas in the CPA most commonly present with hearing loss (100%) and less commonly with facial paresis (20%), while facial paresis and palsy are the most common initial symptoms when the tumor is in the distal segments of the nerve.
112. The most common initial symptoms in chordoma and chondrosarcoma are double vision and headache.
113. Pulsatile tinnitus and hearing loss are the most common initial symptoms of paraganglioma and occur in about 75%.
114. Rhabdomyosarcoma is the most common malignant tumor of childhood that invades the skull base from the orbit.
115. The most common sacral neoplasm in general is metastasis, while the most common malignant primary bone tumor of the sacrum is chordoma.
116. Carotid paragangliomas are the most common head and neck paragangliomas, followed by jugular paragangliomas.
117. The most common metastasis site of paragangliomas is the regional lymph nodes (69%).
118. The most common signs and symptoms of hormonally active paragangliomas include palpitations, headaches, perspiration, facial flushing, and hypertension.
119. The most common primary sites of sinonasal tumors are the nasal cavity (43.9%) and maxillary sinus (35.9%).
120. The most common histological types of sinonasal tumors are squamous cell carcinoma, adenocarcinoma, olfactory neuroblastoma, and adenoid cystic carcinoma.
121. The most common symptoms of sinonasal tumors are nasal obstruction (mostly unilateral), followed by nasal discharge, facial pain, and epistaxis.
122. The most common location of trigeminal schwannomas is the middle cranial fossa (Jefferson classification type A), followed by the posterior fossa (Jefferson classification type B).
123. The most common site of juvenile nasopharyngeal angiofibroma is the superior margin of the sphenopalatine foramen.
124. The most common presenting symptoms of juvenile nasopharyngeal angiofibroma are nasal obstruction and epistaxis.

125. The most common primary orbital tumors in adults include cavernous hemangiomas, lymphoid tumors, and meningiomas, whereas dermoid cysts, capillary hemangiomas, and rhabdomyosarcoma are the most common in children.
126. The most common tumors that extend into the orbit are meningiomas and sinonasal carcinomas.
127. The most common initial presentation of an orbital mass is proptosis.
128. The most common primary skull lesion is osteoma, and they are most frequently located in the frontal sinus, followed by the ethmoid sinus.
129. The most common site of chondromas at the skull base is the sphenoid bone or around the foramen lacerum.
130. Metastases are the most common neoplasms of the calvarium, with carcinomas of the breast, lung, and prostate being the three most common primary tumors causing skull metastasis, respectively.
131. Neuroblastoma is the most common skull metastasis found in children.
132. The most common malignant bone tumor in childhood is osteosarcoma, followed by Ewing's sarcoma.
133. The most common solid tumors in children are brain tumors. Neuroblastoma is the second most common solid tumor in children and the most common in infants.
134. The skull is the second most common location after the pelvis for Paget's disease of bone.
135. The monostotic type is the most common form of fibrous dysplasia, accounting for about 70% of cases. The other two types are polyostotic and McCune-Albright syndrome.
136. The most commonly involved bone in Langerhans cell histiocytosis (LCH) is the skull.
137. Basal cell carcinoma is the most common type of skin cancer, followed by squamous cell carcinoma.
138. The middle fossa or sylvian fissure is the most common site for intracranial arachnoid cysts across all age groups.
139. The most common symptom of arachnoid cysts is a unilateral headache in the supraorbital or temporal region that is exacerbated with physical exertion.
140. The most common type of middle fossa arachnoid cyst is Galassi type 1 (approximately 68%).
141. Brain cancer is the second most common type of cancer after leukemia in the pediatric age group.
142. The most common malignant childhood brain tumor is medulloblastoma.

143. The most common cytogenetic alteration in patients with medulloblastoma is the loss of chromosome 17p and gain of 17q (30–40%).
144. The most common genomic alteration in ependymoma is the loss of chromosome 22, found in up to 71% of cases.
145. Subependymal giant cell astrocytomas (SEGAs) are the most common brain tumors in tuberous sclerosis complex (TSC) patients.
146. The posterior fossa (comprising 67% of cases) is the most frequent site for childhood brain tumors. The three most common types, each with equal incidence, are medulloblastoma, cerebellar (pilocytic) astrocytoma, and brainstem gliomas, with each accounting for 27%.
147. The most common infantile brain tumors (0–2 years of age) are choroid plexus papillomas, desmoplastic infantile astrocytomas, teratomas, PNETs, and atypical teratoid/rhabdoid tumors.
148. The most common thalamic tumors are juvenile pilocytic astrocytomas or fibrillary astrocytomas.
149. The most common presentation of choroid plexus tumors is related to increased ICP due to obstructive hydrocephalus and/or CSF overproduction.
150. Craniopharyngioma is the most common non-glial tumor of childhood.
151. The most common complication after treatment of craniopharyngioma is tumor recurrence.
152. The most common site of pediatric high-grade gliomas is within the brainstem (nearly 50%).
153. Diffuse intrinsic pontine gliomas (DIPGs) are the most common type of pediatric brainstem glioma, accounting for 80% of cases.
154. The most common spinal epidural tumors in the pediatric population are neuroblastomas, lymphomas, chloromas (myelogenous leukemia), and metastases.
155. The most common extracranial tumor in the pediatric population is neuroblastoma (15%).
156. The most common metastatic spinal tumors in the pediatric age group are Ewing's sarcoma and neuroblastoma.
157. The most commonly encountered spinal cord tumor in children is intramedullary astrocytoma, followed by ganglioglioma.
158. The most common spinal intramedullary tumor found in adults is ependymoma.
159. Schwannomas (neurilemomas) are the most common peripheral nerve tumors.

25

160. Meningiomas are the most common non-glial intracranial neoplasms in adults.
161. Nonfunctioning adenomas are the most common form of pituitary macroadenoma.
162. Among adults, the most frequent spinal extradural tumors are metastases, while intradural extramedullary tumors are often meningiomas, and intramedullary spinal cord tumors typically manifest as ependymomas.
163. Multiple myeloma, chordoma, chondrosarcoma, osteogenic sarcoma, and Ewing's sarcoma are the most common primary malignant neoplasms of the axial skeleton.
164. The most common benign vertebral column tumor in adults is vertebral hemangioma, most commonly found in the thoracic and lumbar spine.
165. In adults, multiple myelomas represent the most prevalent malignant bone neoplasms, with the spine being affected in 30–50% of cases, primarily the thoracic spine.
166. The sacrum is the most common site for giant cell tumors.
167. The most common site of osteochondromas is the cervical spine, with the axis (C2) being the most common.
168. The most common osseous spinal tumors involving the posterior elements are benign tumors such as aneurysmal bone cysts, osteoblastoma, and osteoid osteoma.
169. The most common malignant primary tumors of the spine in adults are multiple myeloma, plasmacytoma, chordoma, osteosarcoma, and chondrosarcoma in descending order.
170. The most common site of Ewing's sarcoma of the spine is the sacrococcygeal area.
171. The most common histologic subtype of spinal meningioma is the psammomatous variant.
172. The most common intradural spinal tumors (both intra- and extramedullary) are meningiomas.
173. The most common lesion of the filum terminale in adults is myxopapillary ependymoma.
174. The vertebral body is the most common site for skeletal metastasis.
175. The most common CNS tumor to cause precocious puberty is hypothalamic hamartoma. Other causes include other CNS tumors (astrocytoma, ependymoma, pineal tumors, optic pathway hypothalamic gliomas), CNS XRT, hydrocephalus, septo-optic dysplasia, and chronic hypothyroidism.

176. Gelastic seizures (episodes of unprovoked laughter) are the most common type and the earliest seizure manifestation (92%) in patients with hypothalamic hamartoma.

177. The most common site of spinal arachnoid cysts is the thoracic spine.

178. In the pediatric age group, astrocytomas are the most common supratentorial tumors.

179. In neonates, teratomas are the most common type of brain tumor.

180. In NF1, the most commonly associated intramedullary spinal cord tumor is astrocytoma, while in NF2, it is ependymoma.

181. The most common site of pilocytic astrocytoma in NF1 is the optic nerve (optic glioma).

182. The most common site of ependymomas is the posterior fossa in children and the intramedullary spinal cord in adults.

183. The most common pineal region tumor is germinoma followed by astrocytoma, teratoma, and pineoblastoma.

184. Meningiomas are the most common primary intracranial tumors.

185. The most common primary posterior fossa tumor in adults is hemangioblastoma.

186. The retina is the second most common location for hemangioblastomas after the cerebellum in VHL patients.

187. Renal cell carcinoma (RCC) is the most common malignant tumor in VHL.

188. The most common presenting symptom of Langerhans cell histiocytosis of the skull is a tender, enlarging skull mass (>90%), with the parietal bone being the most common site.

189. The most common tumor of the posterior pituitary (neurohypophysis) is metastasis.

190. Granular cell tumor of the sellar region (pituicytoma WHO grade I) is the most common primary tumor of the neurohypophysis and pituitary stalk/infundibulum. The most common presenting symptom is visual field defect.

191. The most common benign tumor of the skull is osteoma. Osteosarcoma is the most common malignant tumor of the skull.

192. The most common sites of spinal cord tumors are extradural (55%), intradural extramedullary (40%), and intramedullary (5%).

193. The most common sites of spinal ependymomas are the lower spinal cord, conus, and filum. The cervical spinal cord is the second most common.

194. Vertebral hemangioma is the most prevalent primary spine tumor, and it most commonly occurs in the lumbar and lower thoracic spine.

25

195. The most common type of foramen magnum lesion is foramen magnum meningioma (46%).
196. In adults, cavernous hemangioma is the most common benign primary intraorbital neoplasm, while melanoma is the most common primary malignancy. In children, the dermoid cyst is the most common benign lesion, and rhabdomyosarcoma is the most common malignant tumor of the orbit.
197. The most common site for atypical teratoid/rhabdoid tumors is the posterior fossa (75%).
198. Adjustment disorder and acute stress disorder are the most common psychiatric diagnoses in patients with brain tumors.
199. The most common presenting features in oligodendroglioma are seizures rather than functional deficits.
200. Mutations in the isocitrate dehydrogenase gene 1 (IDH1; chromosome 2q) or 2 (IDH2; chromosome 15q) are the most common genetic mutations (90%) in glial brain tumors.

Printed in the United States
by Baker & Taylor Publisher Services